Congenital Adrenal Hyperplasia

Congenital Adrenal Hyperplasia

Edited by
Members of the Division of Pediatric Endocrinology
The Johns Hopkins University School of Medicine

Peter A. Lee, Ph.D., M.D.
Associate Professor

Leslie P. Plotnick, M.D.
Assistant Professor

A. Avinoam Kowarski, M.D.
Associate Professor

Claude J. Migeon, M.D.
Professor

University Park Press
Baltimore · London · Tokyo

UNIVERSITY PARK PRESS
International Publishers in Science and Medicine
Chamber of Commerce Building
Baltimore, Maryland 21202

Typeset by The Composing Room of Michigan, Inc.
Manufactured in the United States of America by Universal Lithographers, Inc.,
and The Optic Bindery Incorporated.

Proceedings of "Treatment of Congenital Adrenal Hyperplasia: A Quarter of a
Century Later," an international symposium held at The Johns Hopkins Hospital, Baltimore, Maryland, October 20–24, 1975.

Library of Congress Cataloging in Publication Data

Main entry under title:

Congenital adrenal hyperplasia.

Proceedings of a symposium held at Johns Hopkins
Hospital, Oct. 20–24, 1975.
Includes index.
1. Adrenogenital syndrome—Congresses.
2. Pediatric endocrinology—Congresses. I. Lee,
Peter Allen, 1939–   II. Johns Hopkins University.
Division of Pediatric Endocrinology.
RJ420.A3C66   618.9'24'5   76-30549
ISBN 0-8391-0974-1

Contents

HISTORICAL ASPECTS

PATHOPHYSIOLOGY

HORMONE MEASUREMENT IN DIAGNOSIS AND MANAGEMENT

LONG-RANGE FOLLOW-UP

SURGICAL CORRECTION AND SEXUAL MATURATION

Contributors

Thomas Aceto, Jr., M.D.
Professor and Chairman
Department of Pediatrics and
  Adolescent Medicine
School of Medicine
The University of South Dakota
McKennan Hospital
Sioux Falls, South Dakota 57101

Fatui Ademola Akesode, M.D.
Fellow in Pediatric Endocrinology
Department of Pediatrics
The Johns Hopkins University School
  of Medicine
Baltimore, Maryland 21205

James A. Amrhein, M.D.
Assistant Professor
Department of Pediatrics
The Johns Hopkins University School
  of Medicine
Baltimore, Maryland 21205

Andrea Attanasio, M.D.
Department of Diagnostic
  Endocrinology
University Children's Hospital
University of Tübingen
Tübingen, Federal Republic of
  Germany

Susan W. Baker, B.A.
Departments of Psychiatry and
  Pediatrics
Children's Hospital
219 Bryant Street
Buffalo, New York 14222

Frederic C. Bartter, M.D.
Hypertension-Endocrine Branch
National Heart, Lung, and Blood
  Institute
National Institutes of Health
Bethesda, Maryland 20014

Joyce B. Baumann, Ph.D.
Department of Endocrinology
University Children's Hospital
Römergasse 8
CH-4005 Basel, Switzerland

Carl Beling, M.D.
Associate Professor
Department of Obstetrics and
  Gynecology
Director, Endocrine Division
Downstate Medical Center
Brooklyn, New York 11203

Jennifer J. Bell, M.D.
Associate Professor of Clinical
  Pediatrics
Department of Pediatrics
Columbia University College of
  Physicians and Surgeons
New York, New York 10032

Jean Bertrand, M.D.
Unité de Recherches Endocriniennes
  et Métaboliques chez l'Enfant
I.N.S.E.R.M. U.34
Hôpital Debrousse
Lyon Cedex 1, France

Frank Bidlingmaier, M.D.
Children's Hospital
University of Munich Medical School
Department of Pediatric
  Endocrinology
D-8 Munich 2
Lindwurmstrasse 4, Federal Republic
  of Germany

Robert M. Blizzard, M.D.
Chairman, Department of Pediatrics
University of Virginia School of
  Medicine
Charlottesville, Virginia 22901

Alfred M. Bongiovanni, M.D.
Professor of Pediatrics
The University of Pennsylvania
Children's Hospital of Philadelphia
Philadelphia, Pennsylvania 19104

Ian Meadows Burr, M.D.
Professor, Department of Pediatrics
Vanderbilt University School of
  Medicine
Nashville, Tennessee 37203

Otfrid Butenandt, M.D.
Children's Hospital

University of Munich Medical School
Department of Pediatric
  Endocrinology
D-8 Munich 2
Lindwurmstrasse 4, Federal Republic
  of Germany
George W. Clayton, M.D.
Professor of Pediatrics
Head, Endocrine Section, Department
  of Pediatrics
Baylor College of Medicine
Texas Medical Center
Houston, Texas 77030
Felix A. Conte, M.D.
Associate Professor
Department of Pediatrics
University of California, San Francisco
San Francisco, California 94143
Jean Daléry, M.D.
Child Neuropsychiatry
Hospices Civils Lyon
Hôpital Neurologique
69374 Lyon, France
Louis David, M.D.
Hôpital Edouard Herriot
Place d'Arsonval
69374 Lyon Cedex 2, France
M. David
Clinical Endocrine Units
Hôpital Debrousse
69322 Lyon Cedex 1, France
Raphael R. David, M.D.
Associate Professor of Pediatrics
New York University School of
  Medicine
New York, New York 10016
Geraldine R. Davis
Division of Pediatric
  Endocrinology
Department of Pediatrics
The Johns Hopkins University
  School of Medicine
Baltimore, Maryland 21205
Allan L. Drash, M.D.
Professor of Pediatrics
Department of Pediatrics
The University of Pittsburgh School of
  Medicine
and Children's Hospital of Pittsburgh
Pittsburgh, Pennsylvania 15213
Anke A. Ehrhardt, Ph.D.
Associate Professor

Departments of Psychiatry and
  Pediatrics
Children's Hospital
Buffalo, New York 14222
Atilla T. A. Fazekas, M.D.
Department of Pediatrics
Endocrinology and Metabolism
University of Ulm
D-79 Ulm/Donau
Federal Republic of Germany
Walter Fleischmann, M.D., Ph.D.
1406 Lynnwood Drive
Johnson City, Tennessee 37601
Thomas P. Foley, M.D.
Assistant Professor of Pediatrics
The University of Pittsburgh School of
  Medicine
and Children's Hospital of Pittsburgh
Pittsburgh, Pennsylvania 15213
Maguelone G. Forest, M.D., Ph.D.
Unité de Recherches Endocriniennes
  et Métaboliques chez l'Enfant
I.N.S.E.R.M. U.34
Hôpital Debrousse
69322 Lyon Cedex 1, France
Professeur R. François
Pavillon S BIS
Service de Pediatrie
Hôpital Edouard Herriot
Place d'Arsonval
69374 Lyon Cedex 2, France
Silvia C. Garcia, M.D.
Division of Reproductive
  Endocrinology
Department of Gynecology and
  Obstetrics
The Johns Hopkins University School
  of Medicine
Baltimore, Maryland 21205
Frank J. Gareis, M.D.
Department of Pediatrics
Naval Regional Medical Center
Oakland, California 94627
Myron Genel, M.D.
Associate Professor of Pediatrics
Director, Children's Clinical Research
  Center
Yale University School of Medicine
New Haven, Connecticut 06510
I. Ghali
Clinical Endocrine Units
Hôpital Debrousse

69322 Lyon Cedex 1, France
P. Gillet
Clinical Endocrine Units
Hôpital Debrousse
69322 Lyon Cedex 1, France
Jürg Girard, M.D.
Department of Endocrinology
University Children's Hospital
Römergasse 8
CH-4005 Basel, Switzerland
Peter Göbel, M.D.
Medical University Policlinic and
Department of Experimental
  Endocrinology
D-Tübingen
Liebermeisterstrasse 14
Federal Republic of Germany
Thomas A. Good, M.D.
Professor of Pediatrics
Medical College of Wisconsin
Milwaukee Children's Hospital
Milwaukee, Wisconsin 53233
Melvin M. Grumbach, M.D.
Chairman and Professor
Department of Pediatrics
University of California, San
  Francisco, School of Medicine
San Francisco, California 94143
Derek Gupta, Ph.D. Med. (Lond.)
Department of Diagnostic Endocrinology
Universitäts-Kinderklinik
Rümelinstrasse 23
74 Tübingen, Federal Republic of
  Germany
James P. Gutai, M.D.
Assistant Professor
Department of Pediatrics
The Children's Hospital of Pittsburgh
Pittsburgh, Pennsylvania 15213
F. Heni
Medical University Policlinic
and Department of Experimental
  Endocrinology
D-Tübingen
Liebermeisterstrasse 14
Federal Republic of Germany
Janos Homoki, M.D.
Department of Pediatrics,
  Endocrinology and Metabolism
University of Ulm
D-79 Ulm/Donau
Federal Republic of Germany

John Eager Howard, M.D.
Professor Emeritus
Department of Medicine
The Johns Hopkins University
  School of Medicine
Baltimore, Maryland 21205
Ieuan A. Hughes, M.D.
Department of Paediatrics
University of Manitoba
Winnipeg, Manitoba, Canada
Carol Huseman, M.D.
Department of Pediatrics
The University of Michigan Medical
  School
Ann Arbor, Michigan 48104
Ruth Illig, M.D.
Department of Pediatrics
Kinderspital
University of Zurich
Steinwiesstrasse 75
8032 Zürich, Switzerland
Alfonso H. Janoski, M.D.
Assistant Professor
Department of Medicine
University of Maryland Hospital
Baltimore, Maryland 21201
Anthony S. Jennings, M.D.
Fellow in Endocrinology
Department of Medicine
Vanderbilt University School of
  Medicine
Nashville, Tennessee 37203
Professeur M. Jeune
Clinical Endocrine Units
Hôpital Debrousse
69322 Lyon Cedex 1, France
Ann Johanson, M.D.
Associate Professor
Department of Pediatrics
University of Virginia Hospital
Charlottesville, Virginia 22901
Georgeanna Seegar Jones, M.D.
Professor and Director
Division of Reproductive
  Endocrinology
Department of Gynecology and
  Obstetrics
The Johns Hopkins University School
  of Medicine
Baltimore, Maryland 21205
Howard W. Jones, Jr., M.D.
Professor, Active Staff

Division of Reproductive
  Endocrinology
Department of Gynecology and
  Obstetrics
The Johns Hopkins University School
  of Medicine
Baltimore, Maryland 21205
Nathalie Josso, M.D.
Unité de Recherches de Genetique
  Medicale
I.N.S.E.R.M.
Hôpital des Enfants Malades
75730 Paris Cedex 15, France
Selna L. Kaplan, M.D., Ph.D.
Professor, Department of Pediatrics
University of California, San Francisco
San Francisco, California 94143
Solomon A. Kaplan, M.D.
Professor, Department of Pediatrics
Center for Health Sciences
UCLA School of Medicine
Los Angeles, California 90024
Bruce S. Keenan, M.D.
Assistant Professor
Department of Pediatrics, Endocrine
  Section
Baylor College of Medicine
Houston, Texas 77030
Frederic M. Kenny, M.D.*
Professor of Pediatrics
The University of Pittsburgh School c
  Medicine
and Children's Hospital of Pittsburgh
Pittsburgh, Pennsylvania 15261
Rebecca T. Kirkland, M.D.
Assistant Professor of Pediatrics
Department of Pediatrics, Endocrine
  Section
Baylor College of Medicine
Houston, Texas 77030
Werner Klemm, M.D.
Department of Diagnostic
  Endocrinology
University Children's Hospital
University of Tübingen
Tübingen, Federal Republic of
  Germany
Georgeanna Jones Klingensmith, M.D.
Assistant Professor

---

*Deceased

Department of Pediatric Endocrinology
The Children's Hospital
Denver, Colorado 80218
Dietrich Knorr, M.D.
Children's Hospital
University of Munich Medical School
Department of Pediatric
  Endocrinology
D-8 Munich 2
Lindwurmstrasse 4, Federal Republic
  of Germany
Elaine E. Kohler, M.D.
The Medical College of Wisconsin
Milwaukee, Wisconsin 53233
Jerry Kolins, M.D.
Laboratory of Pathology
National Cancer Institute
Bethesda, Maryland 20014
Sigrun Korth-Schutz, M.D.
Pediatric Endocrine Fellow
Department of Pediatrics
Division of Pediatric Endocrinology
The New York Hospital—Cornell
  Medical Center
New York, New York 10021
A. Avinoam Kowarski, M.D.
Associate Professor
Division of Pediatric Endocrinology
Department of Pediatrics
The Johns Hopkins University
  School of Medicine
Baltimore, Maryland 21205
Stephen H. LaFranchi, M.D.
Departments of Pediatrics
and Obstetrics and Gynecology
Center for Health Sciences
and Harbor General Hospital
UCLA School of Medicine
Los Angeles, California 90024
Peter A. Lee, M.D., Ph.D.
Associate Professor
Division of Pediatric Endocrinology
Department of Pediatrics
The Johns Hopkins University
  School of Medicine
Baltimore, Maryland 21205
Lenore S. Levine, M.D.
Assistant Professor of Pediatrics
Department of Pediatrics
Division of Pediatric Endocrinology
The New York Hospital—Cornell

Medical Center
New York, New York 10021
Viola G. Lewis, B.S.
Instructor, Medical Psychology
Psychohormonal Research Unit
Department of Psychiatry and
  Behavioral Sciences
The Johns Hopkins University
  School of Medicine
Baltimore, Maryland 21205
Grant W. Liddle, M.D.
Professor and Chairman
Department of Medicine
Vanderbilt University Hospital
Nashville, Tennessee 37232
Jean-Marie Limal, M.D.
Chef de Clinique—Assistant
Hôpital des Enfants Malades
75730 Paris Cedex 15, France
Barbara M. Lippe, M.D.
Departments of Pediatrics
and Obstetrics and Gynecology
Center for Health Sciences
and Harbor General Hospital
UCLA School of Medicine
Los Angeles, California 90024
H. Lansing Lipton, M.D.
Postdoctoral Fellow in Endocrinology
Department of Internal Medicine
Yale University School of Medicine
New Haven, Connecticut 06510
Bernadette Loras, M.D.
Unité de Recherches Endocriniennes
  et Métaboliques chez l'Enfant
I.N.S.E.R.M. U.34
Hôpital Debrousse
69322 Lyon Cedex 1, France
Noel K. MacLaren, M.D.
Associate Professor
Department of Pediatrics
University of Maryland School of
  Medicine
Baltimore, Maryland 21201
Terence J. McKenna, M.B.
Assistant Professor of Medicine
Department of Medicine
Vanderbilt University School of
  Medicine
Nashville, Tennessee 37203
Walter J. Meyer, III, M.D.
Associate Professor

Division of Endocrinology
Department of Pediatrics
University of Texas Medical Branch
Galveston, Texas 77550
Claude J. Migeon, M.D.
Director, Division of Pediatric
  Endocrinology
Professor, Department of Pediatrics
The Johns Hopkins University School
  of Medicine
Baltimore, Maryland 21205
John Money, Ph.D.
Professor of Medical Psychology
Associate Professor of Pediatrics
Director, Psychohormonal Research
  Unit
Department of Psychiatry and
  Behavioral Sciences
and Department of Pediatrics
The Johns Hopkins University School
  of Medicine
Baltimore, Maryland 21205
Anne-Marie Morera
Unité de Recherches Endocriniennes
  et Métaboliques chez l'Enfant
I.N.S.E.R.M. U.34
Hôpital Debrousse
69322 Lyon Cedex 1, France
Akira Morishima, M.D.
Associate Professor of Pediatrics
Columbia University College of
  Physicians and Surgeons
New York, New York 10032
H. David Mosier, Jr., M.D.
Professor and Head, Pediatric
  Endocrinology and Metabolism
Department of Pediatrics
University of California, Irvine
Long Beach, California 90801
Patrick J. Mulrow, M.D.
Professor and Chairman
Department of Medicine
Medical College of Ohio at Toledo
Toledo, Ohio 43614
Maria I. New, M.D.
Professor and Vice-Chairman
Department of Pediatrics
Division of Pedatric Endocrinology
The New York Hospital—Cornell
  Medical Center
New York, New York 10021

Robert Noth, M.D.
Assistant Professor of Medicine
Yale University School of Medicine
New Haven, Connecticut 06510
Songja Pang, M.D.
Research Associate
Department of Pediatrics
Division of Pediatric Endocrinology
The New York Hospital—Cornell
  Medical Center
New York, New York 10021
Albert F. Parlow, Ph.D.
Resident Professor
Department of Obstetrics and
  Gynecology
Harbor General Hospital
UCLA School of Medicine
Torrance, California 90509
Jean-Yves Picard
Unité de Recherches de Genetique
  Medicale
I.N.S.E.R.M.
Hôpital des Enfants Malades
75730 Paris Cedex 15, France
Andrea Prader, M.D.
Professor and Chairman, Department
  of Pediatrics
Kinderspital
University of Zurich
Steinwiesstrasse 75
8032 Zürich, Switzerland
Nezam Radfar, M.D.
Hypertension-Endocrine Branch
National Heart, Lung, and Blood
  Institute
National Institutes of Health
Bethesda, Maryland 20014
Klaus Rager, M.D.
Department of Diagnostic
  Endocrinology
Universitäts- Kinderklinik
Rumelinstrasse 23
74 Tübingen, Federal Republic of
  Germany
Salvatore Raiti, M.D.
Associate Professor
Department of Pediatrics
University of Maryland School of
  Medicine
Baltimore, Maryland 21201

Raphael Rappaport, M.D.
Associate Professor
Hôpital des Enfants Malades
75730 Paris Cedex 15, France
Gail E. Richards, M.D.
Post-doctoral Fellow in Pediatrics
Department of Pediatrics
University of California, San Francisco
San Francisco, California 94143
Arlan Lee Rosenbloom, M.D.
Professor, Division of Genetics,
  Endocrinology, and Metabolism
Department of Pediatrics
Director, General Clinical Research
  Center
University of Florida College of
  Medicine
Gainesville, Florida 32610
Henriette Roux
Unité de Recherches Endocriniennes
  et Métaboliques chez l'Enfant
I.N.S.E.R.M. U.34
Hôpital Debrousse
69322 Lyon Cedex 1, France
Paul Saenger, M.D.
Assistant Professor of Pediatrics
Department of Pediatrics
Division of Pediatric Endocrinology
The New York Hospital—Cornell
  Medical Center
New York, New York 10021
Jose M. Saez, M.D.
Unité de Recherches Endocriniennes
  et Métaboliques chez l'Enfant
I.N.S.E.R.M. U.34
Hôpital Debrousse
69322 Lyon Cedex 1, France
Klaus von Schnakenburg, M.D.
Children's Hospital
University of Kiel Medical School
D-23 Kiel 1
Froebelstrasse 15/17, Federal
  Republic of Germany
Edgar J. Schoen, M.D.
Chief, Department of Pediatrics
Kaiser-Permanente Medical Center
Oakland, California 94611
Mark F. Schwartz, B.S.
Research Associate
Psychohormonal Research Unit

Department of Psychiatry and
Behavioral Sciences
The Johns Hopkins University School
of Medicine
Baltimore, Maryland 21205
Irene L. Solomon, M.D.
Department of Pediatrics
Kaiser-Permanente Medical Center
Oakland, California 94611
Dennis M. Styne, M.D.
Post-doctoral Fellow in Pediatrics
Department of Pediatrics
University of California, San Francisco
San Francisco, California 94143
William J. Sweeney, III, M.D.
Clinical Professor of Obstetrics and
Gynecology
Department of Pediatrics
Department of Obstetrics and
Gynecology
The New York Hospital—Cornell
Medical Center
New York, New York 10021
Siang Y. Tan, M.D.
Assistant Professor of Medicine
Medical College of Ohio at Toledo
Toledo, Ohio 43614
Guy P. E. Tell
Unité de Recherches Endocriniennes
et Métaboliques chez l'Enfant
I.N.S.E.R.M. U. 34
Hôpital Debrousse
69322 Lyon Cedex 1, France
Walter M. Teller, M.D.
Professor of Pediatrics
University of Ulm
D-79 Ulm/Donau
Federal Republic of Germany
Dien Tran
Unité de Recherches de Genetique
Medicale
I.N.S.E.R.M.
Hôpital des Enfants Malades
75730 Paris Cedex 15, France

Madan Varma, Ph.D.
Department of Pediatrics
University of Virginia Medical Center
Charlottesville, Virginia 22901
Wolfgang Wagner
Children's Hospital
University of Munich Medical School
Department of Pediatric
Endocrinology
D-8 Munich 2
Lindwurmstrasse 4, Federal Republic
of Germany
Anne Colston Wentz, M.D.
Division of Reproductive
Endocrinology
Department of Gynecology and
Obstetrics
The Johns Hopkins University School
of Medicine
Baltimore, Maryland 21205
Jeremy S. D. Winter, M.D.
Endocrine-Metabolism Laboratory
Health Sciences Centre
University of Manitoba
Winnipeg, Manitoba, Canada
Robert J. Winter, M.D.
Assistant Professor
Department of Endocrinology
Children's Memorial Hospital
Northwestern University Medical
School
2300 Children's Plaza
Chicago, Illinois 60614
E. Youssefnejadian
Department of Biochemical
Endocrinology
Chelsea Hospital for Women
Dovehouse Street
London, SW3 6LT, England
Milo Zachmann, M.D.
Department of Pediatrics
Kinderspital
University of Zurich
Steinwiesstrasse 75
8032 Zürich, Switzerland

Preface

In the opening lines of his textbook *The Diagnosis and Treatment of Endocrine Disorders in Childhood and Adolescence,* Lawson Wilkins states:

> "Childhood and adolescence are the most interesting periods in which to study the effects of endocrine disorders. In adults hormonal dysfunctions are manifested largely by metabolic disturbances. During embryonic life or childhood these same metabolic disorders may alter the growth and differentiation of tissues causing marked deviations from the usual patterns of somatic or sexual growth and development."

Congenital adrenal hyperplasia, an inborn error of steroid metabolism, certainly illustrates this point. The syndrome with its variants has major effects on the fetus, the infant, and the growing child—which no doubt explains Wilkins' great interest in this endocrine disorder.

It is generally agreed that the scientific history of congenital adrenal hyperplasia started in 1949 with the discovery of the efficacy of cortisone therapy by Wilkins et al. and by Bartter and his colleagues. Both groups observed a rapid decrease of the urinary 17-ketosteroids and the suppression of the metabolic effects of the adrenal androgens. Lawson Wilkins followed through his initial contribution with intensive clinical and laboratory studies of large numbers of affected children. During that time, he trained a series of Fellows who in turn contributed to the elucidation of the biochemical basis for the spectrum of clinical abnormalities associated with the syndrome. He also recognized the importance of psychologic investigation in children with abnormal sex differentiation and he helped nurture the Psychohormonal Clinic at Hopkins.

When this witness to the 25 years of progress in our understanding of the syndrome suggested the possibility of a symposium on "The Treatment of Congenital Adrenal Hyperplasia: A Quarter of a Century Later," the response was uniformly enthusiastic. The Symposium took place in the Turner Auditorium of The Johns Hopkins Hospital on October 20 to 24, 1975, and was part of the celebration of the centennial year of The Johns Hopkins University. There were more than 50 speakers and the proceedings were attended by more than 250 pediatric endocrinologists from the United States and from abroad. For many it was a sort of homecoming, and for all it was a warm as well as instructive encounter. The contents of this book represent a large part of the proceedings of the symposium.

Claude J. Migeon

Acknowledgment

The editors wish to acknowledge the financial support of the Symposium by Dr. Ralph I. Dorfman, President, Syntex Research, Palo Alto, California, and by Mr. Samuel N. Turiel, Director, Department of Professional Education and Communications, Searle Laboratories, Chicago, Illinois.

A great deal of thanks are due to a large number of colleagues at The Johns Hopkins Medical Institutions, particularly Dr. Russell H. Morgan, Dean (Emeritus) of the Medical School, Drs. Georgeanna Seegar Jones, Howard W. Jones, Jr., and Anne C. Wentz of the Department of Obstetrics and Gynecology, Dr. John Money, Director, Psychohormonal Clinic, and Drs. Patrick C. Walsh and Donald S. Coffey, Department of Urology.

The dedicated secretarial help of Mrs. Mary Westervelt and Mrs. Doris Barrington is greatly appreciated.

Dedication

The contributions of Lawson Wilkins to the field of pediatric endocrinology in general and to the syndrome of congenital adrenal hyperplasia in particular have been numerous. However, his greatest achievement may well be the creation of a generation of pediatric endocrinologists in the United States and in the world who either trained with him or obtained an appreciation of this sub-specialty from him.

This book is dedicated to the memory of Lawson Wilkins, a great physician, a magnificent teacher, an investigator with insatiable curiosity, by his Fellows at the Pediatric Endocrine Clinic of The Johns Hopkins Hospital, by the Fellows of his Fellows, and by all those who were influenced by his teaching.

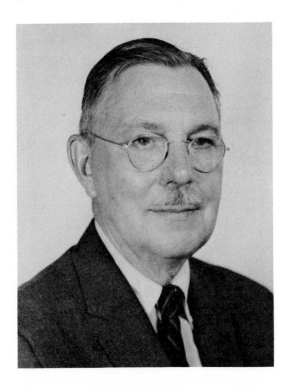

Lawson Wilkins

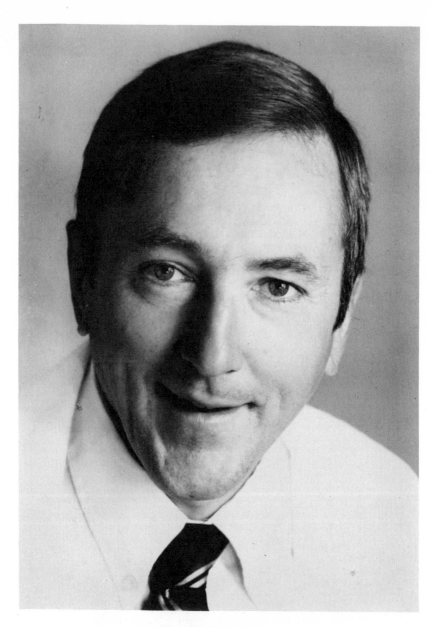

Frederic Marshal Kenny

A Tribute
to Frederic Marshal Kenny

Thomas Aceto, Jr.

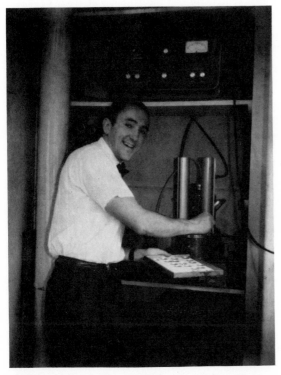

Frederic Marshal Kenny, Professor of Pediatrics, The University of Pittsburgh School of Medicine, died on July 4, 1975. Because of his remarkable contributions as scientist, teacher, and human being, we have prepared this tribute that others may join us in remembering him.

After completing secondary education at Trinity School in Manhattan, Fritz entered Princeton University, where he majored in English and acquired a broad knowledge of literature. Fritz ran for the varsity track team, an experience he enjoyed and often recalled.

He studied medicine and pediatrics at The Johns Hopkins University. There he met medical student Jean Felty, whom he married in 1958. The traditions of The Johns Hopkins Hospital remained with him always, particularly the tradition of the scientist-clinician.

Following two years as a pediatrician at the Naval Hospital in Annapolis, Fritz returned to study pediatric endocrinology at Hopkins with Robert Blizzard, Claude Migeon, and the late Lawson Wilkins, then semi-retired. In 1962, Dr. Richard Day invited Fritz to succeed Robert Klein at The Children's Hospital of Pittsburgh as pediatric endocrinologist. Fritz worked there until his death.

During those thirteen years at The Children's Hospital of Pittsburgh, Fritz headed and further developed The Pediatric Endocrine Unit. He co-authored almost one hundred papers and made forty presentations at scientific meetings, both in this country and abroad.

There were scores of collaborators, students, fellows, and leading investigators in pediatric endocrinology and in other disciplines. Fritz enjoyed research and writing. He often referred to the tedious work as "fun."

Dr. Allen Drash, Fritz's colleague at the University of Pittsburgh, comments:

"Probably the most significant permanent monument to Fritz's life are the contributions—past, present, and future—of the young men and women who received training with him. He touched the lives of many medical students, over 100 of whom spent elective time with him in the endocrine clinic. Under his sure guidance and gentle direction, 11 of these students co-authored publications with him. All of them learned from him that an inquiring, scientific approach to medical problems was perfectly compatible with a primary concern for, and understanding of, the sick child and his family. Fritz was particularly proud of the fellows who received training in pediatric endocrinology with him. The impressive list totals 23 individuals. Of this group, 15 hold full-time academic appointments and several are already demonstrating their leadership in our field."

His peers became increasingly aware of Fritz's accomplishments. He was president of the Mid-Western Society for Pediatric Research in 1973. He frequently reviewed papers for pediatric and endocrine journals, he chaired many scientific sessions of the Society for Pediatric Research, and he served on the Drug Committee of the Academy of Pediatrics.

What drew a host of people to this man? So many spoke enthusiastically about him. One hardly ever heard a word against him. Why did one never tire of his company? We had fun with him and gained reassurance. He listened carefully to problems, pointed out the humorous aspects, put the problem in perspective by describing some parallel situation in history, the theatre, or his own experience, and predicted an optimistic outcome. Rarely did he criticize or gossip. Fritz genuinely enjoyed the successes of his friends and former fellows and often pointed out to them evidence of new achievements. Fritz appreciated the efforts that people made in his behalf and often spoke about them long after the effort had been made. He readily expressed his admiration and appreciation. His criticisms were kind and constructive.

Throughout his life, Fritz maintained many constant interests. He enjoyed sports: sailing, skiing, swimming, jogging, and hiking. He read non-medical literature at the end of each day, including plays, novels, poetry, and religious works. He painted oils and watercolors. Fritz also enjoyed classical and popular music and had a considerable knowledge of opera. He was talented in writing and wrote easily, as evidenced by his many scientific papers and letters to friends. Fritz enjoyed traveling and described in long letters what he had seen. He liked living near the water, as he and Jean had done in Annapolis, and more recently in a summer cottage on Lake Pymatuning, which is close to Pittsburgh. He was very constant in his enthusiasm for his successful marriage of 18 years and for Jean's scientific accomplishments. He attended church regularly.

Frederic Marshal Kenny lived a rich life. He had achieved what he wished: a solid marriage, professional success, accomplished disciples, close friends, wisdom, and "fun."

Congenital
Adrenal
Hyperplasia

HISTORICAL ASPECTS

Early Days of the Wilkins Clinic

Walter Fleischmann

Dr. Lawson Wilkins used to call his fellows and associates his "boys" with a certain pride. As the oldest of these boys, I am pleased to write of the early days of the Wilkins Clinic.

The Pediatric Endocrine Clinic owed its existence to the foresight of Dr. Edwards Park, who was anxious to place Lawson Wilkins at the head of some important section of the department and offered him the directorship of the endocrine clinic in 1935. So Wilkins became the first director of the newly created Pediatric Endocrine Clinic. He was eminently suited for this position. He had graduated from the Johns Hopkins Medical School while with the army in France in World War I. Upon discharge from the army, he served an internship at Yale, followed by advanced training in pediatrics at the Harriet Lane Home under Dr. Howland. After this, he went very successfully into the private practice of pediatrics in Baltimore. But despite his increasing practice, he found time for clinical investigation. His paper on the growth and osseous and mental development in cretins as a guide to thyroid treatment is still a classic (Wilkins, 1938).

When did he find time for these activities? Generally between 10:00 p.m. and 2:00 a.m., and I was a rather unwilling witness of this nocturnal activity. I became used to Lawson calling me at midnight, and in his low-pitched, gruff voice asking me, for instance, "Was A. G.'s last cholesterol 174 or 147 mg%? I am just working on her chart." I would answer, rubbing my eyes, "147, Dr. Wilkins." Lawson would say, "Thank you," and I would go back to bed.

Lawson Wilkins recognized very early the need for visual representation of his studies and developed a method for representing the results of these longitudinal studies on charts (Wilkins, 1938). According to Money (1965), Dr. Park stated many years later: "Lawson's method of study by means of his painstaking graphic analysis certainly deserves a very special comment. I think that his were the most beautiful graphic charts I have ever seen. Moreover, the charts were perfect models for the study of chronic disease. It used to be thought that only in private practice could long-term studies be established. Lawson's work showed that a special clinic, like the endocrine clinic, where complicated data can be systematically obtained, is the ideal place for such a study."

Lawson's success was also due to his perfectionism. He was only content with the very best. For example, we were very much interested in creatine excretion initially only in thyroid disease and as an effect of thyroid medication. At this time, a friendly but vociferous argument was going on between our excellent technician, Ed Smetana, and me, on the one side, and Dr. Anthony Albanese, a gifted biochemist working with Emmett Holt, on the other side, about the method of determining creatine. Dr. Wilkins sent me to New York to seek advice from Dr. Dubos, who was at that time very much interested in the methodology of creatine determination. Dr. Dubos, not yet famous, not yet the Nobel Prize winner, very graciously gave me all the needed information. Dr. Dubos also let us have a small amount of the enzyme creatininase, which he had recently isolated. This was of value for identifying the substance in urine which gave the Folin reaction. After concluding the study on the effects of thyroid medication on creatine excretion in patients with thyroid disease, Dr. Wilkins initiated studies on the treatment of dwarfed boys and girls. The suppressing effect of testosterone propionate on creatine excretion was well known, but we chose to use methyl testosterone for our studies, as it could be given by mouth. Observing the effect of androgens on dwarfed children included observations on sexual development, growth, bone development, balance studies of nitrogen, urinary excretion of 17-ketosteroids, serum cholesterol, non-protein nitrogen, Ca and P, and phosphatase.

Dr. Wilkins also wanted to include studies of creatine and creatinine excretion. I was reluctant and said that there was no reason to suspect that methyl testosterone would have a different effect from testosterone propionate, but Lawson was the boss and so I grudgingly started to include creatine and creatinine studies. To our great surprise, oral administration of methyl testosterone caused a marked increase in creatine excretion in sexually underdeveloped dwarfs (Wilkins, Fleischmann, and Howard, 1941). This unexpected finding was soon confirmed by others. I do not wish to claim that this was an important discovery, but it certainly was a case of serendipity.

The syndrome of sexual infantilism with ovarian agenesis and associated defects was of special interest to us (Wilkins and Fleischmann, 1944), and I may have contributed to this line of research by a joke. We had three patients with the characteristic appearance of Turner's syndrome on the metabolism ward, and Lawson said one day, "We ought to do more tests on these girls." Whereupon I asked, "How do we know they are girls; maybe they are boys." Lawson only laughed. However, a few years later it was found (Wilkins, Grumbach, and Van Wyk, 1959) that most of the patients with Turner's syndrome actually had male chromosomal patterns, as judged by Barr's (1954) skin biopsy test of chromosomal sex. Now *I* could laugh.

Dr. Wilkins' interest in the basic sciences was in morphology and biochemistry. Psychology was not his cup of tea, but he was broadminded enough to encourage me to chart the physical and chemical changes in a 13-year-old hypothyroid boy on thyroid medication for 2 years. This study was done in conjunction with Dr. Horsly Gantt of the Phipps Clinic. Dr. Gantt had spent some years in Russia with Professor Pavlov. Dr. Gantt followed the changes of the patient's higher nervous activity by Pavlov's conditional reflex method. He could show that the patient's ability to form and differentiate conditional reflexes ran parallel to the changes in basal metabolic rate and serum cholesterol, which showed a marked improvement within several weeks of therapy. In contrast, the IQ, dependent upon an accumulation of learning, showed a marked stability. The IQ behaves quite differently from the conditional reflex, which is a delicate measure of higher nervous function practically independent of education but related in this patient specifically to metabolic changes (Gantt and Fleischmann, 1948).

I have discussed this study of one case not because I feel it to be a major contribution, but because it shows that the interest of the Wilkins clinic encompassed many facets of endocrinology. The full psychological implications of the various types of abnormal sexual development came later, with the establishment of a new psychohormonal unit under John Money, which greatly and fundamentally has increased our knowledge of the psychology of hermaphroditism and related disorders.

I have very arbitrarily limited the scope of this chapter to the period when I was a full-time member of this clinic (1938–1946). However, I attended the Saturday sessions of the Pediatric Endocrine Clinic until 1952, when I left Baltimore. On one of these Saturdays, I was told by Lawson in confidence about his discovery (made together with Roger Lewis, Bob Klein, and Genia Rosemberg) that cortisone markedly decreased the output of urinary 17-ketosteroids and biologically active androgen in congenital adrenal hyperplasia (Wilkins et al., 1950).

If I may sum up the qualities which led to the success of the Wilkins Clinic, they were absolute integrity in research and the greatest concern or empathy for the patient. This is a rare combination.

I am very grateful that I had the good fortune to be associated with Wilkins for a number of years and consider these years the highlight of my scientific career.

REFERENCES

Barr, M. L. 1954. An interim note on the application of the skin biopsy test of chromosomal sex to hermaphroditism. Surg. Gynecol. Obstet. 99:184–186.

Gantt, W. H., and W. Fleischmann. 1948. Effect of thyroid therapy on the conditional reflex function in hypothyroidism. Am. J. Psychol. 104:673–681.

Money, J. 1965. *In* L. Wilkins (ed.), Diagnosis and Treatment of Endocrine Diseases in Childhood and Adolescence, Ed. 3, page IX. Charles C. Thomas, Springfield, Illinois.

Wilkins, L. 1938. The rates of growth, osseous development and mental development in cretins as a guide to thyroid treatment. J. Pediatr. 12:429–438.

Wilkins, L., R. A. Lewis, R. Klein, and E. Rosemberg. 1950. The suppression of
androgen secretion by cortisone in a case of congenital adrenal hyperplasia.
Bull. Johns Hopkins Hosp. 86:249–252.

Wilkins, L., and W. Fleischmann. 1944. Ovarian agenesis: pathology, associated
clinical symptoms and the bearing on the theories of sex differentiation. J.
Clin. Endocrinol. 4:357–375.

Wilkins, L., W. Fleischmann, and J. E. Howard. 1941. Creatinuria induced by
methyl testosterone in the treatment of dwarfed boys and girls. Bull. Johns
Hopkins Hosp. 69:493–503.

Wilkins, L., M. M. Grumbach, and J. J. Van Wyk. 1959. Chromosomal sex in
"ovarian agenesis." J. Clin. Endocrinol. Metab. 14:1270–1271.

Early Report of a Salt-losing Patient

John Eager Howard

My remarks are purely of historical and anecdotal nature, reflecting on one of the many instances of my close relationship with Lawson Wilkins, always most pleasant and instructive (Wilkins, Fleischmann, and Howard, 1940).

It was an evening in the fall of 1938 that I received an urgent call from Lawson to meet him at some time the next morning in the Harriet Lane Home to see a most bizarre child. The boy, about 4 years old, had been referred from Florida to Dr. T. Campbell Goodwin, a close friend to both of us. He presented a most unusual picture. Large and well muscled for his age, his voice was coarse and rasping, the skin of a dusky, sand-brown hue even in unexposed areas; and there were patches of pigmentation on the buccal membranes, though he was clearly a blond. The genitalia were the size of a midadolescent, including the prostate which was readily outlined; and there was modest pubic hair. Testes were large, smooth, and of a rubbery consistency. A mental defect was clearly present, with speech only a sort of snarl. Yet he had been able, it turned out later, to make his wishes—and smart wishes they were—clear to his mother, a circumstance which had permitted him to live as long as he had.

The urine and blood morphology were normal, but the non-protein nitrogen was 99. His dietary idiosyncracies were not then known. He had been on ward diet for 3 days, which was for the most part refused; and when forced to eat, he had vomited. When we saw him he had lost 2.5 kilos over a 3-day period.

The history recorded that the patient had had enlarged genitalia at birth; acne had developed at 5 months and pubic hair began to grow at 1 year.

We were completely baffled by the situation. Clearly some sort of prerenal azotemia existed for his phenolsulfonphthalein excretion was normal. He had many features of Addison's disease, yet lacked anemia and hypotension. How did this fit in with the precocious puberty, enormous gonads, and the mental retardation? It was only after his sudden unexpected death 3 days later that, from the postmortem examination, a serum sodium value of 112 mEq returned from the laboratory 1 week later on postmortem blood, and the mother's vivid story, we were able to piece the thing together as an example of one type of familial enzymatic defect.

Dr. W. G. MacCallum's postmortem examination disclosed marked cortical adrenal hyperplasia and, to everyone's astonishment, the large gonads consisted of the same tissue throughout. There were no reproductive cells at all.

From his mother's beautifully kept diaries, it was later learned that the patient had learned early that he had a taste for salty foods and was able to communicate his craving to her. This native gift, resembling exactly that displayed by Richter's adrenalectomized rats, was vividly described in a later manuscript by Wilkins and Richter (1940).

Had we known these important historical facts about the boy, he might have survived by a high-salt diet alone, plus 11-deoxycorticosterone acetate, until cortisone became available; and then the entire metabolic abnormality could have been overcome. However, it is almost certain his existence would have been a miserable one, even had we known then everything we know now.

REFERENCES

Wilkins, L., W. Fleischmann, and J. E. Howard. 1940. Macrogenitosomia precox associated with hyperplasia of the adrenogenic tissue of the adrenal and death from corticoadrenal insufficiency. Endocrinology 26:385–395.

Wilkins, L., and C. P. Richter. 1940. A great craving for salt by a child with cortico-adrenal insufficiency. J.A.M.A. 114:886.

Adrenogenital Syndromes
From Physiology to Chemistry (1950-1975)

Frederic C. Bartter

As our knowledge of the adrenogenital syndromes resulting from adrenal cortical hyperplasia has proceeded from one of disordered physiology to one of precise biochemical defects, it is apparent that this group of "experiments of nature" has taught us an enormous amount about the function of the kidneys, the adrenals, and, indeed, the whole endocrine system. Repeatedly, we advance from a new physiological fact through a new chemical fact to a new and better hypothesis.

In 1949 we had two syndromes of adrenal hyperplasia, the adrenogenital syndrome and Cushing's syndrome, the first producing a precociously muscular child known as an "infant Hercules," the second, a short, fat, weak patient with thin skin and bruises. Presumably, the adrenogenital syndrome resulted from too much nitrogen-retaining hormone (known in prechemical times as "N-hormone" for physiological purposes), reflected in the urine as 17-ketosteroids. Cushing's syndrome, on the other hand, was presumed to result from too much nitrogen-losing hormone (known as "S-hormone" for gluconeogenesis from amino acids), reflected in the urine as 11-hydroxy or 11,17-dihydroxy or Porter-Silber corticosteroids (Figure 1). The hypothesis (hypothesis 1) proposed that both syn-

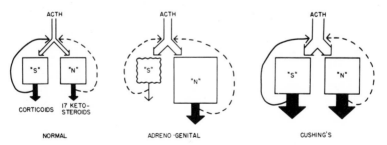

Figure 1. The effect of ACTH on the production of steroids from the adrenal glands in normal subjects, in patients with the adrenogenital syndrome, and in patients with Cushing's syndrome.

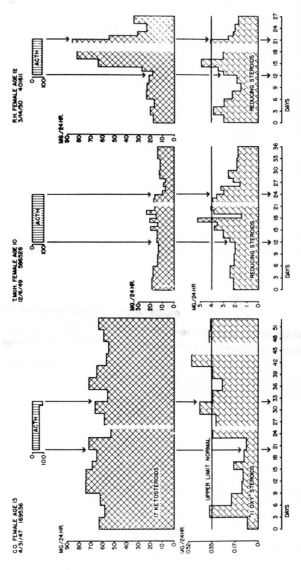

Figure 2. The effect of ACTH on the urinary excretion of 17-ketosteroids and 11-oxysteroids in three patients with the adrenogenital syndrome.

dromes, involving hyperplasia of all adrenal cortical tissue, must result from too much adrenocorticotropic hormone (ACTH). One objection to this conclusion was noted early: Porter-Silber steroid output may be actually low in the adrenogenital syndrome.

In 1948 ACTH was isolated and purified. The adrenogenital syndrome responded abnormally to ACTH (Figure 2), which caused little rise in urinary S-hormone metabolites and little loss of nitrogen. Indeed, in large doses it caused nitrogen retention (Figure 3). A new hypothesis (hypothesis 2) evolved: because the adrenogenital syndrome makes S-hormone very poorly in response to ACTH

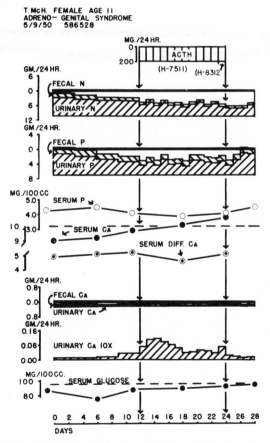

Figure 3. The effect of ACTH on the balance of nitrogen (N), phosphorus (P), and calcium (Ca), and on serum phosphorus, calcium, diffusible calcium, and glucose in a patient with the adrenogenital syndrome. Balance data are plotted so that positive balance is shown by a clear area below the zero line. Reprinted with permission from J. Clin. Invest. 30:237–251 (1951).

and makes N-hormone too well, the S-hormone must be a better inhibitor of ACTH than N-hormone.

Shortly thereafter, cortisol was shown to be the S-hormone in man. A third hypothesis clearly followed: cortisol should lower ACTH, and thus N-hormone secretion, in the adrenogenital syndrome. The physiological experiment illustrated in Figure 4 was carried out simultaneously in Baltimore and Boston (Bartter et al., 1951; Bartter, Forbes, and Leaf, 1950; Wilkins et al., 1950) and supported this hypothesis.

The demonstration that adrenal extracts caused more sodium retention than that explained by known steroids led to another chemical event, the isolation and structural characterization of aldosterone (Simpson and Tait, 1953). The fifth chemical "discovery" was in reality the fruit of many laboratories—the clarification of the biogenetic pathways for cortisol and aldosterone (Figure 5). This in turn led to hypothesis 4, which concluded that most cases of the adrenogenital syndrome result from a 21-hydroxylase deficiency in steroidogenesis (Jailer, 1953). This has, of course, found universal acceptance.

The isolation of aldosterone immediately suggested hypothesis 5: salt-losing patients with the adrenogenital syndrome lack aldosterone (Figure 6). This conclusion resulted from a physiological experiment (salt deprivation in the adrenogenital syndrome) performed simultaneously in Baltimore and Bethesda (Blizzard et al., 1959; Bryan, Kliman, and Bartter, 1965).

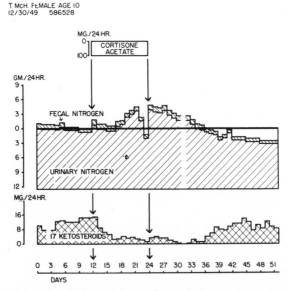

Figure 4. The effect of cortisone acetate on nitrogen balance and on urinary 17-ketosteroid excretion in a patient with the adrenogenital syndrome.

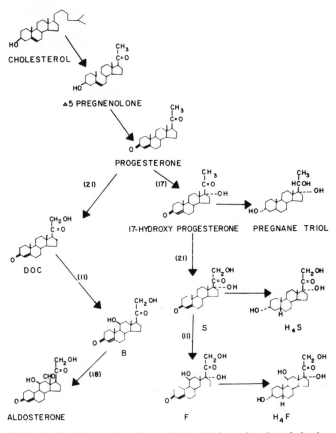

Figure 5. The biogenetic pathway of steroids from the adrenal gland.

The delineation of the biosynthetic pathways of adrenal steroids clarified, and was clarified by, the appearance of three new syndromes. First, Prader noted in 1955 (Prader, Spahr, and Neher, 1955) adrenal "lipoid" hyperplasia without virilization—indeed, virtually without steroid production. His hypothesis (hypothesis 6) stated that this must represent a failure of the desmolase necessary for conversion of cholesterol to Δ5-pregnenolone and could, indeed, be confirmed on tissues of patients with this lethal defect.

In 1956, Bongiovanni and Eberlein made the second important discovery: a few patients with the adrenogenital syndrome were hypertensive (Bongiovanni and Eberlein, 1958). Furthermore, these patients excreted abundant urinary Porter-Silber steroids.

The advance in chemistry that provided the solution was a third discovery: these Porter-Silber steroids represented tetrahydro "S," not tetrahydrocortisol.

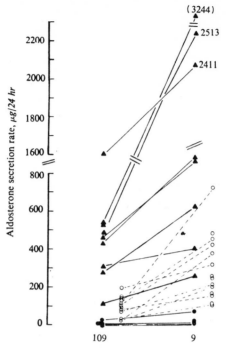

Figure 6. The aldosterone secretion rates on normal (109 mEq) sodium intakes and after 4 days on low (9 mEq) sodium intakes in three groups of patients: o, normal subjects; •, patients with salt-losing form of adrenogenital syndrome; ▲, patients with nonsalt-losing form of adrenogenital syndrome. Reprinted with permission from Kidney International 6:272–280 (1974).

Hypothesis 7, which reconciled all these findings—that of an 11-hydroxylase defect—was readily confirmed (Bongiovanni and Root, 1963). The cause of the hypertension was shown to be an excess of the non-11-oxygenated steroid deoxycorticosterone, which could be made by both zona glomerulosa and zona fasciculata cells. Presumably, most of it arose from the zona fasciculata, where it could not be converted to aldosterone.

The fourth "new" syndrome of adrenal hyperplasia, that of a mutation often fatal in fetal or infant life, with only moderate virilization, was thought by Bongiovanni (Bongiovanni and Root, 1963) in a new hypothesis to result from a defect in 3β-ol-dehydrogenase. This would allow Δ5-steroids (but not Δ4-steroids) to proceed down the biosynthetic pathways; cortisol could not be produced, but dehydroisoandrosterone could.

(In this short chronicle, the syndromes of 17-ketosteroid reductase, C-21 desmolase, and 5α-reductase deficiencies will not be discussed. This is not to denigrate their importance, but only to highlight the syndromes that have taught us the most about physiology.)

The next physiological event that required explanation concerned aldosterone biogenesis in the non-salt-losers. It was found in Baltimore (Kowarski et al., 1965) and in Bethesda (Bartter, Henkin, and Bryan, 1968) simultaneously that these patients, clearly different from salt losers genetically, secreted abnormal amounts of aldosterone—very large amounts indeed—which became still larger with salt deprivation (Figure 6). This finding led to a rejection of the earlier hypothesis (hypothesis 4) (Bongiovanni and Eberlein, 1958) that non-salt-losers differ from salt losers only in the severity of the 21-hydroxylase deficiency (Figure 7). Were this the case, aldosterone secretion should be limited even in non-salt-losers; clearly it was not. It could be explained by a different hypothesis (hypothesis 2) (Figure 7): the 21-hydroxylases for progesterone and for 17-hydroxyprogesterone are different (Bartter, Henkin, and Bryan, 1968),

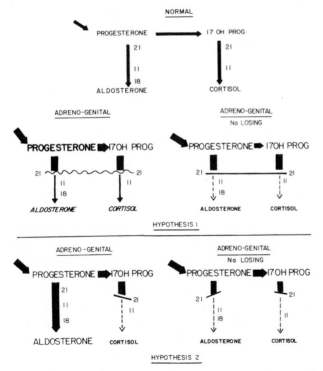

Figure 7. Hypotheses for the difference in aldosterone secretion between salt-losers and non-salt-losers: in Hypothesis 1, non-salt-losers have a mild defect of 21-hydroxylase for progesterone; in Hypothesis 2, they do not.

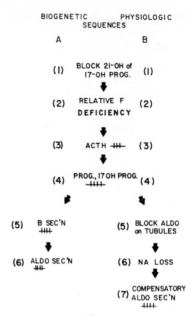

Figure 8. Two possible hypotheses (*A*—Biogenetic, *B*—Physiologic) to explain the excessive production of aldosterone in the non-salt-losing form of adrenogenital syndrome.

and salt losers have both defects, while non-salt-losers have only one, that for 17-hydroxyprogesterone.

Thus, the aldosterone excess might result (hypothesis 9A) from the vis-a-tergo provided by the accumulation of progesterone (Figure 8*A*). However, this hypothesis had to be rejected because of our final physiological "event"—the consistent observation that blood pressure, plasma potassium, and plasma bicarbonate were normal in the non-salt-losers. Primary excess of aldosterone of this magnitude clearly produced hypertension and hypokalemic alkalosis; therefore, the aldosteronism in this syndrome must be secondary. We suggested (hypothesis 9B) that it could be secondary to sodium loss, resulting in turn from excessive production of the weak sodium-excreting steroids, 17-hydroxyprogesterone and progesterone (George, Saucier, and Bartter, 1965) (Figure 8*B*).

One final physiological consequence should follow: "obligatory" salt loss, such as that produced by diuretics or by lack of aldosterone, or sodium-excreting steroids should increase plasma renin activity. Plasma renin is regularly high (for the sodium intake) in non-salt-losers as it is in salt losers. Finally, this suggested a possible explanation (hypothesis 10) (Simopoulos et al., 1971) for the findings in a patient whose salt loss and normal aldosterone secretion might have suggested that his was a case transitional between salt losers and non-salt-losers. Thus, in contrast to the very high aldosterone secretion rates and

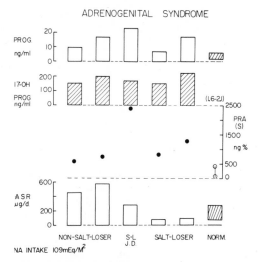

Figure 9. Serum progesterone (Prog), 17-hydroxyprogesterone (17 OH Prog), plasma renin activity (PRA), and aldosterone secretion rate (ASR) in patients with the non-salt-losing and salt-losing forms of the adrenogenital syndrome and in normal subjects. Patient J.D. is a salt-loser with normal aldosterone secretion rate.

moderately high plasma renin values of two non-salt-losers (Figure 9) and the very low aldosterone secretion rates despite high renin values of two salt losers, in this case of a moderate salt loser, normal aldosterone rates were achieved in spite of extremely high plasma renin values, perhaps high enough to stimulate even a defective 21-hydroxylase system for progesterone to produce normal amounts of aldosterone.

In summary, the adrenogenital syndrome has been a splendid teacher for the past 25 years. It is clear that it has not stopped teaching us; indeed, it is in the process of correcting our past mistakes.

REFERENCES

Bartter, F. C., F. Albright, A. P. Forbes, A. Leaf, E. Dempsey, and E. Carroll. 1951. The effects of adrenocorticotropic hormone and cortisone in the adrenogenital syndrome associated with congenital adrenal hyperplasia: an attempt to explain and correct its disordered hormonal pattern. J. Clin. Invest. 30:237–251.

Bartter, F. C., A. P. Forbes, and A. Leaf. 1950. Congenital adrenal hyperplasia associated with the adrenogenital syndrome: an attempt to correct its disordered hormonal pattern. J. Clin. Invest. 29:797 (Abstr.).

Bartter, F. C., R. I. Henkin, and G. T. Bryan. 1968. Aldosterone hypersecretion in "non-salt-losing" congenital adrenal hyperplasia. J. Clin. Invest. 47: 1742–1752.

Blizzard, R. M., G. W. Liddle, C. J. Migeon, and L. Wilkins. 1959. Aldosterone excretion in virilizing adrenal hyperplasia. J. Clin. Invest. 38:1442–1451.

Bongiovanni, A. M., and W. R. Eberlein. 1958. Defective steroidal biogenesis in congenital adrenal hyperplasia. Pediatrics 21:661–672.

Bongiovanni, A. M., and A. W. Root. 1963. The adrenogenital syndrome. N. Engl. J. Med. 268:1283–1289.

Bryan, G. T., B. Kliman, and F. C. Bartter. 1965. Impaired aldosterone production in "salt-losing" congenital adrenal hyperplasia. J. Clin. Invest. 44: 957–965.

George, J. M., G. Saucier, and F. C. Bartter. 1965. Is there a potent, naturally occurring sodium-losing steroid hormone? J. Clin. Endocrinol. Metab. 25: 621–627.

Jailer, J. W. 1953. Virilism. Bull. N. Y. Acad. Med. 29:377–394.

Kowarski, A., J. W. Finkelstein, J. S. Spaulding, G. H. Holman, and C. J. Migeon. 1965. Aldosterone secretion rate in congenital adrenal hyperplasia. A discussion of the theories on the pathogenesis of the salt-losing form of the syndrome. J. Clin. Invest. 44:1505–1513.

Prader, A., A. Spahr, and R. Neher. 1955. Erhöhte aldosteron-ausscheidung beim kongenitalen adrenogenitalen syndrom. Schweiz. Med. Wochenschr. 85: 1085–1088.

Simopoulos, A. P., J. R. Marshall, C. S. Delea, and F. C. Bartter. 1971. Studies on the deficiency of 21-hydroxylation in patients with congenital adrenal hyperplasia. J. Clin. Endocrinol. Metab. 32:438–443.

Simpson, S. A., and J. F. Tait. 1953. Physico-chemical methods of detection of a previously unidentified adrenal hormone. Memories of the Society of Endocrinology (Lond.) 2:9–24.

Wilkins, L., R. A. Lewis, R. Klein, and E. Rosemberg. 1950. The suppression of androgen secretion by cortisone in a case of congenital adrenal hyperplasia. Bull. Johns Hopkins Hosp. 86:249–255.

Reminiscence
A View from Europe

Andrea Prader

Lawson Wilkins has advanced and stimulated the development of pediatric endocrinology more than anyone else. He achieved his leadership not by sophisticated laboratory investigations, but mainly by clinical observation and application of common sense. He had a great talent for analyzing his experiences and for learning from them. He was a superb clinician devoted to his patients and a master in the doctor-parent and the doctor-patient relationship. Above all, he was an enthusiastic permanent student and a forceful teacher. It is a privilege and a great pleasure to recall our relations between 1950 and 1963, the year of his death, and to show his influence on the development of pediatric endocrinology in Europe.

I met him for the first time in Zürich in 1950 at the Sixth International Congress of Pediatrics. He was 56 years old and had just published a note on the first patient successfully treated for congenital adrenal hyperplasia with cortisone (Wilkins et al., 1950). His book, which was to become the classic text for pediatric endocrinology, was not yet published, but its illustrations were on exhibition at the congress. Both the exhibit and the man were a great success. It was the first comprehensive review of pediatric endocrinology, and Lawson Wilkins stood in front of his exhibit each day for many hours to answer questions. It was there that I asked him to see a young baby in our hospital who had ambiguous genitalia and the salt-losing form of congenital adrenal hyperplasia. He examined the baby and spent about 3 hours with me explaining his new concepts of pathogenesis and treatment. That baby was the first patient in our hospital and possibly the first patient in our country to be treated with cortisone. We had only a very small amount, just sufficient for a treatment period of 6 days. However, with the help of DOCA and salt, the baby survived. I was not experienced enough at that time to convince the parents that the baby was a girl. She grew up as a boy, received no cortisone, and later had penile reconstruction and ovariectomy. At 11, his height was 147 cm, and his bone age was adult. At 20, he was a very short but muscular young man who had to shave every other day.

After the congress, I moved to New York to complete my pediatric training with Dr. Emmett Holt at Bellevue Hospital. There I met Dr. Edwards Park, the famous teacher and friend of Dr. Holt and Dr. Wilkins, both of whom admired him greatly. In the early summer of the following year, 1951, I visited Baltimore for the first time. I had the great privilege to stay at Dr. Park's lovely home and to spend about 3 weeks with Lawson Wilkins and his associates at the Harriet Lane Home. This short period was for me truly exciting and most fruitful. Dr. Park's knowledge, wisdom, and friendliness impressed me greatly. We had long evening talks about scientific and social aspects of pediatrics, and he told me his memories of European pediatrics in the years after the first world war. During the days, I went through a pleasant and most intensive training with Lawson Wilkins and his group. I had previously studied his book carefully and had a long list of questions which he answered with patience and enthusiasm. His associates were Lytt Gardner, who demonstrated to me the Allen blue test to estimate dehydroepiandrosterone; John Crigler, who showed me the practical problems of his long-term study of the salt-losing form of congenital adrenal hyperplasia; and Claude Migeon, who had arrived from France the year before and who was studying the effect of cortisone on thyroid function.

Between 1951 and 1963, I met Lawson Wilkins several times again. I especially recall a Ciba Foundation Colloquium in London in 1954. I was unable to grasp the steroid pathway presented by one of the speakers and asked for the slide to copy after the session. To my surprise, Lawson wanted to do the same, and we sat together in the empty meeting room copying the projected slide. In his deep voice he commented bluntly how damned difficult it was to understand the steroid specialists.

Lawson was highly interested in my presentation of an adult male with congenital adrenal hyperplasia. The patient, aged 37, was of small stature, but otherwise healthy and unremarkable with the exception of grossly enlarged testes. The testicular volume was 60 and 120 ml. Under cortisone treatment it decreased to 20 and 40 ml. We felt this to be good indirect evidence that the testicular enlargement was due to adrenocortical tissue.

In 1955 and 1958 my colleagues and I published two papers on congenital lipoid adrenal hyperplasia, which we felt was a newly recognized adrenal disorder, and I was looking forward with some pride to discussing this with Lawson. It was difficult to stimulate his interest, however. He simply said, "You may be right, but I have never seen it." I was rather disappointed by this sceptical comment, but today I think it was a friendly compliment. It was hard for him to accept something he had never seen in his huge experience, but he wanted to show at least his friendly feelings.

I also recall with great pleasure the Lawson Wilkins party in Copenhagen in 1960 on the occasion of the First International Congress of Endocrinology. Lawson and several of his former associates attended that congress. Lawson was depressed because of the recent death of his wife, but he did enjoy the delightful party organized by Henning Andersen for him, his associates, and friends. At this and many other occasions I was accepted by him and his former associates as a former fellow, which filled me with pride.

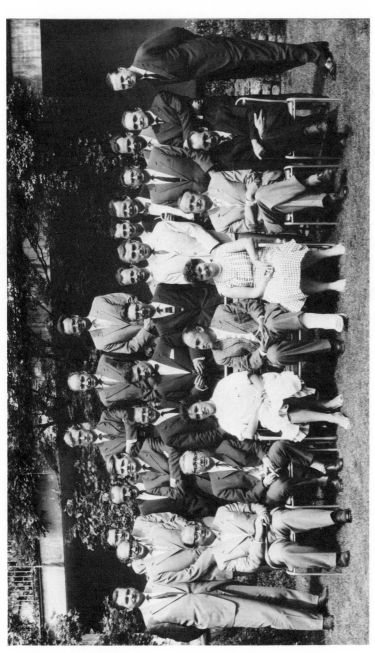

Figure 1. Pediatric Endocrinology Meeting in Zürich in July, 1962, later regarded as the first meeting of the European Society for Pediatric Endocrinology. From left to right, front row: Henning J. Andersen, Copenhagen, Denmark; Andrea Prader, Zürich, Switzerland; Ruth Illig, Zürich, Switzerland; Hans Habich, Steffisburg-Bern, Switzerland; Gertrud Mürset, Zürich, Switzerland; Alfred Schwenk, Köln, West Germany; Carl-Gustaf Bergstrand, Stockholm, Sweden. Second row: Egon Werner, Berlin-Charlottenburg, West Germany; Robert Steendijk, Amsterdam, The Netherlands; Hendrick K. A. Visser, Groningen, The Netherlands; Pierre Ferrier, Genève, Switzerland; Jacob J. Van der Werff ten Bosch, Leiden, The Netherlands; Lucien Corbeel, Louvain, Belgium; René Francois, Lyon, France; Markus F. Vest, Basel, Switzerland; Dietrich Knorr, München, West Germany; André Spahr, Sion, Switzerland; Andreas Fanconi, Zürich, Switzerland; Jürgen R. Bierich, Hamburg, West Germany; Zvi Laron, Petah Tiqva, Israel; Karl Schärer, Aarau, Switzerland; F. J. Huix, Oss, The Netherlands; José M. Francés-Antonin, Barcelona, Spain (deceased). Third row: Lars Nilsson, Göteborg, Sweden (deceased); Gerhard Stalder, Basel, Switzerland; Emile Gautier, Bern, Switzerland.

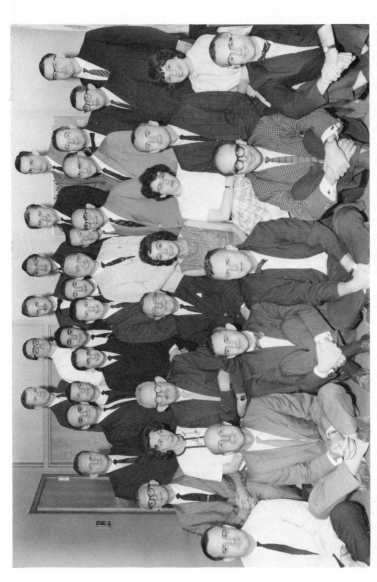

Figure 2. Reunion of the Pediatric Endocrine Fellows (for names, see Figure 3), Harriet Lane Home, Johns Hopkins Hospital, Baltimore, June 11, 1963. This group was the precursor of the Lawson Wilkins Pediatric Endocrine Society, founded in 1971.

Between 1950 and 1960, the Harriet Lane Home had become a mecca for pediatric endocrinology. Many of the leading pediatric endocrinologists in the United States, Latin America, and Europe received their training there. Among the European fellows, I mention Henning Andersen, Jean Bertrand, and Raphael Rappaport. After Lawson's death, pediatric endocrinology at the Johns Hopkins Hospital continued to be a center of excellence under the leadership of Claude Migeon, Robert Blizzard, and John Money. With time, Lawson's indirect influence became much greater than his direct influence. Through his book and through his students, all pediatric endocrinologists of today have been influenced by this great pioneer. He is also the spiritual father of two societies: The Lawson Wilkins Pediatric Endocrine Society in the United States and the European Society for Pediatric Endocrinology.

In 1962 we organized in Zürich a small informal meeting for the few pediatricians from various European countries who attended the Acta Endocrinologica Congress in Geneva. Because all of us felt indebted directly or indirectly to Lawson Wilkins, we sent him our picture (Figure 1) and a message signed by all of us, expressing our gratitude and affection. This meeting created

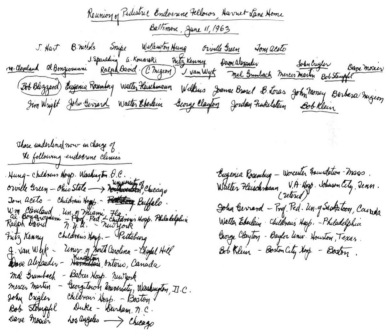

Figure 3. List of names of Fellows shown in Figure 2, as handwritten by Dr. Lawson Wilkins. Seven of these Fellows are or have been Chairmen of Departments of Pediatrics (Drs. Aceto, Blizzard, Bongiovanni, Cleveland, Gerrard, Grumbach, and Stempfel). Dr. Wilkins was Chairman of Pediatrics at Hopkins, 1954–1956.

much enthusiasm. A similar one followed the next year in the Netherlands, where we organized as the European Society for Pediatric Endocrinology (ESPE) with annual meetings. Lawson was proud of his spiritual role in the creation of our society and was moved by our affection. In return, shortly before his death he sent me the picture of the 1963 reunion with his "boys" (Figure 2) and a detailed list in his own handwriting of the names and the professional positions of each one (Figure 3).

The European Society for Pediatric Endocrinology has been very successful in its 13 years of existence and has greatly stimulated the development of pediatric endocrinology in Europe. The close spiritual relationship with Lawson Wilkins and the friendly support in the following years from many of his former associates in the United States have been a great help and encouragement. Today there are many personal links of friendship between the Lawson Wilkins Pediatric Endocrine Society in this country and the European Society for Pediatric Endocrinology. These and the fact that both societies regard Lawson Wilkins as their spiritual father promise a continuous close and friendly relationship between our two societies.

REFERENCES

Wilkins, L., R. A. Lewis, R. Klein, and E. Rosemberg. 1950. The suppression of androgen secretion by cortisone in a case of congenital adrenal hyperplasia. Bull. Johns Hopkins Hosp. 86:249–255.

PATHOPHYSIOLOGY

Congenital Adrenal Hyperplasia and Enzymatic Transactions in the Biosynthesis of Cortisol

Alfred M. Bongiovanni

This chapter gives a brief account of the chronology of the deficiencies in the several distinct enzymatic transactions in the biosynthesis of cortisol associated with congenital adrenal hyperplasia in man. Defects in the train of biochemical events leading to the production of cortisol (or aldosterone) in the adrenal gland are expressed in clinical manifestations arising either from a deficiency of a critical hormone or from the inappropriate biological activity of an excessive precursor. Sometimes these two effects occur simultaneously, as in the virilized female with the salt-losing syndrome. Certain of the enzymes are similar to, if not identical with, those in the gonads for the synthesis of sex steroids. Early blocks in this train of events preclude the synthesis of any active compounds whatsoever, and, in some forms of the disease outlined below, the defect is shared by the gonads so that a genotypic male may demonstrate incomplete embryological masculinization as well as adrenocortical insufficiency. The number of observations in diseased humans of this last variety is sufficient to suggest strongly that the defective enzymatic step is shared by both gonads and adrenals and is probably attributable to a single gene.

The association of large adrenal glands with abnormal genitalia seems to explain the introduction of the term "adrenogenital syndrome." Because genital changes in both sexes in the most common form of the disease are those of masculinization, it was early supposed that large quantities of androgens were coming from the adrenal glands. This was later supported by tests of urine employing group chemical reactions and bioassay of urine from affected subjects. For a long time it was supposed that the adrenal gland was senselessly pouring forth large quantities of androgenic hormones.

The classic work of Hechter and Pincus (1954) on the step-wise hydroxylation of the steroid molecule to its final product, cortisol, by beef adrenal perfusion opened the door to the examination of the individual transactions in human disease.

In 1950, the discovery that was made independently by Wilkins et al. (1950) and by Bartter, Forbes, and Leaf (1950) that cortisone suppressed the elevated urinary 17-ketosteroids provided the first clue that the true basis of the disease was inadequate corticoid production. And in 1951, Bartter et al. demonstrated that the urinary corticoids in this condition did not respond well to the administration of adrenocorticotropic hormone (ACTH). It should be noted that in this last work the method employed gave rather high baseline levels of urinary corticoids, and in all probability, because of the nonspecificity of the reaction, there was included a number of compounds which are elevated in this disease. Between 1952 and 1955, several investigators measured the blood levels of corticoids by more specific chemical means and showed that they were often abnormally low or within the low normal range and demonstrated little, if any, response to ACTH (Bongiovanni, Eberlein, and Cara, 1954; Christy, Wallace, and Jailer, 1955; Kelley, Ely, and Raile, 1952, 1953).

Around the same time, in examining the Hechter schema of cortisol biogenesis, Jailer (1953) predicted a block at 17-hydroxyprogesterone. He arrived at this conclusion because some of the earlier bioassays suggested that this steroid was a potent androgen, although later studies, in particular those of Migeon's group (Camacho and Migeon, 1966), revealed that it was in all probability testosterone itself, a much more potent androgen, that explained the virilizing manifestations. Precise evidence for a block at this site in the usual form of the disease followed several lines of laboratory investigation.

Among the early explorations by the giants of steroid chemistry was the investigation of urine from a variety of clinical oddities in the pursuit of novel steroid compounds. Butler and Marrian (1937) and again Mason and Kepler (1945) isolated and characterized pregnanetriol from the urine of a few virilized adults. These classic investigations made it possible to show that large amounts of this "abnormal" steroid were present in the majority of cases of this disease studied at that time (Bongiovanni, 1953). Lieberman and Dobriner (1945) reported large amounts of 17-hydroxypregnenolone in the urine of a patient with congenital adrenal hyperplasia. Furthermore, Finkelstein, von Euw, and Reichstein (1953) found urinary 11-ketopregnanetriol to be high. It is to be noted that these compounds lack an hydroxyl function at position 21. Thus, there was firm if indirect evidence that in the most common form of this disease there was a deficiency of 21-hydroxylation. Bongiovanni (1958) was able to demonstrate directly the absence of this enzyme activity in the adrenal glands from two cases of this disease. It remains unsettled whether or not there might be two different enzymes for 21-hydroxylation, one intended for the biogenesis of cortisol and the other for aldosterone. Such a thesis is attractive as a means of explaining those patients with this form of disease who have the salt-losing complication. Bartter, Henkin, and Bryan (1952) presented evidence in favor of this hypothesis.

It had been known for some years that rare cases of congenital adrenal hyperplasia were associated with high blood pressure. Eberlein and Bongiovanni (1956) studied in detail the steroid hormones in the blood and urine of such a subject. They found excessive levels of steroids lacking the hydroxyl function at position C-11. This has been confirmed in a number of similar studies. Here and there, an instance of this form with the expected steroidal pattern has been described, but supposedly without the hypertension. This raises the question that there may be various degrees of enzyme deficiency. Eberlein and Bongiovanni (1958) demonstrated the variable degrees of 21-hydroxylation deficiency and were able to show some correlation with the salt-losing syndrome. Further study is needed on the 11-hydroxylase deficiency in order to explain the variable hypertension.

Prader and Gurtener (1955) and Prader and Siebermann (1957) recognized a variety of adrenal hyperplasia wherein the urine was virtually devoid of steroids. This syndrome was exceptional in that affected males were not normally masculinized. Based on the large amounts of cholesterol in these adrenal glands, they suggested 20,22-cholesterol desmolase deficiency, which over the years has been better defined by further indirect evidence. Degenhart et al. (1972) studied the adrenal activity from one case and found no cleavage of cholesterol, although 20α-cholesterol was appropriately converted. This suggests a deficiency of 20α-cholesterol hydroxylase as the basis. A separate defect, not truly within this narrow theme, namely 17,20-desmolase deficiency, has been proposed recently by Zachmann et al. (1972) after the study of a male pseudohermaphrodite. In this case it appeared that cortisol and aldosterone synthesis were entirely normal, but there was no production of C-19 compounds, including testosterone.

Bongiovanni (1962) studied several cases of congenital adrenal hyperplasia in which the males were incompletely masculinized at birth. The urinary pattern consisted almost entirely of a large assortment of 5-ene-3β-hydroxysteroids in the face of inadequate cortisol production. He proposed a 3β-hydroxysteroid dehydrogenase deficiency. In collaboration with the Prader group, it was possible to demonstrate directly the absence of this enzyme from the adrenal tissue and from the gonads of affected cases (Goldman et al., 1964).

Biglieri, Herron, and Brust (1966) delineated yet another subgroup in a phenotypic, genotypic female adult with hypogonadism, no secondary sexual characteristics, and hypertension. Cortisol production was virtually nil, and the major secretory product was corticosterone with increased deoxycorticosterone. Thus, good evidence was provided for 17-hydroxylase deficiency, and this has been confirmed by the studies of others. Such a deficiency should preclude the formation not only of estrogens, but of androgens as well, and thus an affected male should be incompletely masculinized. This conclusion was confirmed by a careful, detailed study by New (1970) of an appropriate male subject with ambiguous genitalia.

Thus, virtually each point of attack on the steroid molecule in the course of the formation of cortisol has been found faulty in a variety of human disorders, and each has been accompanied by the expected clinical manifestations attributed to the overproduction or the underproduction of active steroid hormones. Other enzymatic defects in the biosynthesis of steroid hormones have been described in man, certain of them related to inadequate aldosterone or testosterone production, but these do not directly relate to congenital adrenal hyperplasia.

Perhaps the variations of enzymatic defects are exhausted. The exact nature of the several deficient enzymatic activities is still not known—whether it be deformity of an enzyme or a critical cofactor or some other related abnormality. Each of the disorders studied in sufficient numbers appears to indicate a Mendelian recessive gene. Surely a more precise understanding of these conditions will emerge with further investigation and continued support for such research.

REFERENCES

Bartter, F. C., F. Albright, A. P. Forbes, A. Leaf, E. Dempsey, and E. Carroll. 1951. The effects of adrenocorticotropic hormone and cortisone in the adrenogenital syndrome associated with congenital adrenal hyperplasia: an attempt to explain and correct its disordered hormonal pattern. J. Clin. Invest. 30:237–251.

Bartter, F. C., A. P. Forbes, and A. Leaf. 1950. Congenital adrenal hyperplasia associated with the adrenogenital syndrome: an attempt to correct its disordered hormonal pattern. J. Clin. Invest. 29:797–802.

Bartter, F. C., R. I. Henkin, and G. T. Bryan. 1952. Aldosterone hypersecretion in "non-salt-losing" congenital adrenal hyperplasia. J. Clin. Invest. 47:1742–1752.

Biglieri, E. G., M. A. Herron, and N. Brust. 1966. 17-Hydroxylation deficiency in man. J. Clin. Invest. 45:1946–1957.

Bongiovanni, A. M. 1953. Detection of pregnandiol and pregnantriol in urine of patients with adrenal hyperplasia: suppression with cortisone: preliminary report. Bull. Johns Hopkins Hosp. 92:244–257.

Bongiovanni, A. M. 1958. In vitro hydroxylation of steroids by whole adrenal homogenates of beef, normal man, and patients with adrenogenital syndrome. J. Clin. Invest. 37:1342–1347.

Bongiovanni, A. M. 1962. Adrenogenital syndrome with deficiency of 3β-hydroxysteroid dehydrogenase. J. Clin. Invest. 41:2086–2092.

Bongiovanni, A. M., W. R. Eberlein, and J. Cara. 1954. Studies on metabolism of adrenal steroids in adrenogenital syndrome. J. Clin. Endocrinol. 14:409–422.

Butler, G. C., and G. F. Marrian. 1937. Isolation of pregnane-3,17,20-triol from urine of women showing adrenogenital syndrome. J. Biol. Chem. 119:565–575.

Camacho, A. M., and C. J. Migeon. 1966. Testosterone excretion and production rate in normal adults and patients with congenital adrenal hyperplasia. J. Clin. Endocrinol. 26:893–896.

Christy, N. P., E. Z. Wallace, and J. W. Jailer. 1955. Effect of intravenously administered ACTH on plasma 17,21-dihydroxy-20-ketosteroids in normal individuals and in patients with disorders of adrenal cortex. J. Clin. Invest. 34:899–909.

Degenhart, H. J., H. K. Visser, H. Boon, and N. J. O'Doherty. 1972. Evidence for deficient 20-cholesterol-hydroxylase activity in lipoid adrenal hyperplasia. Acta Endocrinol. (Kbh) 71:512–520.

Eberlein, W. R., and A. M. Bongiovanni. 1956. Plasma and urinary corticosteroids in hypertensive form of congenital adrenal hyperplasia. J. Biol. Chem. 223:85–94.

Eberlein, W. R., and A. M. Bongiovanni. 1958. Defective steroidal biogenesis in congenital adrenal hyperplasia. Pediatrics 21:661–672.

Finkelstein, M., J. von Euw, and T. Reichstein. 1953. Isolierung von $3\alpha,17,20\alpha$-trioxy-pregnanon-11 aus pathologischen menschlichen Harn. Helv. Chim. Acta 36:1266–1274.

Goldman, A. S., A. M. Bongiovanni, W. C. Yakovac, and A. Prader. 1964. Study of 3β-hydroxysteroid dehydrogenase in normal, hyperplastic and neoplastic adrenal cortical tissue. J. Clin. Endocrinol. 24:894–909.

Hechter, O., and G. Pincus. 1954. Genesis of the adrenocortical secretion. Physiol. Rev. 34:459–496.

Jailer, J. W. 1953. Virilism. Bull. N. Y. Acad. Med. 29:377–387.

Kelley, V. C., R. S. Ely, and R. B. Raile. 1952. Metabolic studies in patients with congenital adrenal hyperplasia: effects of cortisone therapy. J. Clin. Endocrinol. 12:1140–1148.

Kelley, V. C., R. S. Ely, and R. B. Raile. 1953. Hormone patterns with congenital adrenal hyperplasia. Pediatrics 12:541–550.

Lieberman, S., and K. Dobriner. 1945. Isolation of pregnanediol-3α,17-one-20 from human urine. J. Biol. Chem. 161:269–278.

Mason, H. L., and E. J. Kepler. 1945. Isolation of steroids from urine of patients with adrenal cortical tumors and adrenal cortical hyperplasia: new 17-ketosteroid, androstane-$3(\alpha)$,11-diol-17-one. J. Biol. Chem. 161:235–257.

New, M. 1970. Male pseudohermaphroditism due to 17α-hydroxylase deficiency. J. Clin. Invest. 49:1930–1939.

Prader, A., and H. P. Gurtener. 1955. Das Syndrom des Pseudo-hermaphroditismus masculinus bei kongenitaler Nebennierenrinden Hyperplasie ohne Androgenuberproduktion. Helv. Paediatr. Acta 10:397–408.

Prader, A., and R. E. Siebermann. 1957. Nebenniereninsuffizienz bei kongenitaler Lipoidhyperplasie der Nebennieren. Helv. Paediatr. Acta 12:509–522.

Wilkins, L., R. A. Lewis, K. Klein, and E. Rosemberg. 1950. Suppression of androgen secretion by cortisone in case of congenital adrenal hyperplasia: preliminary report. Bull. Johns Hopkins Hosp. 86:249–255.

Zachmann, M., J. A. Vellmin, W. Hamilton, and A. Prader. 1972. Steroid 17,20-desmolase deficiency. Clin. Endocrinol. 1:369–388.

Mechanism of Action of Adrenocorticotropic Hormone

Guy P. E. Tell, Anne-Marie Morera, and Jose M. Saez

The primordial role of adrenocorticotropic hormone (ACTH) for the maintenance of the adrenal cortex structure and function has been known for over 40 years (Smith, 1930), but its mechanism of action at the molecular level is still not perfectly understood.

During the last 10 years, several monographs (Eisenstein, 1967; McKerns, 1968) and general reviews (Bransome, 1968; Garren, 1968; Garren et al., 1971; Gill, 1972; Hilf, 1965; Kowal, 1970b; Schulster, 1974a) by authors specializing in the field of ACTH study have delineated the progress achieved in understanding the role of ACTH.

ACTH has multiple effects on the adrenal cortex. The main functions which ACTH controls are steroidogenesis, RNA and protein synthesis, cell multiplication, and cell differentiation.

However, it is not yet clearly defined whether ACTH controls all these functions through the same initial biochemical pathway and whether the same sequence of the hormone molecule is responsible for all its effects.

This chapter presents an overview of the literature on the mechanism of action of ACTH on steroidogenesis and cell growth principally. The biochemical abnormalities which can be responsible for the insensitivity of some human adrenal cortical tumors to ACTH are also discussed.

STRUCTURE OF ACTH

ACTH is a peptide of 39 amino acids (Figure 1). The primary structure of different ACTHs of several species has been elucidated (Jöhl, Riniker, and Schenkel-Hulliger, 1974; Li, 1972; Li and Oelofsen, 1967; Riniker et al., 1972). The sequences of the NH_2-terminal$_{1-24}$ amino acids and the COOH-terminal$_{34-39}$ amino acids are identical for all ACTHs. The 25–33 sequence is different for each species and is probably responsible for the antigenic specific-

Some of the original work described in this review was supported by grants from Centre National de la Recherche Scientifique (42 9904), Institut National de la Santé et de la Recherche Medicale (ATP 74-5-432-36), and Délégation Générale à la Recherche Scientifique et Technique (75-7-0802).

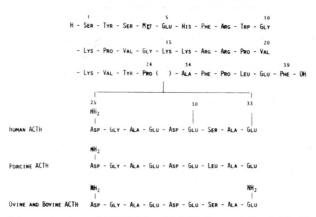

Figure 1. Primary structure of ACTH (after Jöhl, Riniker, and Shenkel-Hulliger, 1974).

ity. In addition, the study of the biological activity, namely the steroidogenic activity, of synthetic peptides has revealed that it is not affected, provided that the sequence of the first 18 amino acids is present (Ide et al., 1972; Ramachandran and Li, 1967; Seelig and Sayers, 1973).

The ACTH of the plasma and the pituitary gland exists in two forms: a little ACTH with a molecular weight identical with that of the 1–39 peptide and a big ACTH with a higher molecular weight (Yalow, 1974). The big ACTH is virtually devoid of biological activity, but a moderate tryptic digestion converts it into a peptide with physicochemical and biological properties similar to those of the little ACTH. In normal human plasma, there are large variations in the relative distribution of big and little ACTHs. In patients with Addison's disease, little ACTH is the major component, but in patients with ectopic ACTH production, big ACTH predominates (Yalow, 1974). More recently, it has been reported that there are differences among those ACTHs extracted from the pituitary gland of various species. In man, monkey, sheep, dog, cat, and guinea pig the predominant form is little ACTH; in rabbit, rat, mouse, and hamster, it is an intermediate-sized ACTH; and in cattle, there is both little and intermediate ACTH (Coslovsky and Yalow, 1974). Because, in the first group, cortisol is the main glucocorticoid secreted, whereas, in the second group, corticosterone is the principal glucocorticoid, and because bovine adrenal secretes both steroids, Coslovsky and Yalow (1974) have suggested that the molecular form of ACTH could be an important factor regulating the cortisol to corticosterone ratio in mammalian adrenal secretion.

Eipper and Maines (1975) and Maines and Eipper (1975) have confirmed the existence of an intermediate ACTH (MW 6,500–9,000) in mouse pituitary and in a mouse pituitary tumor cell line. In addition, they have demonstrated in the

same tissues two other forms of ACTH, the molecular weights of which are
20,000–30,000 (big) and 4,000–5,000 (little).

ACTH AND CONTROL OF STEROIDOGENESIS

The synthesis of adrenal steroids from cholesterol is achieved by a series of
enzymes associated with different intracellular loci (Figure 2). Three enzymatic
reactions are located within the mitochondria, i.e., conversion of cholesterol into
pregnenolone, 11β-hydroxylation, and 18-hydroxylation–all of which require
NADPH. The other reactions involved in the synthesis of the steroids occur
either in the cytosol or in the microsomes.

The cellular mechanism of action of ACTH is illustrated in Figure 3. The
different steps can be described as follows:

1. Binding of ACTH to a specific component of the plasma membrane of the
adrenal cells (Hofmann, Wingender, and Finn, 1970; Lefkowitz, Roth, and
Pastan, 1971; Lefkowitz et al., 1970; McIlhinney and Schulster, 1975; Richardson and Schulster, 1972; Saez et al., 1974; Schimmer, Aeda, and Sato, 1968;
Selinger and Civen, 1971; Wolfsen, McIntyre, and Odell, 1972).
2. Stimulation of the plasma membrane-bound adenylate cyclase and increase of
intracellular cyclic adenosine $3':5'$-monophosphate (cAMP) concentration
(Dazord, Gallet, and Saez, 1975; Finn et al., 1975; Finn, Widness, and Hofmann,
1972; Glossman and Gips, 1974; Kelly and Koritz, 1971; Satre et al., 1971;
Schimmer, 1972; Schorr et al., 1971; Taunton, Roth, and Pastan, 1969).
3. Binding of cAMP to the regulatory subunit of a cAMP-dependent protein
kinase and liberation of the catalytic subunit (Garren et al., 1971; Gill, 1972).
This activated protein kinase then phosphorylates several intracellular substrates,
i.e., ribosomal proteins (Roos, 1973; Walton and Gill, 1973), the cholesterol side
chain cleavage enzyme (Caron et al., 1975), and the cholesterol esterase (Boyd
and Trzeciak, 1974; Naghshineh et al., 1974).
4. Translocation of free cholesterol from lipid droplets to mitochondria and its
transformation into pregnenolone (Garren et al., 1971; Mahafee, Reitz, and Ney,
1974).

Our understanding of ACTH action on steroidogenesis is based on the
following results. First, the rate-limiting step of steroidogenesis is the conversion
of cholesterol into pregnenolone; ACTH acts at this level (Constantopoulos and
Tchen, 1961; Kahnt et al., 1974; Stone and Hechter, 1954). Second, the
steroidogenic effect of ACTH is inhibited by protein synthesis inhibitors, but
not by RNA synthesis inhibitors (Ferguson, 1968; Garren, Ney, and Davis, 1965;
Mostafapour and Tchen, 1972; Schulster et al., 1970; Schulster, Richardson, and
Palfreyman, 1974). In addition, protein synthesis inhibitors have no early action
on cAMP synthesis (Boyd and Trzeciak, 1974; Ichii, 1972), protein kinase
activity (Boyd and Trzeciak, 1974), or cholesterol side chain cleavage enzyme

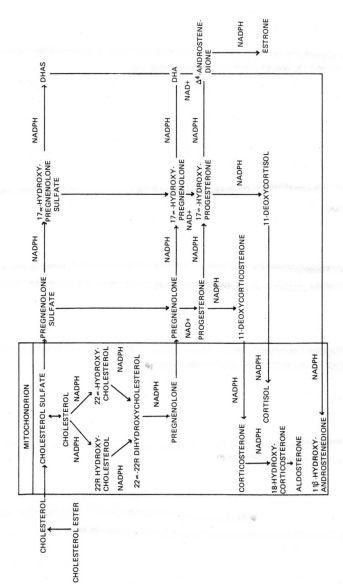

Figure 2. Main pathways of the biosynthesis of adrenal steroids.

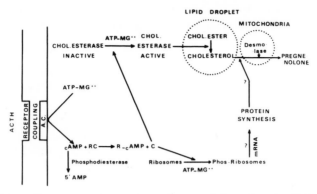

Figure 3. Schematic representation of the mechanism of the action of ACTH on steroidogenesis.

activity (Garren et al., 1971). Conversely, protein synthesis inhibitors do block the transfer of cholesterol from lipid droplets to mitochondria (Garren et al., 1971; Mahafee, Reitz, and Ney, 1974).

Numerous hypotheses have been proposed in the past which could explain the stimulatory effect of ACTH on steroidogenesis. They have been recently reviewed (Bransome, 1968; Eisenstein, 1967; Hilf, 1965; McKerns, 1968). Because NADPH is required for some of the enzymatic steps of steroidogenesis, the hypothetic role of ACTH on NADPH production has been considered by several authors. Haynes and Berthet (1957) demonstrated that ACTH induces an activation of glycogen phosphorylase in the bovine adrenal; therefore, they proposed that this increased enzymatic activity would in turn augment the production of glucose 6-phosphate, which would accelerate the NADPH production by the pentose phosphate pathway. However, there is much doubt about any relationship between phosphorylase activity and steroidogenesis. The rat adrenal phosphorylase is not stimulated by ACTH (Ferguson, 1963), and ACTH is capable of stimulating steroidogenesis even after the adrenal glycogen has been depleted (Vance, Girard, and Gahill, 1962). More recently, McKerns (1968) has proposed that ACTH would stimulate steroidogenesis by an increase of the extramitochondrial NADPH related to an activation of the glucose-6-phosphate dehydrogenase activity. The main argument against this latter hypothesis lies in the facts that the generation of NADPH occurs outside the mitochondria and that pyridine nucleotides cannot cross the mitochondrial membranes. Exogenous NADPH stimulates steroidogenesis in adrenal slices (Halkerston, Feinstein, and Hechter, 1968). However, the nucleotide seems to stimulate only damaged cells, whereas ACTH stimulates intact cells (Halkerston, 1968; Halkerston, Feinstein, and Hechter, 1968). Neher and Milani (1974), using isolated adrenal cell preparations, have presented data which strongly suggest that the

steps stimulated by cAMP and NADPH are different. Finally, since cycloheximide does not inhibit the steroidogenic response to NADPH (Garren et al.,
1971), it can be concluded that this effect of the nucleotide is not related to the
steroidogenic action of ACTH.

A second hypothesis for the mechanism of action of ACTH on steroidogenesis stimulation implies a cAMP-mediated modification of the mitochondrial
membrane permeability (Koritz and Kumar, 1970). Such a change could affect
steroidogenesis in two ways—by facilitating the transfer of externally produced
NADPH into the mitochondria and by increasing the output of pregnenolone
from the mitochondria. Koritz (1968) has actually shown that both processes
can be accelerated by substances which induce mitochondrial swelling. In addition, such substances can stimulate pregnenolone production. Because pregnenolone is an inhibitor of its own synthesis, and because the inhibitory effect of
cycloheximide on the steroidogenic action of ACTH is not related to a decrease
of the total activity of any known enzyme of the steroidogenesis pathway,
Koritz (1968) and Koritz and Kumer (1970) postulated the existence of a labile
protein required for ACTH action which would control the mitochondrial
membrane permeability to the efflux of pregnenolone. This hypothesis is not in
agreement with data presented by Garren et al. (1971), who have shown that
cycloheximide increased unconjugated cholesterol accumulation in the lipid
droplets and not in the mitochondria, as suggested by Koritz's hypothesis. In
addition, Farese (1971a) has shown that in the presence of cyanoketone, which
inhibits the conversion of pregnenolone to progesterone, both ACTH and cAMP
stimulated pregnenolone synthesis despite its accumulation within the adrenal
tissue.

Conversion of Cholesterol to Pregnenolone

The rate-limiting step of ACTH-stimulated steroidogenesis was shown to occur at
the conversion of cholesterol to pregnenolone (Constantopoulos and Tchen,
1961; Kahnt et al., 1974; Stone and Hechter, 1954). Further studies have
indicated that it is more precisely located at the conversion of cholesterol to
(20S)-20-hydroxycholesterol (Hall and Young, 1968; Koritz, 1962). Moreover,
Sharma (1973a) has shown that ACTH also stimulates the conversion of (20S)-
20-hydroxycholesterol into corticosterone by isolated adrenal cells, but this
conversion is not inhibited by cycloheximide. Burstein and Gut (1971), using
acetone-dried preparations of human, bovine, and guinea pig adrenals, found
that the conversion of cholesterol to (22R)-22-hydroxycholesterol is 3- to
20-fold greater than to (20S)-20-hydroxycholesterol. These results are in agreement with the concentrations of (20S)-20-hydroxycholesterol, (22R)-22-
hydroxycholesterol, and (20S,22R)-20,22-dihydroxycholesterol observed in bovine adrenal glands, i.e., 100 μg, 1.5 mg, and 2.2 mg/kg of tissue, respectively
(Dixon, Furutachi, and Lieberman, 1970; Roberts, Banby, and Lieberman,
1969). More recently, Kraaipoel et al. (1975) have suggested that the conversion

of cholesterol to pregnenolone mainly corresponds to the following pathway: Δ20,22-cholesterol $\rightarrow$ 20,22-epoxycholesterol $\rightarrow$ (20S,22R)-20,22-dihydroxy-cholesterol.

Hydroxylation of cholesterol requires NADPH and oxygen. It has been proposed that cytochrome P-450 serves as the terminal oxidase for the electron transport system from NADPH to oxygen (Burstein and Gut, 1973; Omura et al., 1966; Simpson et al., 1972). After its transport to the side chain cleavage enzyme, cholesterol is bound to cytochrome P-450 and produces a change in this enzyme from a low spin to a high spin state (Bell, Cheng, and Harding, 1973). The transfer of electrons to the cytochrome P-450 associated with the side chain cleavage system (Figure 4) is characterized by a rapid change from a high spin to a low spin state (Simpson, Jefcoate, and Boyd, 1971). It has thus been postulated that cytochrome P-450, responsible for cholesterol side chain cleavage, exists in at least two forms; one is an active high spin enzyme-cholesterol complex and the other is a low spin state not bound to cholesterol (Jefcoate et al., 1973). ACTH administered in vivo brings about an increase in the amount of high spin enzyme-cholesterol complex in adrenal mitochondria, this increase being more important in the inner zones of the adrenal cortex. Cycloheximide prevents the ACTH-induced increase of the high spin form of the enzyme (Brownie et al., 1973). Despite the fact that not all enzymatic steps involved in the conversion of cholesterol to pregnenolone are fully understood, kinetic studies in vitro suggest that the rate of access of the substrate to the intramitochondrial enzyme compartment is the proper rate-limiting step, because this process is slower than the rates of the enzymatic reactions involved in the actual conversion of cholesterol to pregnenolone (Burstein and Gut, 1973; Kahnt et al., 1974; Simpson et al., 1972).

Interaction of ACTH with
Its Adrenal Receptor: Structure-Function Relationship

The first step which can be described for the cellular mechanism of action of ACTH is the recognition by the hormone of specific receptors on the outer plasma membrane of the target cell. The existence of such structures has been shown directly and indirectly.

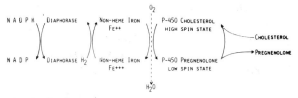

Figure 4. Postulated role of cytochrome P-450 in the conversion of cholesterol to pregnenolone inside the mitochondrion.

Schimmer, Aeda, and Sato (1968) first demonstrated that cellulose-bound ACTH stimulates steroidogenesis of cultured adrenal tumor cells. Similarly, Selinger and Civen (1971) and Richardson and Schulster (1972) reported that ACTH coupled to agarose or to polyacrylamide stimulates steroidogenesis in isolated adrenal cells. Both groups of investigators have provided data suggesting that the biological activity of the complex is not due to free peptides liberated from the ACTH polymers. However, such an approach, directed toward the localization of the interaction at the surface of the cell, has been criticized; on the one hand, it is difficult to reject definitively the possibility of a leakage of hormone from the complex (Butcher et al., 1973; Katzen and Vlahakes, 1973; Kolb et al., 1975), and, on the other hand, the liberated hormone could have a greater biological activity than the native form (Oka and Topper, 1974; Vonderhaar and Topper, 1974; Wilchek, Oka, and Topper, 1975). Another type of indirect approach consisted of studying the distribution of radioactivity in the adrenal tissue after administration of radiolabeled ^{125}I-ACTH$_{1-24}$. Golder and Boyns (1972) have shown that the radioactivity is preferentially concentrated in the reticular zone and at the frontier between reticularis and fasciculata. Previous administration of dexamethasone increases the bound radioactivity to both zones, whereas ACTH inhibits it. However, such studies did not precisely determine the subcellular localization or the molecular form of the adrenal-bound radioactivity.

Binding Direct evidence for specific ACTH receptors was obtained in solubilized extracts of a mouse adrenal tumor which specifically bound ^{125}I-ACTH (Hofmann, Wingender, and Finn, 1970; Lefkowitz, Roth, and Pastan, 1971; Lefkowitz et al., 1970) and in a particulate fraction of bovine adrenal which bound [^{14}C]Phe$_7$-ACTH$_{1-20}$ (Hofmann, Wingender, and Finn, 1970). In addition, such studies demonstrated that the binding of ACTH is linked to an activation of adenylate cyclase. Specific ACTH binding was subsequently found in particulate fractions containing plasma membrane obtained from humans, from several other species (Saez et al., 1974; Wolfsen, McIntyre, and Odell, 1972), and from isolated adrenal cells of rats (McIlhinney and Schulster, 1975).

Studying the interaction of [^{14}C]Phe$_7$-ACTH$_{1-20}$ amide and several ACTH analogues with a bovine adrenal particulate fraction, Hofmann, Wingender, and Finn (1970) have shown that the binding site of the ACTH molecule is located in the COOH-terminal sequence, i.e., the 11–20 sequence of ACTH; and that the ε-amino groups of lysines 11, 15, and 16 are involved in the binding process. Formylation of these lysines, which eliminates the positive charges of the ε-amino groups, inhibits the binding of ACTH$_{1-20}$ amide. Replacing Lys-11 with an amino acid lacking the positive charge greatly reduces the biological activity of ACTH, probably by lowering the binding affinity (Geiger and Schröder, 1973).

Further information concerning the relationship between the structure of ACTH and its binding ability has been obtained with the use of pure monoiodo derivatives of $ACTH_{1-24}$, its o-nitrophenylsulfenyl (NPS) derivative (NPS-$ACTH_{1-24}$), and $ACTH_{11-24}$ (Saez et al., 1974). The binding affinity of $ACTH_{1-24}$ is similar to that of NPS-$ACTH_{1-24}$, but about 10 times higher than that of $ACTH_{11-24}$ (Figures 5 and 6). Because high concentrations of $ACTH_{1-10}$ can displace ^{125}I-$ACTH_{1-24}$, but not ^{125}I-$ACTH_{11-24}$, and because the affinity of the COOH-terminal sequences of ACTH ($ACTH_{11-20}$ amide) (Hofmann, Wingender, and Finn, 1970) and $ACTH_{11-24}$ (Figures 5 and 6) for the adrenal receptor is much lower than for the sequences of $ACTH_{1-20}$ amide and $ACTH_{1-24}$, respectively, it has been suggested (Saez et al., 1974) that the NH_2-terminal sequence (1−10 amino acids) contributes also to the binding by increasing the binding affinity of the ACTH molecule. The binding affinity of (2-phenylalanine,4-(4,5-dehydro)-norvaline)-$ACTH_{1-24}$ is 10 times lower than that of $ACTH_{1-24}$ (Lang et al., 1974); therefore, Tyr_2 or Met_4 or both must play a role in the binding process. On the other hand, Trp_9 is probably inactive, because the affinities of (Phe_9)-$ACTH_{1-20}$ amide (Hofmann, Wingender, and Finn, 1970) and NPS-$ACTH_{1-24}$ (Figures 5 and 6) are similar to those of $ACTH_{1-20}$ amide and $ACTH_{11-24}$, respectively.

Biological Activity Studies on the relationship between the structure and the biological activity of several ACTH analogues have shown that the NH_2-terminal sequence is essential for the steroidogenic action (Ramachandran and Li, 1967). The COOH-terminal sequence lacks any steroidogenic activity, but, as shown before, it is important for the binding.

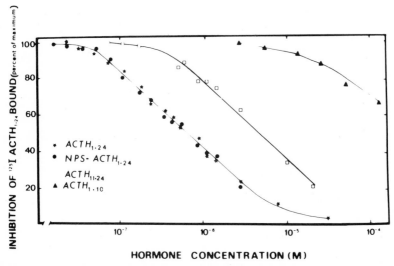

Figure 5. Displacement of ^{125}I-$ACTH_{1-24}$ bound to adrenal plasma membranes by ACTH analogues. From Saez et al. (1975b). Reproduced with permission from J. Biol. Chem. 250:1683–1689.

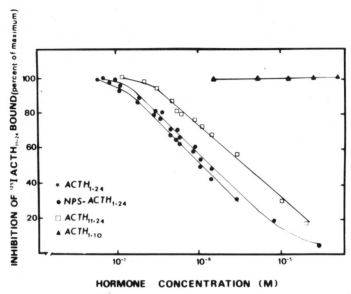

HORMONE CONCENTRATION (M)

Figure 6. Displacement of ^{125}I-ACTH$_{11-24}$bound to adrenal plasma membranes by ACTH analogues. From Saez et al. (1975b). Reproduced with permission from J. Biol. Chem. 250:1683–1689.

The maximal stimulation of corticosterone production by isolated adrenal cells incubated with ACTH$_{1-10}$ and ACTH$_{4-10}$ is similar to that obtained during incubation with ACTH$_{1-24}$; however, molar concentrations required for the former peptides are many times higher than that for ACTH$_{1-24}$ (Schwyzer et al., 1971; Seelig and Sayers, 1973). Since both ACTH$_{4-23}$ amide and ACTH$_{5-24}$ have a relatively high degree of steroidogenic activity in vivo (Fujimo, Hatanaka, and Nishimura, 1971) and in vitro (Sayers et al., 1974), whereas ACTH$_{7-23}$ amide has none, it has been proposed that the "active core" of the molecule for steroidogenesis is located within the region of the 4–10 amino acids in the ACTH peptide. Modifications of the primary structure of the 4–10 sequence lead to a diminution of biological activity. Met$_4$ appears to participate in a hydrophobic interaction of the molecule with its receptor (Draper, Merrifield, and Rizack, 1973; Ramachandran and Li, 1967), and its oxidation or its replacement by α-aminoisobutyric acid leads to some loss of biological activity (Ramachandran and Li, 1967). In addition, intrinsic activities of ACTH$_{5-10}$ and ACTH$_{5-24}$ are lower than those of ACTH$_{4-10}$ and ACTH$_{4-24}$, respectively (Sayers et al., 1974; Schwyzer et al., 1971). Glu$_5$ also seems to have a definite role, because its replacement by glutamine leads to a 70% loss of the steroidogenic activity of ACTH$_{1-19}$ (Li and Hemmasi, 1972) and because the biological activity of ACTH$_{6-24}$ is several times lower than that of ACTH$_{5-24}$ (Fujimo,

Hatanaka, and Nishimura, 1971; Sayers et al., 1974). However, the replacement of Glu_5 by Lys or Arg is followed by a 4-fold increase of the lipolytic activity of $ACTH_{4-10}$ on rabbit adipose cells (Draper, Merrifield, and Rizack, 1973; Draper, Rizack, and Merrifield, 1975); these results suggest that the amino acid Glu_5 plays an important role as a "spacer" in the peptide, this role being independent from the nature of the side chain of the amino acid. The replacement of His_6 by Phe is responsible for a dramatic loss of steroidogenic activity of $ACTH_{1-19}$ (Blake and Li, 1972); in addition, $ACTH_{7-23}$ amide lacks all biological ativity, although it still binds to the receptor (Sayers et al., 1974). A primordial role has been shown for Phe_7, because its replacement by D-Phe leads to more than a 30-fold decrease of steroidogenic activity of $ACTH_{1-19}$ amide (Ide et al., 1972). Substitution of Arg_8 by ornithine or by lysine diminishes the steroidogenic and lipolytic activities of ACTH, but after its replacement by homoarginine an important biological activity persists (Tesser et al., 1973). This suggests that the guanidine residue is essential, whereas the length of the alipathic chain is less important. The role of Trp_9 appears to be fundamental for the steroidogenic activity. Its substitution by phenylalanine (Hofmann, Motibeller, and Finn, 1974; Hofmann, Wingender, and Finn, 1970), by naphtylalanine (Blake and Li, 1975), by pentamethyl-phenylalanine (Vannipsen and Tesser, 1975), and by leucine (Kumar, 1975) or its blockade by a methyl or an o-nitrophenylsulfenyl group (as for $NPS-ACTH_{1-24}$) (Hofmann, Motibeller, and Finn, 1974; Moyle, Kong, and Ramachandran, 1973; Saez et al., 1974; Seelig and Sayers, 1973) abolishes or greatly diminishes the biological activity of the hormone. It is important to stress that the binding affinities of (Phe_9)-$ACTH_{1-20}$ amide (Hofmann, Wingender, and Finn, 1970) and of NPS-$ACTH_{1-24}$ (Figures 5 and 6) are similar to those of $ACTH_{1-20}$ amide and $ACTH_{1-24}$, respectively. This suggests that Trp_9, although essential for the biological activity, is not involved in the binding process.

The 4-10 sequence of ACTH is also biologically active in the central nervous system. $ACTH_{4-10}$ is essential for prolonging the retention of a conditioned avoidance task in the rat; but its analogue $(D-Phe_7)-ACTH_{4-10}$ has effects on behavior which are opposite to those of the native peptide (de Wied, 1973).

The role of the 1-3 amino acids of the NH_2-terminal sequence is not yet clearly defined. The biological activity of $ACTH_{4-10}$ is slightly greater than that of $ACTH_{1-10}$ (Schwyzer et al., 1971; Seelig and Sayers, 1973), whereas the biological activity of $ACTH_{4-23}$ amide is lower than that of $ACTH_{1-24}$ (Fujimo, Hatanaka, and Nishimura, 1971; Sayers et al., 1974). Such contradictory results could be explained by the fact that $ACTH_{1-10}$ is less soluble in aqueous solutions than $ACTH_{4-10}$ (W. Rittel and P. A. Desaulles, personal communication). The free α-amino group is important for high adrenocorticotropic activity (Ramachandran and Li, 1967); the removal of Ser_1 (Geiger and Schroeder, 1974) or the addition of alanine at the NH_2-terminal (Blake, Wang, and Li, 1972) lowers the biological activity of ACTH. The chain length of the

NH_2-terminal sequence also seems to be an important factor, because substitution of the NH_2-terminal dipeptide (Ser_1-Tyr_2) by α-aminovaleric acid and substitution of the NH_2-terminal tripeptide ($Ser_1-Tyr_2-Ser_3$) by ω-amino-caprylic acid maintain and even increase the steroidogenic activity of the hormone (Blake and Li, 1974). The intrinsic activity of $ACTH_{4-23}$ amide for corticosterone and cAMP productions is similar to that of $ACTH_{1-24}$, but its dissociation constant is lower (Sayers et al., 1974). Therefore, it could be suggested that the main contribution of the NH_2-terminal tripeptide of ACTH to the properties of the hormone is to increase its binding affinity. In addition, it has recently been shown that the NH_2-terminal tetrapeptide of ACTH can potentiate the natriuretic action of vasopressin (Cort et al., 1974).

Degradation of ACTH Inactivation of ACTH by plasma and by various tissue homogenates has been described for many years (Geschwind and Li, 1952; Meakin and Nelson, 1960; Meakin, Tingey, and Nelson, 1960). It has recently been shown that the interaction of ACTH with adrenal plasma membranes is characterized by two simultaneous processes—the binding of the hormone to its receptors and its degradation (Saez et al., 1975b). Only unbound ACTH is degraded, whereas bound hormone is protected from degradation. It has also been shown that the two phenomena are independent and that the ACTH sequences which inhibit the binding and the degradation of ^{125}I-$ACTH_{1-24}$ are different (Figure 7). ACTH is also degraded by isolated adrenal cells (Bennett et al., 1974; and unpublished personal data), but the time course and products of degradation are different from those observed with adrenal plasma membranes.

The physiological significance of ACTH degradation is not known. It is important to take this phenomenon into account for the calculation of the binding affinity constant of radiolabeled ACTH. It has been reported that the apparent affinity constants of ^{125}I-$ACTH_{1-24}$ and ^{125}I-$ACTH_{11-24}$ are about 6×10^{-7} M and 4×10^{-6} M, respectively (Saez et al., 1974). However, if the degradations of both ACTHs are considered, the values obtained are about 10^{-8} M and 10^{-7} M, respectively.

The rate-limiting step of ACTH degradation is the hydrolysis of Ser_1. Once Ser has been removed, Tyr_2 is rapidly liberated (White, 1955). Replacement of Ser_1 by other amino acids which are more resistant to enzymatic degradation (i.e., D-Ser, β-Ala, and α-aminoisobutyric acid) increases the biological activity of ACTH in vivo. Alternatively, substitution of L-Ser_1 by Gly decreases the steroidogenic activity (Ide et al., 1972).

Role of cAMP

The cAMP content of a cell is under the control of at least two enzymes. One is adenylate cyclase, which catalyzes the formation of cAMP from ATP; the other is cAMP-phosphodiesterase, which degrades cAMP (Figure 3).

Adenylate Cyclase Adrenal adenylate cyclase is associated with the particulate fraction of the tissue (Dazord, Gallet, and Saez, 1975; Finn et al., 1975;

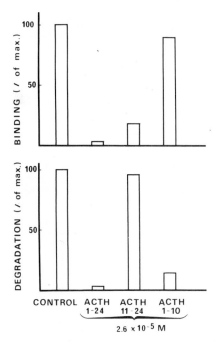

Figure 7. Inhibition of binding and degradation of ^{125}I-ACTH$_{1-24}$ by ACTH analogues.

Finn, Widness, and Hofmann, 1972; Glossman and Gips, 1974; Kelly and Koritz, 1971; Satre et al., 1971; Schimmer, 1972; Schorr et al., 1971; Taunton, Roth, and Pastan, 1969), but its distribution depends, as for other tissues, upon the type of homogenization used. Finn, Widness, and Hofmann (1972) and Saez et al. (1974) have shown that highly purified plasma membranes (with electron microscopic control) retain the highest adenylate cyclase basal, NaF-stimulated, and ACTH-stimulated activities, as well as the capacity to bind ^{125}I-ACTH$_{1-24}$ (Figure 8). Maximal stimulation of human adrenal adenylate cyclase is obtained with 10^{-5} M ACTH, higher concentrations of the hormone leading to a reversal of the stimulation. The apparent concentration required for half-maximal stimulation of the enzyme is about 5×10^{-7} M (Dazord, Gallet, and Saez, 1975; Ide et al., 1972; Lefkowitz et al., 1970; Taunton, Roth, and Pastan, 1969). However, because the hormone is degraded in the experimental conditions for adenylate cyclase assay (Dazord, Gallet, and Saez, 1975), the true K_m must be lower. Nevertheless, these concentrations remain much higher than those required for eliciting half-maximal response of steroidogenesis with isolated adrenal cells (Kitabchi and Sharma, 1974; Moyle, Kong, and Ramachandran, 1973; Richardson and Schulster, 1973; Sayers et al., 1974; Schwyzer et al., 1971; Seelig and Sayers, 1973) and then with physiological, circulating levels of ACTH in the

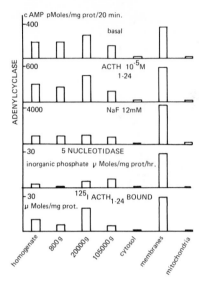

Figure 8. Distribution of adenylate cyclase, 5'-nucleotidase, and ACTH binding activities in different subcellular fractions of adrenal cortex.

blood (Berson and Yalow, 1968). A quantitative difference between the apparent affinities of the hormone for intact and ruptured cells could be due to either a modification of the receptor during homogenization—as suggested for the oxytocin receptors of the toad bladder (Bar et al., 1970; Roy et al., 1973)—or an increased degradation by the broken cells (unpublished personal data). In addition, it has been shown that concentrations required for maximal production of cAMP in isolated adrenal cells are one order of magnitude higher than those needed for maximal stimulation of corticosteroid production (Sayers et al., 1974; Seelig and Sayers, 1973).

The relationship between the hormone structure and its stimulatory effect on adenylate cyclase has been extensively studied (Finn et al., 1975; Finn, Widness, and Hofmann, 1972; Hofmann, Motibeller, and Finn, 1974; Ide et al., 1972; Saez et al., 1974). Results are in agreement with those obtained for the isolated cell. The 1–10 COOH-terminal sequence of ACTH and NPS-ACTH can stimulate the enzyme, but less than $ACTH_{1-24}$ can (Figure 9). On the contrary, $ACTH_{11-24}$ and $ACTH_{11-20}$ amide have no stimulatory effect on the enzyme, but they are able to competitively inhibit the stimulation by $ACTH_{11-24}$. Seelig et al. (1971) have shown that very high concentrations of $ACTH_{11-24}$ can antagonize $ACTH_{1-10}$; however, in the adenylate cyclase assay, $ACTH_{11-24}$ has no antagonistic effects toward the $ACTH_{1-10}$ stimulation (unpublished personal data). This last finding is in agreement with data obtained from binding

ADENYL CYCLASE ACTIVITY IN HUMAN ADRENALS

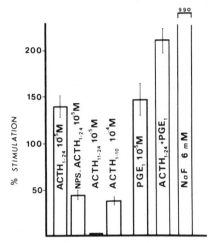

Figure 9. Percentage of stimulation of human adrenal adenylate cyclase by several ACTH analogues, PGE_1, and NaF at maximal concentrations.

studies in which $ACTH_{1-10}$ did not displace bound labeled $ACTH_{11-24}$ (Figure 6).

Human and ovine adrenal adenylate cyclases are also stimulated by prostaglandins E_1 and E_2 (PGE_1 and PGE_2) (Dazord et al., 1974); the stimulation is additive to that of ACTH (Figure 9). This suggests either the existence of two distinct pools of adenylate cyclase within the same cell or the coexistence, in the particulate fraction, of membrane elements originated from two different cell populations. However, since the stimulation of steroidogenesis by PGE_1 is not additive to that by ACTH (Saruta and Kaplan, 1972), it is more likely that both receptors are present in the same cell.

Angiotensin II does not stimulate adrenal adenylate cyclase, although it increases cAMP and steroid production in ovine adrenal slices and isolated cells (Saruta, Cook, and Kaplan, 1972; Peytreman et al., 1973a). In addition, receptor sites for angiotensin II have been shown on both particulate fraction (Glossman, Baukal, and Catt, 1974; Lin and Goodfriend, 1970) and isolated cells (Brecher et al., 1973).

In kinetics characteristic of adrenal adenylate cyclase stimulation, the roles of ions and of guanylnucleotides have been studied more recently (Dazord, Gallet, and Saez, 1975; Finn et al., 1975; Finn, Widness, and Hofmann, 1972; Glossman and Gips, 1974; Halmi, Halmi, and Anderson, 1974; Kelly and Koritz, 1971; Menon, Giese, and Jaffe, 1973; Satre et al., 1971; Schimmer, 1972; Schorr et al., 1971; Taunton, Roth, and Pastan, 1969).

Phosphodiesterases The distribution of these enzymes is ubiquitous, as in the case of adenylate cyclase. Phosphodiesterases are the primary agents responsible for the degradation of cyclic nucleotides into 5'-mononucleotides. Methylxanthines inhibit the action of phosphodiesterases, thus favoring intracellular cAMP accumulation (Applemann, Thompson, and Russell, 1973). Their potentiating effect on hormonal stimulation of the target cell was an argument for the demonstration that some hormones exert their effects via adenylate cyclase (Robison, Butcher, and Sutherland, 1971). In most tissues, at least two types of phosphodiesterases can be found. One of high affinity for cAMP is associated with the plasma membrane particulate fraction; the other of lower affinity for cAMP is soluble (Applemann, Thompson, and Russell, 1973). In the adrenal, most of the phosphodiesterase activity is soluble (Klotz, Vapaatalo, and Stolk, 1972), but plasma membrane preparations also contain a phosphodiesterase activity (Saez, Dazord, and Gallet, 1975a). Although data by Sharma (1972) suggest that the rat adrenal has only one phosphodiesterase with the same affinity for cAMP and cyclic guanosine 3':5'-monophosphate (cGMP), results by Gallant, Kauffman, and Brownie (1974) show to the contrary that there exist at least two types of phosphodiesterase. In addition, this group has measured an activity 10 times higher in the glomerulosa than in the fasciculata reticularis. In rat adrenal cells isolated by tryptic digestion, the phosphodiesterase activity is very low (Kitabchi, Wilson, and Sharma, 1971); this might explain why methylxanthines do not enhance the ACTH-stimulated steroidogenesis of such cells. However, Peytreman et al. (1973b) have shown in vivo and in vitro a potentiating effect of methylxanthines on the ACTH-stimulated production of cAMP and corticosteroids.

Role of cAMP in Mechanism of Action of ACTH on Steroidogenesis After the formation of cAMP, the first event in the action of this cyclic nucleotide is its binding to a protein kinase (Langen, 1973). Like protein kinases of many other tissues, the cAMP-dependent protein kinase consists of two subunits, a regulatory unit and a catalytic kinase (Brostrom et al., 1970). Binding of cAMP to the regulatory unit results in a dissociation of the cAMP-bound receptor from the fully activated kinase (Brostrom et al., 1970; Gill and Garren, 1970). The role of the kinase is to transfer the γ (terminal)-phosphate of ATP onto Ser and Thr residues of proteins. Several specific substrates for the cAMP-dependent protein kinase have been found in different tissues; their phosphorylation is followed by marked changes in their activities (Langen, 1973). However, in the adrenal, the only specific substrate activity which changes after phosphorylation is that of a cholesterol esterase (Boyd and Trzeciak, 1974; Naghshineh et al., 1974). ACTH stimulates the conversion of esterified cholesterol to unconjugated cholesterol which occurs inside the lipid droplet. Therefore, this regulation involves cAMP and activation of the kinase, but is not prevented by the inhibitors of protein synthesis. The other postulated specific substrates for the protein kinase are ribosomal proteins. The in vitro phosphorylation of adrenal ribosomes by the cAMP-dependent protein kinase has already been demon-strated (Garren et al., 1971; Walton and Gill, 1973). In addition, in vivo ACTH administration stimulates adrenal ribosomal phosphorylation (Ichii, 1972; Mura-kami and Ichii, 1973). Roos (1973) has also shown that ACTH increased the phosphorylation of ribosomes of cultured mouse adrenal tumor cells. This phosphorylation of ribosomes has not yet been correlated to any functional changes.

cAMP has been proposed as an obligatory mediator for the mechanism of action of many hormones, including ACTH (Robison, Butcher, and Sutherland, 1971). In favor of this hypothesis are the following arguments: 1) the increase of intracellular cAMP following administration of high concentrations of ACTH precedes the stimulation of steroidogenesis (Grahame-Smith et al., 1967; Peytre-man et al., 1973a; Robison, Butcher, and Sutherland, 1971); 2) cAMP and its active derivatives stimulate adrenal steroidogenesis in vivo and in vitro (Kitabchi and Sharma, 1971; Ney, 1969; Schulster et al., 1970), although other cyclic nucleotides cGMP and cyclic inosine $3':5'$-monophosphate (cIMP) are also able to stimulate steroidogenesis (Kitabchi and Sharma, 1974); 3) all substances which stimulate adrenal steroidogenesis (angiotensin II, prostaglandins E_1 and E_2, cholera toxin) also increase the cAMP production (Donta, King, and Sloper, 1973; Saruta and Kaplan, 1972; Peytreman et al., 1973a; Wolf, Temple, and Cook, 1973); 4) in some experimental and human adrenocortical tumors in which ACTH is unable to stimulate steroidogenesis, the hormone is not able to increase the cAMP production (Saez, Dazord, and Gallet, 1975a; Schimmer, 1969; Schimmer, 1972).

Alternatively, the main arguments against an obligatory role of cAMP for the steroidogenic action of ACTH are the following: 1) a lack of correlation exists between cAMP and steroid production at low concentrations of ACTH (Ide et al., 1972; Mackie, Richardson, and Schulster, 1972; Moyle, Kong, and Rama-chandran, 1973; Peytreman et al., 1973a; Sayers et al., 1974; Sharma et al., 1974); 2) some ACTH analogues are able to produce maximal steroidogenesis without any significant increase in cAMP (Moyle, Kong, and Ramachandran, 1973; Sayers et al., 1974; Seelig and Sayers, 1973). Nevertheless, these findings neither support nor disprove that cAMP may have an obligatory role. Seelig and Sayers (1973) and Sayers et al. (1974) have shown that maximal steroid production is obtained before the increase of cAMP production reaches 20% of its subsequent maximal level and that half-maximal production of steroids is obtained when the cAMP concentration is still less than 1% of the maximal value. In addition, Richardson and Schulster (1973) have shown that submaxi-mal concentrations of ACTH capable of steroidogenesis stimulation in isolated cells do not significantly modify the protein kinase activity. Several hypotheses have been proposed to explain the lack of correlation between steroid produc-tion on the one hand and cAMP production and protein kinase activation on the other hand (Richardson and Schulster, 1973; Sayers et al., 1974; Seelig and

Sayers, 1973): 1) cAMP could be distributed in multiple intracellular compartments, only one of which is involved in the steroidogenic action; 2) the steroidogenic action of ACTH could be mediated by a small fraction of the total cAMP protein kinase; 3) the ACTH effect could be mediated by a factor other than cAMP.

Recently, Sharma et al. (1974) have shown that low concentrations of ACTH increased cGMP rather than cAMP, whereas high concentrations of the hormone increased cAMP but not cGMP. Because cGMP itself also increases the adrenal steroid production, these authors have suggested that ACTH controls steroidogenesis by a process involving both cAMP and cGMP. In addition, it has been reported that the steroidogenic effect of cGMP is inhibited by actinomycin D (Sharma, 1974a); its mechanism of action would therefore be located at both transcriptional and translational levels. The following arguments against an obligatory role for cGMP in steroidogenesis can be listed: 1) ACTH does not stimulate adrenal guanylate cyclase (McMillan, Ney, and Schorr, 1971); 2) if cGMP is able to stimulate steroidogenesis in isolated adrenal cells, the concentrations required are 4–5 times higher than those of cAMP (Kitabchi and Sharma, 1971); 3) no specific cGMP-dependent protein kinase has been found in rat (Sharma, 1974a) or in human adrenals (D. Evain and J. M. Saez, unpublished data); although cGMP can activate the adrenal protein kinase, its activation constant is about 10 times higher than that of cAMP; 4) the steroidogenic effect of ACTH is not inhibited by actinomycin D (Ferguson, 1968; Garren, Ney, and Davis, 1965; Schulster, 1974b; Schulster et al., 1970). Moreover, in the perfused rat adrenals, this inhibitor potentiates the effect of the hormone during at least 6 hr (Mostafapour and Tchen, 1972); this contrasts with the inhibitory effect of the antibiotic on cGMP-induced steroidogenesis, which is seen after 1 hr (Sharma, 1974a).

Finally, present data strongly suggest that cAMP is an obligatory intermediate for ACTH-induced steroidogenesis, but is not the only one since the nucleotide is unable to mimic all the hormonal effects on steroidogenesis, as well as on growth and cell multiplication (Ney, 1969; Nussdorfer, Mazzocchi, and Rebuffat, 1973; Roos, 1974).

Cholesterol Carrier Protein

As previously discussed, the rate-limiting step of steroidogenesis is the translocation of cholesterol from lipid droplets to mitochondria. This step is stimulated by ACTH, but this ACTH action is blocked by protein synthesis inhibitors (Ferguson, 1968; Garren, Ney, and Davis, 1965; Schulster et al., 1970). Garren et al. (1971) have considered the existence of a protein with rapid turnover which would translocate cholesterol and whose synthesis would be stimulated by ACTH. A sterol carrier protein (SCP) has been described in liver 105,000 $\times$ g supernatant (Ritter and Dempsey, 1971; Scallen, Schuster, and Dhar, 1971). SCP is a ubiquitous protein which binds sterols and other water-insoluble precursors to cholesterol by microsomal enzymes. SCP is also present in cytosols of heart, kidney, brain (Johnson and Shan, 1974), and placenta (Astruc et al., 1974). More recent studies have shown that SCP comprises three components (Scallen et al., 1975): SCP, which binds squalene, desmoterol, and cholesterol, but is capable of activating only the microsomal conversion of squalene to lanosterol; SCP_2, which is required for the microsomal conversion of 4,4-di-methyl-Δ^8-cholesterol to C-27-sterol precursors of cholesterol; and SCP_3, which is necessary for the microsomal conversion of 7-dehydrocholesterol to cholesterol. It has been suggested that this last protein is similar to the one described in the liver by Dempsey (1974).

Kan et al. (1972) have reported that a heat-stable liver SCP stimulates the conversion of cholesterol to pregnenolone catalyzed by an acetone powder enzyme extracted from adrenal mitochondria in the presence of NADPH. The same investigators (Kan and Ungar, 1973; Ungar, Kan, and McCoy, 1973) have shown that a similar SCP can be obtained by heating the soluble enzyme extract of acetone powder of adrenal mitochondria ("adrenal activator") at 100°C for 2 min. This adrenal SCP has characteristics similar to those of liver SCP. The adrenal SCP is also present in the cytosol, but not in the microsomes. It specifically binds cholesterol (Kan and Ungar, 1973; Ungar, Kan, and McCoy, 1973). However, the gel filtration on a Sephadex G-25 column used for binding measurements apparently is not an accurate method, because in our experience [^{3}H] cholesterol in buffer alone is eluted in the void volume of several types of Sepharose (G-25, G-50, and G-200). This can probably be attributed to the tendency of cholesterol to form micelles when it is manipulated at 25°C at concentrations of 25–40 nм (Haberland and Reynolds, 1973). With the use of a more specific method for measuring the binding of sterols to a heat-stable adrenal SCP, it appears that the protein recognizes only the side chain of cholesterol (A. Lefevre and J. M. Saez, unpublished data). Figure 10 shows that the sedimentation coefficient of heat-stable adrenal SCP is about 3 and that the binding of [^{3}H] cholesterol is inhibited by several cholesterol analogues but not by more hydroxylated steroids.

The relationship between the adrenal SCP and the protein proposed as a requisite for ACTH action (Garren et al., 1971) remains to be established.

Role of Calcium in Mechanism of Action of ACTH

Ca^{2+} requirements for the steroidogenic effects of ACTH have been known for many years (Birmingham, Elliot, and Valere, 1953). The role of this ion has since been diversely implicated in each step of the stimulatory process: binding of ACTH to membrane receptors (Lefkowitz, Roth, and Pastan, 1970; Saez et al., 1974); activation of adenylate cyclase (Bar and Hechter, 1969; Dazord, Gallet, and Saez, 1975; Taunton, Roth, and Pastan, 1969); conversion of cholesterol to pregnenolone (Simpson et al., 1974); release of steroids from the adrenal (Jaanus, Rosenstein, and Rubin, 1970; Rubin, Carchman, and Jaanus,

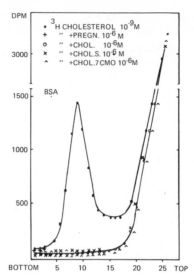

Figure 10. Sucrose gradient centrifugation pattern of heated adrenal cytosol after incubation with [^{3}H]cholesterol in the presence or in the absence of nonradioactive steroids. *Pregn.,* pregnenolone; *Chol.,* cholesterol; *Chol.-S.,* cholesterol sulfate; *Chol. 7-CMO,* cholesterol-7-carboxymethyloxime.

1972); protein synthesis (Farese, 1971b, 1971c, 1971d); protein release (Laychock and Rubin, 1974; Rubin et al., 1974); and RNA (Bransome and Cadwgan, 1968; Castells, Addo, and Kwateng, 1973a) and DNA synthesis (Masui and Garren, 1970).

When steroidogenesis is stimulated with low concentrations of ACTH there is an absolute requirement for Ca^{2+} (optimal concentrations 2–7 mM Ca^{2+}), but this requirement diminishes when higher concentrations of ACTH are used. This is not the case for the stimulation by dibutyryl cAMP, in which the requirement for Ca^{2+} does not change as the concentrations of the nucleotide are increased (Haksar and Peron, 1972; Haksar and Peron, 1973; Sayers, Beall, and Seelig, 1972). Ca^{2+} is also required for the steroidogenic action of cholera toxin (Kowal, Meldolesi, and Macchia, 1974). In addition, both peptides, ACTH and cholera toxin, require calcium for the stimulation of cAMP production (Kowal, Meldolesi, and Macchia, 1974; Sayers, Beall, and Seelig, 1972). These results are in contrast to those presented by Rubin, Carchman, and Jaanus (1972), who reported increased intracellular cAMP levels associated with decreased steroidogenesis in cat adrenals perfused with calcium medium.

Ca^{2+} at concentrations greater than 1 mM depresses the binding of ^{125}I-ACTH to adrenal plasma membranes (Lefkowitz, Roth, and Pastan, 1970; Saez et al., 1974), but has apparently no effect on the binding of the hormone to intact adrenal cells (Kowal, Srinivasan, and Saito, 1974). On the other hand, the stimulation of membrane-bound adenylate cyclase by ACTH is optimal in the presence of 0.1 mM $CaCl_2$, but is inhibited for concentrations of Ca^{2+} higher than 0.5 mM. This diverse effect of Ca^{2+} in particulate fractions and in intact cells can be explained by the fact that in intact cells the Ca^{2+} concentrations near the internally located adenylate cyclase might remain constant despite wide fluctuations of extracellular calcium concentrations, whereas in broken cell membrane preparations the enzyme is directly exposed to the calcium of the medium. Alternatively, Sayers, Beall, and Seelig (1972) have proposed that in intact cells Ca^{2+} amplifies the signal initiated by the ACTH-receptor interaction and transmitted to adenylate cyclase.

If calcium is required for the steroidogenic effect of ACTH, both ACTH and dibutyryl cAMP in turn increase the intracellular concentrations of calcium (Leier and Jugmann, 1973). The degree of stimulation of CA^{2+} uptake and of glucocorticoid production by ACTH and dibutyryl cAMP is dependent upon Ca^{2+} concentrations in the medium and upon amounts of hormone or nucleotide tested. Finally, calcium uptake, like steroidogenesis, is inhibited by cycloheximide but not by actinomycin.

ACTH AND PROTEIN AND RNA SYNTHESIS

At the present time, it seems well established that protein synthesis is an obligatory step in ACTH-stimulated steroidogenesis (Ferguson, 1968; Garren et al., 1971; Gill, 1972; Schulster, 1974a). Ferguson (1962) first reported that the in vitro stimulation of steroidogenesis by ACTH is blocked by puromycin. This inhibition parallels that of protein synthesis. Some puromycin analogues which do not inhibit protein synthesis are also ineffective on ACTH-induced steroidogenesis (Ferguson, 1963). Garren, Ney, and Davis (1965) have obtained in vivo the same results as Ferguson (1962). They have, in addition, presented many arguments in favor of the existence of an ACTH-controlled protein with very fast turnover. Kowal (1970a), using cultured tumor cells, and Schulster et al. (1970), using superfused adrenal slices, have also concluded that protein synthesis is necessary for the steroidogenic action of ACTH. However, inhibitors of RNA synthesis such as actinomycin do not block this ACTH effect, although they inhibit general protein synthesis (Ferguson, Morita, and Mendelsohn, 1967; Garren, Ney, and Davis, 1965). Thus, it had been concluded that ACTH must stimulate the translation of a messenger RNA (mRNA) (Gill, 1972). The half-life of this mRNA is about 6 hr (Kowal, 1970a).

The half-life of the labile protein whose synthesis is stimulated by ACTH is short, i.e., 10 min in vivo, 2–4 min in isolated cells, and 45–49 min in perfused tissues (Ferguson, 1962; Ferguson, Morita, and Mendelsohn, 1967; Mackie, Richardson, and Schulster, 1972). Its synthesis is very rapid, less than 3 min, which represents the lag time observed between the addition of ACTH and the initiation of steroidogenesis (Ferguson, Morita, and Mendelsohn, 1967). Because the average time needed for the ribosomes of eukaryotic cells to translate a mRNA has been estimated at 1–2 min (Palmiter, 1972), and because the lag time which low concentrations of ACTH take to initiate steroidogenesis is longer (Schulster, Richardson, and Palfreyman, 1974), it has been suggested that ACTH could activate a pre-existing labile protein rather than induce its synthesis (Schulster, Richardson, and Palfreyman, 1974).

Although it is commonly accepted that long-term administration of ACTH in vivo stimulates protein synthesis, a possible immediate role in vitro on amino acid incorporation remains controversial. Several investigators have reported an inhibitory effect of ACTH on protein synthesis (Ferguson, Morita, and Mendelsohn, 1967; Halkerston, Feinstein, and Hechter, 1964; Morrow, Burrow, and Mulrow, 1967), although this has not been found by others (Koritz, Peron, and Dorfman, 1957; Nicola, Clayman, and Johnstone, 1968). The inhibitory effect of ACTH on protein synthesis would probably be due to a secondary elevation of intracellular glucocorticoid levels which, under maximal hormonal stimulation, can reach concentrations of 400 μM (Clayman, Tsang, and Johnstone, 1970). It has actually been shown that the blockage of steroidogenesis by aminoglutethimide suppresses the inhibitory effect of ACTH (Farese, 1969). Grower and Bransome (1970), using polyacrylamide gel electrophoresis, have shown changes in the protein pattern after stimulation by ACTH and cAMP. Such modifications are apparent for 15–30 min after addition of the stimulants, but are no longer observed after 60 min.

The contradictory results concerning in vitro acute effects of ACTH on adrenal protein synthesis have recently been explained by Farese (1971b, 1971c, 1971d). This author has shown that Ca^{2+} alone stimulates adrenal protein synthesis by increasing the transfer of the amino acids from the aminoacyl-tRNA to proteins. ACTH and cAMP significantly increase the incorporation of amino acids into protein only if Ca^{2+} concentrations of the medium are moderate; for instance, when 2.2 mM Ca^{2+} is used there is no significant effect of cAMP or ACTH because protein synthesis is already maximally stimulated by Ca^{2+} alone. On the contrary, after preincubating the cells in a calcium-free medium, the addition of the hormone and of 1 mM Ca^{2+} markedly stimulates protein synthesis. Because ACTH increased the ^{45}Ca-adrenal uptake (Leier and Jugmann, 1973), Farese suggested that Ca^{2+} could be the mediator of enzyme activation by ACTH; however, Ca^{2+} alone does not stimulate steroidogenesis (see under "Role of cAMP"). Thus, it seems more likely that the property of this ion would be a general rather than a regulatory one and that its potentiating effect on ACTH action seems necessary for the stimulation of protein synthesis. Rubin et al. (1974) and Laychock and Rubin (1974) have recently reported that ACTH stimulates the synthesis and the release of two proteins (MW 48,000 and 58,000) by perfused cat adrenal. Their precise role has not yet been defined.

Long-term administration of ACTH increases the RNA content of the adrenals. After 24 hr the increase is about 50% (Farese, 1968; Imrie et al.,

1965). Stimulation of labeled uridine incorporation into adrenal RNA has been observed within 30 min following ACTH injection (Bransome and Cadwgan, 1968). Contrasting with these in vivo effects are those reported for in vitro studies, in which it has been shown that ACTH can be inhibitory (Ferguson, 1962; Ferguson, Morita, and Mendelsohn, 1967; Halkerston, Feinstein, and Hechter, 1964), stimulatory (Bransome and Reddy, 1963), or without effect (Farese, 1968). It has actually been suggested that the inhibitory effects of ACTH or cAMP or both on RNA synthesis are due to an intracellular accumulation of cAMP degradation products, namely $5'$-AMP (Tsang and Johnstone, 1973). With the use of a perfusion system which prevents the accumulation of end products, Castells, Addo, and Kwateng (1973a) have shown that ACTH stimulates a fast incorporation of labeled uridine into cytoplasmic RNA and that the rate of incorporation is constant for at least the first 60 min. These investigators also reported that a 30-min incubation with ACTH increases labeled uridine incorporation in all RNA species, but more markedly in fraction 18S (Castells, Addo, and Kwateng, 1973b). It is likely that this stimulatory effect of ACTH on RNA synthesis is the expression of the trophic property of the hormone on its target organ. As previously discussed, RNA synthesis is not necessary for the immediate action of ACTH on the stimulation of steroidogenesis; in fact, RNA synthesis inhibitors in vitro potentiate the steroidogenic effect of the hormone and delay the onset of the refractory phase in perfused rat adrenals (Mostafapour and Tchen, 1972). However, data presented by Mostafapour and Tchen (1971, 1973) show that for a prolonged hormonal stimulation the presence of mRNA, whose half-life is about 7 hr and whose synthesis is stimulated by ACTH, is necessary. It has been suggested that this mRNA codes for the steroidogenic protein postulated by Garren, Ney, and Davis (1965).

ACTH AND CELL GROWTH

The in vivo effects of ACTH on adrenal cell growth have been well documented. After hypophysectomy the adrenal cortex undergoes an involution, but administration of exogenous ACTH can then maintain weight and DNA content of the gland. Excess ACTH from endogenous or exogenous origin leads to cortical adrenal hyperplasia. Farese and Reddy (1963) have reported that ACTH administration for 7 days increased the DNA content of the rat adrenal. Imrie et al. (1965) also found that prolonged ACTH administration increased adrenal DNA. More recently, Masui and Garren (1970) have shown that the guinea pig adrenal DNA content was significantly increased 48 hr after ACTH administration. It continued to rise in response to further ACTH administration. However, stimulation of DNA synthesis, measured by incorporation of [^{3}H] thymidine into DNA, was detected as early as 16 hr after ACTH was given. Concomitantly, an increase of DNA polymerase and thymidine kinase activities (Garren et al., 1971; Masui and Garren, 1970) was shown.

The in vitro effects of ACTH on adrenal cell replication are contradictory. Masui and Garren (1971) have reported that ACTH, as well as several nucleotides (dibutyryl cAMP, cAMP, 5'-AMP, ADP, and ATP), inhibits DNA synthesis and cell replication in cultured mouse adrenal tumor cells (Y-1 tumor). This same effect of ACTH and dibutyryl cAMP has also been observed in cultured normal adrenal cells of the rat (Ramachandran and Suyama, 1975). The biochemical pathway by which ACTH inhibits the cell replication in vitro is not clearly understood. Because ACTH increased cAMP production in all adrenal cell lines studied and because this cyclic nucleotide inhibited replication in many cell lines (Pastan and Johnson, 1974; Pastan, Johnson, and Anderson, 1975; Ryan and Heidrick, 1974; Whitfield et al., 1973), including adrenal cells (Masui and Garren, 1971; Ramachandran and Suyama, 1975), it has been suggested that the inhibitory effect of ACTH on cell growth is mediated by cAMP. Against this hypothesis are the results obtained with NPS-ACTH (see under "Binding"). This ACTH derivative mimics the native hormone effects on steroidogenesis and cell multiplication, although it weakly stimulates cAMP production. In addition, Roos (1974) reported that cAMP is ineffective on cultured human fetal adrenal cells.

A role for glucocorticoids as mediators of the inhibitory effect of ACTH on cell replication could be considered, because glucocorticoids inhibit the multiplication of certain cells (Gospodarowicz and Gospodarowicz, 1974; Sibley et al., 1974), and their production in the adrenal cells is stimulated by ACTH. However, this explanation does not seem very likely in the case of the Y-1 tumor, because 1) the adrenal tissue does not produce glucocorticoids, 2) the blockade of steroidogenesis by aminoglutethimide does not affect the inhibitory action of ACTH on cell growth (Masui and Garren, 1971), and 3) glucocorticoids added to incubation media do not modify the [^{3}H] thymidine incorporation into DNA. However, glucocorticoids inhibit DNA synthesis in normal rat adrenal cells in culture, but their inhibitory effect is much less important than that caused by ACTH (Ramachandran and Suyama, 1975).

In vivo effects of glucocorticoids on DNA synthesis are described in Figure 11, which summarizes the responses of plasma corticosterone, [^{3}H] thymidine incorporation into DNA, and DNA polymerase activity of the rat adrenal after in vivo administration of ACTH, dexamethasone, and aminoglutethimide. Long-acting ACTH alone increases all three parameters studied. The opposite effect is observed with dexamethasone. Aminoglutethimide decreases plasma corticosterone, but increases both [^{3}H] thymidine incorporation and DNA polymerase activity. Because aminoglutethimide inhibits steroidogenesis, the secondary elevation of endogenous ACTH could explain the increases of thymidine incorporation and of DNA polymerase activity. Moreover, when aminoglutethimide and high doses of long-acting ACTH are administered simultaneously, very small changes of plasma corticosterone are observed, whereas thymidine incorporation and DNA polymerase activity are significantly higher than those obtained with

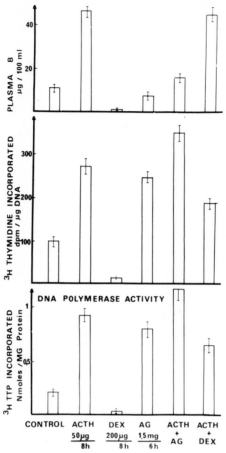

Figure 11. Adenylate cyclase activity of crude membrane preparation (pellet of 20,000 × *g* (*middle*), and adrenal DNA polymerase activity (*bottom*) were measured 24 hr after administration of dexamethasone (*Dex*), aminoglutethimide (*Ag*), and ACTH to 27-day-old male rats.

aminoglutethimide or ACTH separately. In addition, these effects of aminoglutethimide on the same two parameters are completely blocked by dexamethasone. These data, therefore, suggest that the effects of ACTH on the replication of adrenal cells are partially blocked by the increase of glucocorticoids in response to ACTH. This hypothesis is confirmed by results obtained when ACTH and dexamethasone are injected simultaneously. Dexamethasone partially blocks the effect of ACTH on DNA synthesis, although plasma corticosterone levels are similar to those obtained after administration of ACTH alone. A recent report by Takasugi, Takeuchi, and Taguchi (1975) also describes an inhibitory effect of cortisone on the growth of experimentally induced mouse adrenal tumor. Consequently, it appears that glucocorticoids exert a double control over adrenal cell growth—indirectly, by inhibiting the secretions of corticotrophin-releasing factor and ACTH (Sato et al., 1975) and directly, at the adrenal cell level. This phenomenon could explain the larger size of the adrenals in congenital adrenal hyperplasia than in Cushing's syndrome. The ACTH secretion in congenital adrenal hyperplasia is not markedly elevated as in Cushing's syndrome (Fukushima et al., 1975), but in the latter, along with the ACTH hypersecretion, there is also a hypersecretion of cortisol, which in turn partially blocks the trophic action of ACTH on the adrenals. On the contrary, in congenital adrenal hyperplasia the absence of hypersecretion of cortisol will allow the full trophic activity of ACTH. In addition, such an inhibitory role of glucocorticoids on cell replication could also partially explain why ACTH administration inhibits the growth of cortical adrenal tumors transplanted into nonadrenalectomized isogenic mice (Fiala and Fiala, 1968; Masui and La Porte, 1973).

Data presented so far have shown that cAMP and its metabolites on one hand and glucocorticoids on the other hand seem to inhibit the in vitro replication of normal adrenal cells. This could explain the apparently contradictory effects of ACTH in vivo and in vitro. The hormone stimulates in vitro the accumulation of both cAMP ($\cong 10^{-6}$ M) and glucocorticoids ($\cong 10^{-5}$ M) in the incubation media. The in vivo situation might be different, because the secretion of these compounds into the blood circulation would in turn prevent their accumulation.

It has also been demonstrated that ACTH has an in vitro effect on cell differentiation (Kahri, 1966; Kahri, Huhtaniemi, and Salmenpera, 1975; Ramachandran and Suyama, 1975). Fetal rat adrenal cells cultured in ACTH-free medium maintain a nondifferentiated ultrastructural aspect. The addition of ACTH induces the cell differentiation with acquisition of ultrastructural and secretory characteristics similar to those observed in adult cells of the fasciculata (Kahri, 1973; Kahri, Huhtaniemi, and Salmenpera, 1975). In addition, glomerulosa cells in culture have a high rate of multiplication and secrete little corticosterone; but in the presence of ACTH the multiplication rate diminishes while the corticosterone production increases (Ramachandran and Suyama, 1975). These results support the centripetal migration theory of adrenocortical cell renewal (Ford and Young, 1963; Wright, 1971). According to this hypothesis, the cells of outer zones of the adrenal cortex are undifferentiated cells which will undergo ACTH-induced progressive differentiation and will move to other zones of the gland's cortex. According to these results, it has been proposed that the major in vitro cAMP-mediated ACTH function is to induce the transformation of undifferentiated cells of the adrenal cortex into functional fasciculata cells, but that the control of cell multiplication may be under factors other than ACTH (Ramachandran and Suyama, 1975).

Such difficulties encountered in the interpretation of mechanism of action of ACTH on cell growth and differentiation—processes which exclude each other—are common with other hormones (luteinizing hormone, thyroid-stimulating hormone (TSH), etc.). These hormones have in vivo a trophic action on their target organs, and at the same time they contribute to their specific function. Luteinizing hormone, however, and cAMP in vitro inhibit the multiplication of corpus luteum cells and induce their differentiation (Channing, 1974; Gospodarowicz and Gospodarowicz, 1974). Contradictory effects produced in vivo and in vitro by these hormones could be explained by two hypotheses: 1) both processes are under cAMP control, with low concentrations of the nucleotide stimulating replication and high concentrations stimulating differentiation, as observed in several cell lines (Pastan, Johnson, and Anderson, 1975; Ryan and Heidrick, 1974; Whitfield et al., 1973), or 2) the two processes are not under the same control, with cAMP regulating differentiation and the specific function of the target cell, while another factor, independent from cAMP, controls cell multiplication. The initiation of these two separate processes would be related to two distinct sequences in the hormone. Such a possibility is documented by a report on catecholamine action on the mouse parotid glands (Durham, Baserga, and Butcher, 1974). The investigators have shown that the functional groups which control cAMP production are different from those which induce cell multiplication.

ADRENOCORTICAL TUMORS INSENSITIVE TO ACTH

It has been known for many years that in most of the human adrenocortical tumors ACTH does not stimulate steroidogenesis (Lipsett, Hertz, and Roos, 1963). The same ACTH insensitivity has also been described in several types of animal adrenal cortical tumors (Ney et al., 1969; Schimmer, 1969; Schimmer, 1972; Schorr and Ney, 1971; Schorr et al., 1971; Sharma, 1973b; Snell and Stewart, 1959). Theoretically, the biochemical event(s) responsible for this failure of ACTH to stimulate steroidogenesis could be located either within the cell plasma membrane, at the site of the interaction of ACTH with its receptor, or in one of the intracellular events following cAMP formation.

A defect in cell membranes has been described by Schimmer (1969, 1972) in some mutant cell lines of mouse adrenal tumor. In these mutants, adenylate cyclase and steroidogenesis were not stimulated by ACTH, but cAMP was capable of stimulating steroid production. However, since no binding studies were performed, it could not be concluded whether the abnormality was located at the binding site of ACTH or in the coupling system between binding site and catalytic subunit of adenylate cyclase. A similar cell plasma membrane defect has been described in a rat thyroid experimentally induced tumor (Macchia, Meldolesi, and Chiariello, 1972). The membrane-bound adenylate cyclase of this

tumor was not stimulated by TSH, but responded to NaF. Further studies have
shown that this TSH insensitivity was due to an anomaly of the TSH binding site
(Mandato, Meldolesi, and Macchia, 1975). In another experimentally induced
adrenal tumor first described by Snell and Stewart (1959), neither ACTH nor
cAMP was able to stimulate steroidogenesis (Ney et al., 1969; Sharma, 1973a
and b) although adenylate cyclase was sensitive to ACTH (Schorr and Ney,
1971). The defect could thus be attributed to a step beyond cAMP formation. In
addition, this tumor presented other anomalies located in the cell plasma
membrane: abnormal presence of receptors to epinephrine and to luteinizing
hormone (Schorr et al., 1971), and intracellularly in the pathway of steroidogenesis (Sharma, 1973a and b; Sharma, 1974b; Sharma and Brush, 1974).

The failure of certain steroid-secreting human adrenal cortical tumors to
respond to ACTH stimulation has been investigated in two laboratories (Hinshaw
and Ney, 1974; Saez, Dazord, and Gallet, 1975a). According to the adenylate
cyclase responses to ACTH and PGE_1, 16 cases of tumor fell into three different
categories (Figure 12).

In the first group, the enzyme was stimulated by the same factors as in
normal adrenals. In three among these seven cases in the first group, there was an
insensitivity to ACTH in vivo; therefore, for these three cases, it could be
considered that the biochemical anomaly was located beyond the cAMP formation. This hypothesis was confirmed for one of them, because the steroidogenesis of isolated cells was not stimulated by ACTH, PGE_1, or dibutyryl cAMP

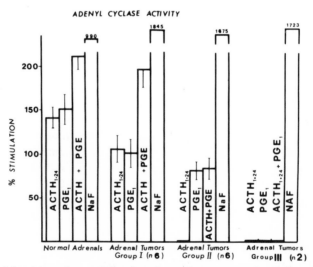

Figure 12. Adenylate cyclase activity of crude membrane preparation (pellet of 20,000 Xgg
centrifugation) of human normal adrenals and human adrenocortical tumors under several
conditions.

Table 1. Cortisol production by isolated cells from human adrenals[a]

| | | Tumors (8 Cases) | | |
Additions	Normal	1 Case	5 Cases	1 Case	1 Case
ACTH, 3×10^{-6} M	+	+	−	−	−
PGE$_1$, 60 nM	+	+	+	−	−
Dibutyryl cAMP, 1 mM	+	+	+	+	−

[a]Incubation 2 hr at 37°C.

(Table 1, column 5). Thus, this case is similar to the 494 adrenocortical tumor of the rat (Richardson and Schulster, 1972; Schorr and Ney, 1971; Sharma, 1973b). In the rat tumor, it has been postulated that an anomaly of the cAMP-dependent protein kinase could be responsible for the steroidogenesis insensitivity to ACTH and cAMP (Sharma, 1973b). Such an anomaly could actually be demonstrated in a human adrenocortical tumor of which the adenylate cyclase was normally stimulated by ACTH (J. P. Riou, D. Evain, and J. M. Saez, unpublished data).

In the second group of tumors, steroidogenesis in vivo and adenylate cyclase activity of membrane preparations were insensitive to ACTH, but the enzyme was stimulated by PGE$_1$ and NaF (Figure 12). This insensitivity to ACTH was confirmed in five among seven cases by the lack of steroidogenic response to ACTH of isolated tumor cells, whereas PGE$_1$ and cAMP were able to increase the cortisol production (Table 1, column 3). Further studies with this group of tumors demonstrated that ^{125}I-ACTH$_{1-24}$ is specifically bound to tumor

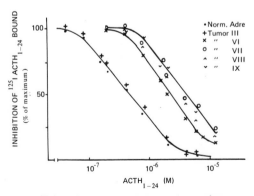

Figure 13. Displacement of bound ^{125}I-ACTH$_{1-24}$ by ACTH$_{1-24}$ in normal human adrenal (●), in a tumor of the first group of ACTH-sensitive tumors (+), and in four tumors of the second group of ACTH-insensitive tumors (x, o, ʌ, and v). From Saez, Dazord, and Gallet (1975). Reproduced with permission from J. Clin. Invest. 56:536–547.

Table 2. Apparent dissociation constants for $ACTH_{1-24}$ and $ACTH_{11-24}$ of crude membranes obtained from normal human adrenals and adrenocortical tumors

	$ACTH_{1-24}$	$ACTH_{11-24}$
Normal adrenal	$3.2 \pm 1.8 \ 10^{-7}$ M	$4.3 \pm 1.6 \ 10^{-6}$ M
Tumor		
Group I	$4.3 \pm 1.9 \ 10^{-7}$ M	$4.7 \pm 1.8 \ 10^{-6}$ M
Group II	$4.2 \pm 1.1 \ 10^{-6}$ M	$5.2 \pm 2.1 \ 10^{-6}$ M

particulate preparations (Saez, Dazord, and Gallet, 1975a); however, the apparent affinity of the binding was about 10 times lower than that measured for the normal adrenal or for the tumors of the first group, i.e., with ACTH-sensitive adenylate cyclase (Figure 13 and Table 2). On the other hand, the binding of ^{125}I-ACTH$_{11-24}$ was similar to that of the other groups (Figure 14 and Table 2) and about 10 times lower than that of ACTH$_{1-24}$ in the normal gland. Because it could be established that ACTH$_{1-10}$ was not able to displace bound ^{125}I-ACTH$_{1-24}$ in one of these tumors of the second group (the reverse of that found in the normal gland), it was suggested that the anomaly could be due to a loss or a modification of the receptor site which binds the NH$_2$-terminal 1–10 sequence of ACTH. This anomaly could explain both the modification of

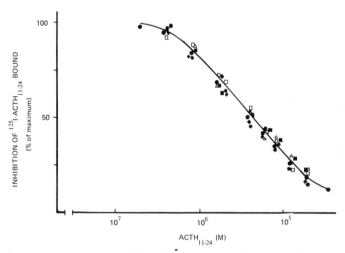

Figure 14. Displacement of bound ^{125}I-ACTH$_{11-24}$ by ACTH$_{11-24}$ in normal human adrenal (●), in a tumor of the first group of ACTH-sensitive tumors (✦), and in four tumors of the second group of ACTH-insensitive tumors (△, □, ■, and ◆). From Saez, Dazord, and Gallet (1975a). Reproduced with permission from J. Clin. Invest. 56:536–547.

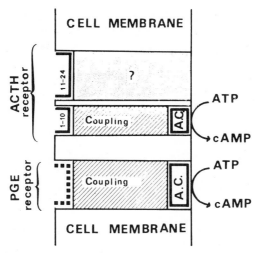

Figure 15. Postulated model for the interaction of ACTH and PGE with their adrenal receptors. From Saez, Dazord, and Gallet (1975a). Reproduced with permission from J. Clin. Invest. 56:536–547.

$ACTH_{1-24}$ binding affinity and the lack of steroidogenic action of this hormone.

The third group encompasses two tumors of which the membrane-bound adenylate cyclase activity and the steroid production by isolated cells were not stimulated either by ACTH or by PGE_1 (Figure 12, group III). Anomalies similar to those of the second group of tumors were found for the ACTH binding sites, but in addition no binding of $[^3H]PGE_1$ could be demonstrated, indicating that the receptor of PGE_1 was also lost or abnormal.

The results obtained in the study of the human adrenal tumor and of the normal gland can be explained by the model presented in Figure 15. It is proposed that the ACTH receptor is composed of two binding sites, one of which binds the 11–24 sequence of the hormone and the other the 1–10 sequence. The COOH-terminal sequence is responsible for the high affinity binding of ACTH and would facilitate the binding of the 1–10 sequence to the second site. Only when this second site is occupied would the adenylate cyclase be stimulated. The loss of this site explains the insensitivity of the second and third group of human tumors to ACTH. The model also suggests that the binding site and the coupling system of PGE_1 are independent of those of ACTH. This hypothesis could explain why ACTH and PGE_1 have additive stimulatory effects on the adenylate cyclase of the normal adrenal and why the adenylate cyclase of the ACTH-insensitive tumor of the second group is still stimulated by PGE_1.

It finally appears from the study of human adrenocortical tumors that the failure of ACTH to stimulate steroidogenesis can be related to a variety of biochemical abnormalities involving the hormone receptor–adenylate cyclase complex or the intracellular steps initiated by the hormone-receptor interaction. Further studies on adrenal tumors should be an important tool to investigate both the fascinating problem of the role of ACTH on cell growth control and whether or not it is the same sequence of ACTH which regulates the specific function and the growth of the adrenal cell.

ACKNOWLEDGMENTS

The authors are indebted to Drs. W. Rittell and P. A. Desaulles for the generous gift of various ACTH analogues. We thank Dr. A. Dazord and Miss D. Gallet de Santerre, who have contributed to various parts of the original work; Dr. J. Bertrand for his interest in this work, and Miss M. Montagnon and Miss J. Bois for secretarial assistance.

REFERENCES

Applemann, M. M., W. J. Thompson, and T. R. Russell. 1973. Cyclic nucleotides phosphodiesterases. Adv. Cyclic Nucleotide Res. 3:65–68.

Astruc, M., C. Tabacik, B. Descomps, and A. Crastes de Paulet. 1974. The binding of squalene by human placental cytosol: role in conversion of squalene to lanosterol. FEBS Lett. 47:66–71.

Bar, H. P., and O. Hechter. 1969. Substrate specificity of adenyl cyclase from rat fat cell ghosts. Biochim. Biophys. Acta 192:141–144.

Bar, H. P., O. Hechter, I. L. Schwartz, and R. Walter. 1970. Neurohypophyseal hormone-sensitive adenyl cyclase of toad urinary bladder. Proc. Natl. Acad. Sci. U.S.A. 67:7–18.

Bell, J. J., S. C. Cheng, and B. W. Harding. 1973. Control of substrate flux and adrenal cytochrome P-450. Ann. N. Y. Acad. Sci. 212:290–306.

Bennett, H. P. J., G. Bullock, P. J. Lowry, C. McMartin, and J. Peters. 1974. Fate of corticotrophins in an isolated adrenal-cell bioassay and decrease of peptide breakdown by cell purification. Biochem. J. 138:185–194.

Berson, S., and R. Yalow. 1968. Radioimmunoassay of ACTH in plasma. J. Clin. Invest. 47:2725–2751.

Birmingham, M. K., F. H. Elliot, and P. H. L. Valere. 1953. The need for the presence of calcium for the stimulation in vitro of rat adrenal glands by adrenocorticotrophic hormone. Endocrinology 53:687–689.

Blake, J., and C. H. Li. 1972. Adrenocorticotropin. Synthesis of [6-phenyl-alanine]-α^{1-19}-adrenocorticotropic hormone and its steroidogenic, melanocyte-stimulating, and lipolytic activity. Biochemistry 11:3459–3461.

Blake, J., and C. H. Li. 1974. Adrenocorticotropin 46. Int. J. Peptide Protein Res. 6:141–144.

Blake, J., and C. H. Li. 1975. Adrenocorticotropin 47. Synthesis and biological activity of adrenocorticotropic peptides modified at the tryptophan position. J. Med. Chem. 18:423–426.

Blake, J., K. T. Wang, and C. H. Li. 1972. Adrenocorticotropin. Solid-phase synthesis of α^{1-19}-adrenocorticotropic hormone, alanyl-α^{1-19}-adrenocorticotropic hormone, and prolyl-α^{1-19}-adrenocorticotropic hormone and their adrenocorticotropic activity. Biochemistry 11:438–441.

Boyd, G. S., and W. H. Trzeciak. 1974. Cholesterol metabolism in the adrenal cortex: studies on the mode of action of ACTH. Ann. N. Y. Acad. Sci. 188:361–377.

Bransome, E. D. 1968. Adrenal cortex. Annu. Rev. Physiol. 30:171–212.

Bransome, E. D., and C. E. Cadwgan. 1968. Cytoplasmic RNA synthesis in adrenal: rapid, selective stimulation by adrenocorticotropic hormone (ACTH). Life Sci. (II) 7:1009–1016.

Bransome, E. D., and W. J. Reddy. 1963. Incorporation of amino acids into rat adrenal nucleic acids: effects of adrenocorticotrophin and growth hormone. Endocrinology 3:540–546.

Brecher, P., M. Tabacchi, H. Y. Pyun, and A. V. Chobanian. 1973. Angiotensin binding to rat adrenal capsular cell suspensions. Biochem. Biophys. Res. Commun. 54:1511–1517.

Brostrom, M. A., E. M. Reimann, D. A. Walsh, and E. G. Krebs. 1970. A cyclic 3',5'-AMP-stimulated protein kinase from cardiac muscle. In G. Weber (ed.), Advances in Enzyme Regulation, Vol. 8, pp. 191–203. Pergamon Press, Oxford.

Brownie, R. C., J. Alfano, C. R. Jefcoate, W. Orme-Johnson, H. Beinert, and E. R. Simpson. 1973. Effect of ACTH on adrenal mitochondral cytochrome P-450 in the rat. Ann. N. Y. Acad. Sci. 212:344–360.

Burstein, S., and M. Gut. 1971. Biosynthesis of pregnenolone. Recent Prog. Horm. Res. 27:303–349.

Burstein, S., and M. Gut. 1973. Kinetic studies on the mechanism of conversion of cholesterol to pregnenolone. Ann. N. Y. Acad. Sci. 212:262–275.

Butcher, R. W., O. B. Crofford, S. Gammeltoff, J. Gliemann, J. R. Gavin, I. D. Goldfine, C. R. Kahn, M. Rodbell, and J. Roth. 1973. Insulin activity: the solid matrix. Science 182:396–397.

Caron, M. G., S. Goldstein, K. Savard, and J. M. Marsh. 1975. Protein kinase stimulation of a reconstituted cholesterol side chain cleavage enzyme system in the bovine corpus luteum. J. Biol. Chem. 250:5137–5143.

Castells S., N. Addo, and K. Kwateng. 1973a. The relationship of rapidly labelled adrenal RNA synthesis to steroidogenesis in a superfusion system: effect of ACTH. Endocrinology 93:285–291.

Castells, S., N. Addo, and K. Kwateng. 1973b. In vitro effects of ACTH on uridine incorporation into rapidly labelled adrenal RNA of normal and dexamethasone-suppressed rats. Steroids 22:171–183.

Channing, C. D. 1974. Temporal effects of LH, hCG, FSH, and dibutyryl cyclic 3',5'-AMP upon luteinization of Rhesus monkey granulosa cells in culture. Endocrinology 94:1215–1223.

Clayman, M., D. Tsang, and R. M. Johnstone. 1970. ACTH, corticosteroids, and inhibition of protein synthesis. Endocrinology 86:931–934.

Constantopoulos, G., and T. T. Tchen. 1961. Cleavage of cholesterol side chain by adrenal cortex. J. Biol. Chem. 236:65–67.

Cort, J. H., J. Cort, J. Novakova, and J. Skopkova. 1974. Interaction of vasopressins and linear N-terminal ACTH fragments in the induction of natriuresis. Eur. J. Clin. Invest. 4:293–298.

Coslovsky, R., and R. S. Yalow. 1974. Influence of the hormonal forms of ACTH on the pattern of corticosteroid secretion. Biochem. Biophys. Res. Commun. 60:1351–1356.

Dazord, A., D. Gallet, and J. M. Saez. 1975. Adrenyl cyclase activity in rat, ovine, and human adrenal preparations. Horm. Metab. Res. 7:184–189.

Dazord, A., A. M. Morera, J. Bertrand, and J. M. Saez. 1974. Prostaglandin receptors in human and ovine adrenal glands: binding and stimulation of adenyl cyclase in subcellular preparations. Endocrinology 95:352–359.

Dempsey, M. E. 1974. Regulation of steroid biosynthesis. Annu. Rev. Biochem. 43:967–990.

deWied, D. 1973. L'hypophyse et le comportement. La Recherche 4:939–948.

Dixon, R., T. Furutachi, and S. Lieberman. 1970. The isolation of crystalline 22R-hydroxycholesterol and 20α,22R-dihydroxycholesterol from bovine adrenals. Biochem. Biophys. Res. Commun. 40:161–165.

Donta, S. T., M. King, and K. Sloper. 1973. Induction of steroidogenesis in tissue culture by cholera enterotoxin. Nature (New Biol.) 243:246–247.

Draper, M. W., R. B. Merrifield, and M. A. Rizack. 1973. Lipolytic activity of Met-Arg-His-Phe-Arg-Trp-Gly, a synthetic analog of the ACTH (4–10) core sequence. J. Med. Chem. 16:1326–1330.

Draper, M. W., M. A. Rizack, and R. B. Merrifield. 1975. Synthetic position 5 analogs of adrenocorticotropin fragments and their in vitro lipolytic activity. Biochemistry 14:2933–2938.

Durham, J. P., R. Baserga, and F. R. Butcher. 1974. Lack of correlation between catecholamine analog effects on cyclic AMP levels and adenylate cyclase activity and the stimulation of DNA synthesis in mouse parotid gland. In B. Clarkson and R. Baserga (eds.), Control of Proliferation in Animal Cells. Cold Spring Harbor Conference on Cell Proliferation, Vol. 1, pp. 595–607.

Eipper, B. A., and R. E. Maines. 1975. High molecular weight forms of adrenocorticotropic hormone in the mouse pituitary and in a mouse pituitary tumor cell line. Biochemistry 14:3836–3846.

Eisenstein, A. B. 1967. The Adrenal Cortex. Little, Brown, Boston.

Farese, R. V. 1968. Regulation of adrenal growth and steroidogenesis by ACTH. In K. W. McKerns (ed.), Functions of the Adrenal Cortex, Vol. 1, pp. 539–583. Appleton-Century-Crofts, New York.

Farese, R. V. 1969. Effects of ACTH and cyclic-AMP in vitro on incorporation of H-leucine and C-orotic acid into protein and RNA in the presence of an inhibitor of cholesterol side chain cleavage. Endocrinology 85:1209–1212.

Farese, R. V. 1971a. Stimulation of pregnenolone synthesis by ACTH in rat adrenal sections. Endocrinology 89:958–962.

Farese, R. V. 1971b. On the requirement for calcium during the steroidogenic effect of ACTH. Endocrinology 89:1057–1063.

Farese, R. V. 1971c. Stimulatory effects of calcium on protein synthesis in adrenal (and thyroidal) cell-free systems as related to trophic hormone action. Endocrinology 89:1064–1074.

Farese, R. V. 1971d. Calcium as a mediator of adrenocorticotrophic hormone action on adrenal protein synthesis. Science 173:447–450.

Farese, R. V., and W. J. Reddy. 1963. Observations on the inter-relations between adrenal protein, RNA, and DNA, during prolonged ACTH administration. Biochim. Biophys. Acta 76:145–148.

Ferguson, J. J. 1962. Puromycin and adrenal responsiveness to adrenocorticotropic hormone. Biochim. Biophys. Acta 57:616–617.

Ferguson, J. J. 1963. Protein synthesis and adrenocorticotropin responsiveness. J. Biol. Chem. 238:2754–2759.

Ferguson, J. J. 1968. Metabolic inhibitors and adrenal function. In K. W. McKerns (ed.), Functions of the Adrenal Cortex, Vol. 1, pp. 463–478. Appleton-Century-Crofts, New York.

Ferguson, J. J., Y. Morita, and L. Mendelsohn. Incorporation in vitro of precursor into protein and RNA of rat adrenal glands. Endocrinology 80: 521—528.

Fiala, S., and A. E. Fiala. 1968. Endocrine factors in the development of transplantable adrenal cortical tumors. I. Inhibition of the growth rate by corticotrophin (ACTH). Int. J. Cancer 3:531—545.

Finn, F. M., J. A. Montibeller, Y. Ushijima, and K. Hofmann. 1975. Adenylate cyclase system of bovine adrenal plasma membranes. J. Biol. Chem. 250: 1186—1192.

Finn, F. M., C. C. Widness, and K. Hofmann. 1972. Localization of an adrenocorticotropic hormone receptor on bovine adrenal cortical membranes. J. Biol. Chem. 247:5695—5702.

Ford, J. K., and R. W. Young. 1963. Cell proliferation and displacement in the adrenal cortex of young rats injected with titrated thymidine. Anat. Rec. 146:125—133.

Fujimo, M., C. Hatanaka, and O. Nishimura. 1971. Synthesis of peptides related to corticotropin (ACTH). VI. Synthesis and biological activity of the peptides corresponding to the amino acid sequence 4—23, 5—23, 6—24, and 7—23 in ACTH. Chem. Pharm. Bull. (Tokyo) 19:1066—1068.

Fukushima, D. K., J. W. Finkelstein, K. Yoshida, R. M. Boyar, and L. Hellman. 1975. Pituitary-adrenal activity in untreated congenital adrenal hyperplasia. J. Clin. Endocrinol. Metab. 40:1—12.

Gallant, S., F. C. Kauffman, and A. C. Brownie. 1974. Cyclic nucleotide phosphodiesterase activity in rat adrenal gland zones. Life Sci. (II) 14: 937—944.

Garren, L. D. 1968. The mechanism of action of adrenocorticotropic hormone. Vitam. Horm. 26:119—145.

Garren, L. D., G. N. Gill, H. Masui, and G. M. Walton. 1971. On the mechanism of action of ACTH. Recent Prog. Horm. Res. 27:433—478.

Garren, L. D., R. L. Ney, and W. W. Davis. 1965. Studies on the role of protein synthesis in the regulation of corticosterone production by adrenocorticotropic hormone in vivo. Proc. Natl. Acad. Sci. U.S.A. 53:1443—1450.

Geiger, R., and H. G. Schröder. 1973. Synthetische analoga des corticotropins. Hoppe Seylers Z. Physiol. Chem. 354:156—162.

Geiger, R., and H. G. Schroeder. 1974. New short-chain synthetic corticotrophin analogues with high corticotrophic activity. In S. Lauda (ed.), Progress in Peptide Research, pp. 273—279. Gordon and Breach, New York.

Geschwind, I. I., and C. H. Li. 1952. Inactivation of adrenocorticotropic hormone in vitro by tissues. Endocrinology 50:226—233.

Gill, G. N. 1972. Mechanism of ACTH action. Metabolism 21:571—588.

Gill, G. N., and L. D. Garren. 1970. A cyclic-3',5'-adenosine monophosphate dependent protein kinase from the adrenal cortex: comparison with a cyclic AMP binding protein. Biochem. Biophys. Res. Commun. 39:335—343.

Glossman, H. 1975. Adrenal cortex adenylate cyclase. Naunyn Schmiedebergs Arch. Pharmacol. 289:99—109.

Glossman, H., A. S. Baukal, and K. J. Catt. 1974. Properties of angiotensin II receptors in the bovine and rat adrenal cortex. J. Biol. Chem. 249:825—834.

Glossman, H., and H. Gips. 1974. Adrenal cortex adenylate cyclase. Naunyn Schmiedebergs Arch. Pharmacol. 286:239—249.

Glossman, H., and H. Gips. 1975. Bovine adrenal cortex adenylate cyclase properties of the particulate enzyme and effects of guanyl nucleotide. Naunyn Schmiedebergs Arch. Pharmacol. 289:77—97.

Golder, M. P., and A. R. Boyns. 1972. Selective uptake of radioactivity by the adrenal cortex of dexamethasone-treated guinea-pigs after the administration of ^{131}I-labelled α^{1-24} adrenocorticotrophin. J. Endocrinol. 53:277–287.

Gospodarowicz, D., and F. Gospodarowicz. 1974. The morphological transformation and inhibition of growth of bovine luteal cells in tissue culture induced by luteinizing hormone and dibutyryl cyclic AMP. Endocrinology 96: 458–467.

Grahame-Smith, D. G., R. Butcher, R. L. Ney, and E. W. Sutherland. 1967. Adenosine 3',5'-monophosphate as the intracellular mediator of the action of adrenocorticotropic hormone on the adrenal cortex. J. Biol. Chem. 242: 5535–5541.

Grower, M. F., and E. D. Bransome. 1970. Adenosine 3',5'-monophosphate, adrenocorticotropic hormone, and adrenocortical cytosol protein synthesis. Science 168:483–485.

Haberland, M. E., and J. A. Reynolds. 1973. Self-association of cholesterol in aqueous solution. Proc. Natl. Acad. Sci. U.S.A. 70:2313–2316.

Haksar, A., and F. G. Peron. 1972. Comparison of the Ca^{++} requirement for the steroidogenic effect of ACTH and dibutyryl cyclic AMP in rat adrenal cell suspensions. Biochem. Biophys. Res. Commun. 47:445–450.

Haksar, A., and F. G. Peron. 1973. The role of calcium in the steroidogenic response of rat adrenal cells to adrenocorticotropic hormone. Biochim. Biophys. Acta 313:363–371.

Halkerston, I. D. K. 1968. Heterogeneity of the response of adrenal cortex tissue slices to adrenocorticotrophin. In K. W. McKerns (ed.), Functions of the Adrenal Cortex, Vol. 1, pp. 399–461. Appleton-Century-Crofts, New York.

Halkerston, I. D. K., M. Feinstein, and O. Hechter. 1964. Inhibition of protein synthesis in rat adrenals by adrenocorticotrophin and cyclic 3',5'-adenosine monophosphate. Endocrinology 74:649–652.

Halkerston, I. D. K., M. Feinstein, and O. Hechter. 1968. Effect of lytic enzymes upon the responsivity of rat adrenals in vitro. I. Effect of trypsin upon the steroidogenic action of reduced triphosphopyridine nucleotide. Endocrinology 83:61–73.

Hall, P. F., and D. G. Young. 1968. Site of action of trophic hormones upon the biosynthetic pathways to steroid hormones. Endocrinology 82:559–568.

Halmi, K. A., N. S. Halmi, and D. J. Anderson. 1974. Effects of ions on adrenocorticotropin-sensitive adenylate cyclase of rat adrenals (38350). Proc. Soc. Exp. Biol. Med. 147:399–402.

Haynes, R. C., and D. Berthet. 1957. Studies on the mechanism of action of the adrenocorticotropic hormone. J. Biol. Chem. 225:115–124.

Hilf, R. 1965. The mechanism of action of ACTH. N. Engl. J. Med. 273: 798–811.

Hinshaw, H. T., and R. L. Ney. 1974. Abnormal hormonal control in the neoplastic adrenal cortex. In K. W. McKerns (ed.), Hormones and Cancer, pp. 309–332. Academic Press, New York.

Hofmann, K., J. A. Montibeller, and F. M. Finn. 1974. ACTH antagonists. Proc. Natl. Acad. Sci. U.S.A. 71:80–83.

Hofmann, K., W. Wingender, and F. M. Finn. 1970. Correlation of adrenocorticotropic activity of ACTH analogs with degree of binding to an adrenal cortical particulate preparation. Proc. Natl. Acad. Sci. U.S.A. 67:829–836.

Ichii, S. 1972. Adenosine 3',5'-monophosphate, adenosine 3',5'-monophosphate binding protein and protein kinase in rats adrenal glands: effect of adrenocorticotropin. Endocrinol. Jap. 19.229–235.

Ide, M., A. Tanaka, M. Nakamura, and T. Kabayashi. 1972. Stimulation by

ACTH analogs of rat adrenal adenyl cyclase activity: correlation with steroidogenic activity. Arch. Biochem. Biophys. 149:189–196.

Imrie, R. C., T. R. Ramaiah, F. Antoni, and W. C. Hutchison. 1965. The effect of adrenocorticotrophin on the nucleic acid metabolism of the rat adrenal gland. J. Endocrinol. 32:303–312.

Jaanus, S. D., M. J. Rosenstein, and R. P. Rubin. 1970. On the mode of action of ACTH on the isolated perfused adrenal gland. J. Physiol. (Lond.) 209: 539–556.

Jefcoate, C. R., E. R. Simpson, G. S. Boyd, R. C. Brownie, and W. H. Orme-Johnson. 1973. The detection of different states of the P-450 cytochromes in adrenal mitochondria; changes induced by ACTH. Ann. N. Y. Acad. Sci. 212:243–261.

Jöhl, A., B. Riniker, and L. Schenkel-Hulliger. 1974. Identity of structure of ovine and bovine ACTH: correction of revised structure of the ovine hormone. FEBS Lett. 45:172–174.

Johnson, R. C., and S. N. Shan. 1974. Microsomal synthesis of cholesterol from squalene, lanosterol, and desmosterol. Arch. Biochem. Biophys. 164:502–510.

Kahnt, F. W., A. Milani, H. Steffen, and R. Neher. 1974. The rate-limiting step of adrenal steroidogenesis and adenosine $3':5'$-monophosphate. Eur. J. Biochem. 44:243–250.

Kahri, A. I. 1966. Histochemical and electron microscopic studies on the cells of the rat adrenal cortex in tissue culture. Acta Endocrinol. 108 (Suppl.):1–96.

Kahri, A. I. 1973. Inhibition of ACTH-induced differentiation of cortical cells and their mitochondria by corticosterone in tissue culture of fetal rat adrenals. Anat. Rec. 176:253–272.

Kahri, A. I., I. Huhtaniemi, and M. Salmenpera. 1975. Functional and morphological differentiation of cortical cells of human fetal adrenals in tissue culture. Acta Endocrinol. 199 (Suppl.):393.

Kan, K. W., M. C. Ritter, F. Ungar, and M. E. Dempsey. 1972. The role of a carrier protein in cholesterol and steroid hormone synthesis by adrenal enzymes, 1, 2. Biochem. Biophys. Res. Commun. 48:423–429.

Kan, K. W., and F. Ungar. 1973. Characterization of an adrenal activator for cholesterol side chain cleavage. J. Biol. Chem. 248:2868–2875.

Katzen, H. M., and G. J. Vlahakes. 1973. Biological activity of insulin-sepharose. Science 179:1142–1143.

Kelly, L. A., and S. B. Koritz. 1971. Bovine adrenal cortical adenyl cyclase and its stimulation by adrenocorticotropic hormone and NaF. Biochim. Biophys. Acta 237:141–155.

Kitabchi, R. E., and R. K. Sharma. 1974. Corticosteroidogenesis in isolated adrenal cells of rats. I. Effect of corticotropins and $3',5'$-cyclic nucleotides on corticosterone production. Endocrinology 88:1109–1116.

Kitabchi, R. E., D. B. Wilson, and R. K. Sharma. 1971. Steroidogenesis in isolated adrenal cells of rat. Biochem. Biophys. Res. Commun. 44:898–904.

Klotz, U., H. Vapaatalo, and K. Stolk. 1972. Rat adrenal cyclic nucleotide-phosphodiesterase; inhibition by drugs known to affect steroidogenesis. Naunyn Schmiedebergs Arch. Pharmacol. 273:376–385.

Kolb, H. J., R. Renner, D. Hepp, L. Weiss, and O. H. Wieland. 1975. Re-evaluation of sepharose-insulin as a tool for the study of insulin action. Proc. Natl. Acad. Sci. U.S.A. 72:248–252.

Koritz, S. B. 1962. The effect of calcium ions and freezing on the in vitro synthesis of pregnenolone by rat adrenal preparations. Biochim. Biophys. Acta 56:63–75.

Koritz, S. B. 1968. On the regulation of pregnenolone synthesis. *In* K. W. McKerns (ed.), Functions of the Adrenal Cortex, Vol. 1, pp. 27–48. Appleton-Century-Crofts, New York.

Koritz, S. B., and A. M. Kumar. 1970. On the mechanism of action of the adrenocorticotrophic hormone. J. Biol. Chem. 245:152–154.

Koritz, S. B., F. G. Peron, and R. I. Dorfman. 1957. Influence of adrenocorticotropic hormone on corticoid production and glycine-1-c incorporation into protein by rat adrenals. J. Biol. Chem. 26:643–650.

Kowal, J. 1970a. Adrenal cells in tissue culture. VII. Effect of inhibitors of protein synthesis on steroidogenesis and glycolysis. Endocrinology 87:951–965.

Kowal, J. 1970b. ACTH and the metabolism of adrenal cell cultures. Recent Prog. Horm. Res. 26:623–676.

Kowal, J., S. Srinivasan, and T. Saito. 1974. Calcium modulation of ACTH and cholera toxin stimulated adrenal steroid and cyclic-AMP biosynthesis. Endocrine Res. Commun. 1:305–319.

Kraaipoel, R. J., H. J. Degenhart, J. G. Leferink, V. Van Beek, H. de Leeuw-Boon, and H. K. A. Visser. 1975. Pregnenolone formation from cholesterol in bovine adrenal cortex mitochondria: proposals of a new mechanism. FEBS Lett. 50:204–209.

Kumar, S. 1975. [9-isoleucine]$ACTH_{1-24}$, a competitive antagonist of $ACTH_{1-24}$, induced cyclic AMP and corticosterone production. Biochem. Biophys. Res. Commun. 66:1063–1068.

Lang, U., G. Karlaganis, R. Vogel, and R. Schwyzer. 1974. Hormone-receptor interactions. Adrenocorticotropic hormone binding site increase in isolated fat. Biochemistry 13:2626–2633.

Langen, T. A. 1973. Protein kinases and protein kinases substrates. Adv. Cyclic Nucleotide Res. 3:99–153.

Laychock, S. G., and R. P. Rubin. 1974. Isolation of ACTH-induced protein from adrenal perfusate. Steroids 24:177–184.

Lefkowitz, R. J., J. Roth, and I. Pastan. 1970. Effects of calcium on ACTH stimulation of the adrenal: separation of hormone binding from adenyl cyclase activation. Nature 228:864–866.

Lefkowitz, R. J., J. Roth, and I. Pastan. 1971. ACTH-receptor interaction in the adrenal: a model for the initial step in the action of hormones that stimulate adenyl cyclase. Ann. N. Y. Acad. Sci. 185:195–209.

Lefkowitz, R. J., J. Roth, W. Pricer, and I. Pastan. 1970. ACTH receptors in the adrenal: specific binding of $ACTH-{}^{125}I$ and its relation to adenyl cyclase. Proc. Natl. Acad. Sci. U.S.A. 65:745–752.

Leier, D. J., and R. A. Jugmann. 1973. Adrenocorticotropic hormone and dibutyryl adenosine cyclic monophosphate-mediated Ca^{2+} uptake by rat adrenal glands. Biochim. Biophys. Acta 329:196–210.

Li, C. H. 1972. Adrenocorticotropin 45. Revised amino acid sequences for sheep and bovine hormones. Biochem. Biophys. Res. Commun. 49:835–839.

Li, C. H., and B. Hemmasi. 1972. Adrenocorticotropin 40. The synthesis of a protected nonapeptide and a biologically active nonadecopeptide related to adrenocorticotropic hormone. [5-6-glutamine]adrenocorticotropin-(1-19). J. Med. Chem. 15:217–219.

Li, C. H., and W. Oelofsen. 1967. The chemistry and biology of ACTH and related peptides. *In* A. B. Eisenstein (ed.), The Adrenal Cortex, pp. 185–201. Little, Brown Co., Boston.

Lin, S. Y., and T. L. Goodfriend. 1970. Angiotensin receptors. Am. J. Physiol. 218:1319–1328.

Lipsett, M. B., R. Hertz, and G. T. Roos. 1963. Clinical and pathophysiologic aspects of adrenocortical carcinoma. Am. J. Med. 35:374–383.

Macchia, V., M. F. Meldolesi, and M. Chiariello. 1972. Adenyl-cyclase in a transplantable thyroid tumor: loss of ability to respond to TSH. Endocrinology 90:1483–1491.

Mackie, C., M. C. Richardson, and D. Schulster. 1972. Kinetics and dose-response characteristics of adenosine $3',5'$-monophosphate production by isolated rat adrenal cells stimulated with adrenocorticotrophic hormone. FEBS Lett. 23:345–348.

Mahafee, D., R. C. Reitz, and R. L. Ney. 1974. The mechanism of action of adrenocorticotropic hormone. J. Biol. Chem. 249:227–233.

Maines, R. E., and B. A. Eipper. 1975. Molecular weight of adrenocorticotropic hormone in extracts of anterior and intermediate posterior lobe of mouse pituitary. Proc. Natl. Acad. Sci. U.S.A. 72:3565–3569.

Mandato, E., M. F. Meldolesi, and V. Macchia. 1975. Diminished binding of thyroid-stimulating hormone in a transplantable rat thyroid tumor as a possible cause of hormone unresponsiveness. Cancer Res. 35:3089–3093.

Masui, H., and L. D. Garren. 1970. On the mechanism of action of adrenocorticotropic hormone. J. Biol. Chem. 245:2627–2632.

Masui, H., and L. D. Garren. 1971. Inhibition of replication in functional mouse adrenal tumor cells by adrenocorticotropic hormone mediated by adenosine $3':5'$-cyclic monophosphate. Proc. Natl. Acad. Sci. U.S.A. 68:3206–3210.

Masui, H., and P. La Porte. 1973. Inhibition of the growth of transplanted functional adrenal tumor cells by adrenocorticotropic hormone (ACTH). Endocrinology 92:A-54.

McIlhinney, R. A. J., and D. Schulster. 1975. Studies on the binding of ^{125}I-labelled corticotrophin to isolated rat adrenocortical cells. J. Endocrinol. 64:175–184.

McKerns, K. W. 1968. Mechanisms of ACTH regulation of the adrenal cortex. In K. W. McKerns (ed.), Functions of the Adrenal Cortex, pp. 479–537. Appleton-Century-Crofts, New York.

McMillan, B. H., R. L. Ney, and I. Schorr. 1971. Guanyl cyclase activity in normal adrenals and a corticosterone producing adrenal cancer of the rat. Endocrinology 89:281–283.

Meakin, J. W., and D. H. Nelson. 1960. The catabolism of adrenocorticotropic hormone: some characteristics of an ACTH-inactivating system in plasma. Endocrinology 66:73–79.

Meakin, J. W., W. H. Tingey, and D. H. Nelson. 1960. The catabolism of adrenocorticotropic hormone: the stability of adrenocorticotropic hormone in blood, plasma, serum, and saline. Endocrinology 66:59–72.

Menon, K. M. J., S. Giese, and R. B. Jaffe. 1973. Hormone and fluoride-sensitive adenylate cyclases in human fetal tissues. Biochim. Biophys. Acta 304:203–204.

Morrow, L. B., G. W. Burrow, and P. J. Mulrow. 1967. Inhibition of adrenal protein synthesis by steroids in vitro. Endocrinology 80:883–888.

Mostafapour, M. K., and T. T. Tchen. 1971. Evidence for another factor in the regulation of corticosterone biosynthesis by ACTH. Biochem. Biophys. Res. Commun. 44:774–778.

Mostafapour, M. K., and T. T. Tchen. 1972. Effects of actinomycin D on hormone-induced steroidogenesis by superfused rat adrenal glands. Biochem. Biophys. Res. Commun. 48:491–495.

Mostafapour, M. K., and T. T. Tchen. 1973. Capacity for steroidogenesis of adrenals in hypophysectomized and adrenocorticotropic hormone-treated hypophysectomized rats. J. Biol. Chem. 248:6674–6678.

Moyle, W. R., Y. L. Kong, and J. Ramachandran. 1973. Steroidogenesis and cyclic adenosine 3',5'-monophosphate accumulation in rat adrenal cells. J. Biol. Chem. 248:2409–2417.

Murakami, N., and S. Ichii. 1973. Effect of ACTH on the phosphorylation of proteins in subcellular fractions of rat adrenal glands. Endocrinol. Jap. 20: 421–424.

Naghshineh, S., C. R. Treadwell, L. Gallo, and G. V. Vahouny. 1974. Activation of adrenal sterol ester hydrolase by dibutyryl cAMP and protein kinase. Biochem. Biophys. Res. Commun. 61:1076–1082.

Neher, R., and A. Milani. 1974. Steroidogenesis in adrenal cells. J. Steroid Biochem. 5:811–816.

Ney, R. L. 1969. Effects of dibutyryl cyclic AMP on adrenal growth and steroidogenic capacity. Endocrinology 84:168–170.

Ney, R. L., N. J. Hochella, D. G. Grahame-Smith, R. N. Dexter, and R. W. Butcher. 1969. Abnormal regulation of adenosine 3',5'-monophosphate and corticosterone formulation in an adrenocortical carcinoma. J. Clin. Invest. 48:1733–1739.

Nicola, A. F., M. Clayman, and R. M. Johnstone. 1968. Hormonal control of ascorbic acid transport in rat adrenal glands. Endocrinology 82:436–446.

Nussdorfer, G. G., G. Mazzocchi, and P. Rebuffat. 1973. An ultrastructural stereologic study of the effects of ACTH and adenosine 3',5'-cyclic monophosphate on the zona glomerulosa of rat adrenal cortex. Endocrinology 92: 141–151.

Oka, T., and Y. J. Topper. 1974. A soluble super-active form of insulin. Proc. Natl. Acad. Sci. U.S.A. 71:1630–1633.

Omura, T., E. Sanders, R. W. Estrabook, D. Y. Cooper, and D. Rosenthal. 1966. Isolation from adrenal cortex of a nonheme iron protein and a flavoprotein functional as a reduced triphosphopyridine nucleotide-cytochrome P-450 reductase. Arch. Biochem. Biophys. 117:660–668.

Palmiter, R. D. 1972. Regulation of protein synthesis in chick oviduct. J. Biol. Chem. 247:6770–6787.

Pastan, I. H., and G. S. Johnson. 1974. Cyclic AMP and the transformation of fibroblasts. Adv. Cancer Res. 19:303–327.

Pastan, I. H., G. G. Johnson, and W. B. Anderson. 1975. Role of cyclic nucleotides in growth control. Annu. Rev. Biochem. 44:491–522.

Peytreman, A., W. E. Nicholson, R. B. Brown, G. W. Liddle, and J. G. Hardman. 1973a. Comparative effects of angiotensin and ACTH on cyclic AMP and steroidogenesis in isolated bovine adrenal cells. J. Clin. Invest. 52:835–842.

Peytreman, A., W. E. Nicholson, G. W. Liddle, J. G. Hardman, and E. W. Sutherland. 1973b. Effects of methylxanthines on adenosine 3',5'-monophosphate and corticosterone in the rat adrenal. Endocrinology 92:525–530.

Ramachandran, J., and C. H. Li. 1967. Structure-activity relationships of the adrenocorticotropins and melanotropins: the synthetic approach. Adv. Enzymol. 29:391–477.

Ramachandran, J., and A. T. Suyama. 1975. Inhibition of replication of normal adrenocortical cells in culture by adrenocorticotropin. Proc. Natl. Acad. Sci. U.S.A. 72:113–117.

Richardson, M. C., and D. Schulster. 1972. Corticosteroidogenesis in isolated adrenal cells: effect of adrenocorticotrophic hormone, adenosine $3',5'$-monophosphate and β_{1-24} adrenocorticotrophic hormone diazotized to polyacrylamide. J. Endocrinol. 55:127−139.

Richardson, M. C., and D. Schulster. 1973. The role of protein kinase activation in the control of steroidogenesis by adrenocorticotrophic hormone in the adrenal cortex. Biochem. J. 136:993−998.

Riniker, B., P. Sieber, W. Rittel, and H. Zuber. 1972. Revised amino-acid sequences for porcine and human adrenocorticotrophic hormone. Nature (New Biol.) 235:114−115.

Ritter, M. C., and M. E. Dempsey. 1971. Specificity and role in cholesterol biosynthesis of a squalene and sterol carrier protein. J. Biol. Chem. 246: 1436−1539.

Roberts, K. D., L. Banby, and S. Lieberman. 1969. The occurrence and metabolism of 20α-hydroxycholesterol in bovine adrenal preparations. Biochemistry 8:1259−1268.

Robison, G. A., R. W. Butcher, and E. W. Sutherland. 1971. Cyclic AMP, p. 41. Academic Press, New York.

Roos, B. A. 1973. ACTH and cAMP stimulation of adrenal ribosomal protein phosphorylation. Endocrinology 93:1287−1293.

Roos, B. A. 1974. Effect of ACTH and cAMP on human adrenocortical growth and function in vitro. Endocrinology 94:685−690.

Roy, C., J. Bockaert, R. Rajerison, and S. Jard. 1973. Oxytocin receptor in frog bladder epithelial cells: relationship of [^{3}H]oxytocin binding to adenylate cyclase activation. FEBS Lett. 30:329−332.

Rubin, R. P., R. A. Carchman, and S. D. Jaanus. 1972. Role of calcium and adenosine cyclic $3',5'$-phosphate in action of adrenocorticotropin. Nature 240:150−152.

Rubin, R. P., B. Sheid, R. McCauley, and S. G. Laychock. 1974. ACTH-induced protein release from the perfused cat adrenal gland: evidence for exocytosis? Endocrinology 95:370−378.

Ryan, W. L., and M. G. Heidrick. 1974. Role of cyclic nucleotides in cancer. Adv. Cyclic Nucleotide Res. 4:81−116.

Saez, J. M., A. Dazord, and D. Gallet. 1975a. ACTH and prostaglandin receptors in human adrenocortical tumors. J. Clin. Invest. 56:536−547.

Saez, J. M., A. Dazord, A. M. Morera, and P. Bataille. 1975b. Interactions of adrenocorticotropic hormone with its adrenal receptors. J. Biol. Chem. 250: 1683−1689.

Saez, J. M., A. M. Morera, A. Dazord, and P. Bataille. 1974. Interactions of ACTH with its adrenal receptors: specific binding of ACTH$_{1-24}$, its O-nitrophenyl sulfenyl derivative and ACTH$_{11-24}$. J. Steroid Biochem. 5:925−933.

Saruta, T., R. Cook, and N. M. Kaplan. 1972. Adrenocortical steroidogenesis: studies on the mechanism of action of angiotensin and electrolytes. J. Clin. Invest. 51:2239−2246.

Saruta, T., and N. M. Kaplan. 1972. Adrenocortical steroidogenesis: the effects of prostaglandins. J. Clin. Invest. 51:2246−2251.

Sato, T., M. Sato, J. Shinsako, and M. F. Dallman. 1975. Corticosterone-induced changes in hypothalamic corticotropin-releasing factor (CRF) content after stress. Endocrinology 97:265−274.

Satre, M., E. M. Chambaz, P. V. Vignais, and S. Idelman. 1971. Intracellular localization of adenyl cyclase and of binding sites for $3',5'$-adenosine monophosphate in adrenal cortex. FEBS Lett. 12:207−211.

Sayers, G., R. J. Beall, and S. Seelig. 1972. Isolated adrenal cells: adrenocortico-tropic hormone, calcium, steroidogenesis, and cyclic adenosine monophos-phate. Science 175:1131–1133.

Sayers, G., S. Seelig, S. Kumar, G. Karlaganis, R. Schwyzer, and M. Fujimo. 1974. Isolated adrenal cortex cells: $ACTH_{4-23}$ (NH_2), $ACTH_{5-24}$, $ACTH_{6-24}$, and $ACTH_{7-23}$ (NH_2); cyclic AMP and corticosterone produc-tion. Proc. Soc. Exp. Biol. Med. 145:176–181.

Scallen, T. J., M. W. Schuster, and R. K. Dhar. 1971. Evidence for a noncatalytic carrier protein in cholesterol biosynthesis. J. Biol. Chem. 246:224–230.

Scallen, T. J., B. Seetharam, M. V. Srikantaiah, E. Hawsbury, and M. K. Lewis. 1975. Sterol carrier protein hypothesis: requirement for three substrate-specific soluble proteins in liver cholesterol biosynthesis. Life Sci. (II) 16: 853–874.

Schimmer, B. P. 1969. Phenotypically variant adrenal tumor cell cultures with biochemical lesions in the ACTH-stimulated steroidogenic pathway. J. Cell. Physiol. 74:115–122.

Schimmer, B. P. 1972. Adenylate cyclase activity in adrenocorticotropic hor-mone-sensitive and mutant adrenocortical tumor cell lines. J. Biol. Chem. 247:3134–3138.

Schimmer, B. P., K. Aeda, and G. H. Sato. 1968. Site of action of adrenocortico-tropic hormone (ACTH) in adrenal cell cultures. Biochem. Biophys. Res. Commun. 32:806–811.

Schorr, I. S., and R. L. Ney. 1971. Abnormal hormone responses of an adreno-cortical cancer adenyl cyclase. J. Clin. Invest. 50:1295–1300.

Schorr, I. S., P. Rathnam, B. B. Saxena, and R. L. Ney. 1971. Multiple specific hormone receptors in the adenylate cyclase of an adrenocortical carcinoma. J. Biol. Chem. 246:5806–5811.

Schulster, D. 1974a. Adrenocorticotrophic hormone and the control of adrenal corticosteroidogenesis. Adv. Steroid Biochem. Pharmacol. 4:233–295.

Schulster, D. 1974b. Corticosteroid and ribonucleic acid synthesis in isolated adrenal cells: inhibition by actinomycin D. Mol. Cell. Endocrinol. 1:55–64.

Schulster, D., M. C. Richardson, and J. W. Palfreyman. 1974. The role of protein synthesis in adrenocorticotrophin action: effects of cycloheximide and puro-mycin on the steroidogenesis response of isolated adrenocortical cells. Mol. Cell. Endocrinol. 2:17–29.

Schulster, D., S. A. S. Tait, J. F. Tait, and J. Mrotek. 1970. Production of steroids by in vitro superfusion of endocrine tissue. III. Corticosterone output from rat adrenals stimulated by adrenocorticotropin or cyclic $3',5'$-adenosine monophosphate and the inhibitory effect of cycloheximide. Endocrinology 86:487–502.

Schwyzer, R., P. Shiller, S. Seelig, and G. Sayers. 1971. Isolated adrenal cells: log dose response curves for steroidogenesis induced by $ACTH_{1-24}$, $ACTH_{1-10}$, $ACTH_{4-10}$, and $ACTH_{5-10}$. FEBS Lett. 19:229–231.

Seelig, S., and G. Sayers. 1973. Isolated adrenal cortex cells: ACTH agonists, partial agonists, antagonists; cyclic AMP and corticosterone production. Arch. Biochem. Biophys. 154:230–239.

Seelig, S., G. Sayers, R. Schwyzer, and D. Schiller. 1971. Isolated adrenal cells: $ACTH_{11-24}$, a competitive antagonist of $ACTH_{1-39}$ and $ACTH_{1-10}$. FEBS Lett. 19:232–234.

Selinger, R. C. L., and M. Civen. 1971. ACTH diazotized to agarose: effects on isolated adrenal cells. Biochem. Biophys. Res. Commun. 43:793–796.

Sharma, R. K. 1972. Studies on adrenocortical carcinoma of rat cyclic nucleotide phosphodiesterase activities. Cancer Res. 32:1734—1736.

Sharma, R. K. 1973a. Regulation of steroidogenesis by adrenocorticotropic hormone in isolated adrenal cells of rat. J. Biol. Chem. 248:5473—5478.

Sharma, R. K. 1973b. Metabolic regulation of steroidogenesis in adrenocortical carcinoma cells of rat: effect of adrenocorticotropin and adenosine cyclic 3':5'-monophosphate on corticosteroidogenesis. Eur. J. Biochem. 32:506—512.

Sharma, R. K. 1974a. Metabolic regulation of steroidogenesis in isolated adrenal cells of rat. Effect of actinomycin D on cGMP-induced steroidogenesis. Biochem. Biophys. Res. Commun. 59:992—1004.

Sharma, R. K. 1974b. Metabolic regulation of steroidogenesis in isolated adrenal and adrenocortical carcinoma cells of rat. Effect of adrenocorticotrophic hormone and adenosine cyclic 3':5'-monophosphate on the plasma membrane. FEBS Lett. 38:197—201.

Sharma, R. K., N. K. Ahmed, L. S. Sutliff, and J. S. Brush. 1974. Metabolic regulation of steroidogenesis in isolated adrenal cells of the rat. ACTH regulation of cGMP and cAMP levels and steroidogenesis. FEBS Lett. 45:107—110.

Sharma, R. K., and J. S. Brush. 1974. Metabolic regulation of steroidogenesis in adrenocortical carcinoma cells of rat. Effect of adrenocorticotropin and adenosine cyclic 3',5'-monophosphate on the incorporation of (20S)-20-hydroxy-[7α-^{3}H]cholesterol into deoxycorticosterone and corticosterone. Biochem. Biophys. Res. Commun. 56:256—263.

Sibley, C., U. Gehring, H. Bourne, and G. M. Tomkins. 1974. Hormonal control of cellular growth. In B. Clarkson and R. Baserga (eds.), Control of Proliferation in Animal Cells. Cold Spring Harbor Conference on Cell Proliferation, Vol. 1, pp. 115—124.

Simpson, E. R., C. R. Jefcoate, and G. S. Boyd. 1971. Spin state changes in cytochrome P-450 associated with cholesterol side chain cleavage in bovine adrenal cortex mitochondria. FEBS Lett. 15:53—58.

Simpson, E. R., C. R. Jefcoate, P. C. Brownie, and G. S. Boyd. 1972. The effect of ether anaesthesia stress on cholesterol-side-chain cleavage and cytochrome P-450 in rat-adrenal mitochondria. Eur. J. Biochem. 28:442—450.

Simpson, E. R., C. R. Jefcoate, J. L. McCarthy, and G. S. Boyd. 1974. Effect of calcium ions on steroid-binding spectra and pregnenolone formation in rat-adrenal mitochondria. Eur. J. Biochem. 45:181—188.

Smith, P. E. 1930. Hypophysectomy and a replacement therapy in the rat. Am. J. Anat. 45:205—209.

Snell, K. C., and H. L. Stewart. 1959. Variations in histologic pattern and functional effects of a transplantable adrenal cortical carcinoma in intact, hypophysectomized, and newborn rats. J. Natl. Cancer Inst. 22:1119—1155.

Stone, D., and O. Hechter. 1954. Studies on ACTH action in perfused bovine adrenals: the site of action of ACTH in corticosteroidogenesis. Arch. Biochem. Biophys. 51:457—469.

Takasugi, N., H. Takeuchi, and O. Taguchi. 1975. Effect of steroid hormones on growth of adrenocortical carcinoma transplants in mice. Gann 66:57—67.

Taunton, O. D., J. Roth, and I. Pastan. 1969. Studies on the adrenocorticotropic hormone-activated adenyl cyclase of a functional adrenal tumor. J. Biol. Chem. 244:247—253.

Tesser, G. I., R. Maier, L. Schenkel-Hullinger, P. L. Barthe, B. Kamer, and W. Rittel. 1973. Biological activity of corticotrophin peptides with homoarginine, lysine, or ornithine substituted for arginine in position 8. Acta Endocrinol. 74:56−66.

Tsang, D., and R. M. Johnstone. 1973. Steroidogenesis and RNA synthesis in rat adrenal gland in vitro. Endocrinology 93:119−126.

Ungar, F., K. W. Kan, and K. E. McCoy. 1973. Activator and inhibitor factors in cholesterol side-chain cleavage. Ann. N. Y. Acad. Sci. 212:276−282.

Vance, V. K., F. Girard, and G. F. Gahill. 1962. Effect of ACTH on glucose metabolism in rat adrenal in vitro. Endocrinology 71:113−119.

Vannipsen, J. W., and G. I. Tesser. 1975. Synthesis and charge-transfer properties of two ACTH analogues containing pentamethylphenylalanine in position 9. Int. J. Peptide Protein Res. 7:57−67.

Vonderhaar, B. K., and Y. J. Topper. 1974. Super-active forms of placental lactogen and prolactin. Biochem. Biophys. Res. Commun. 60:1323−1330.

Walton, G. M., and G. N. Gill. 1973. Adenosine $3',5'$-monophosphate and protein kinase dependent phosphorylation of ribosomal protein. Biochemistry 12:2604−2611.

White, W. F. 1955. Studies on adrenocorticotropin. XII. Action of aminopeptidase on corticotropin-A; effect on biological activity. J. Am. Chem. Soc. 77:4691−4692.

Whitfield, J. F., R. H. Rixon, J. P. MacManus, and S. D. Balk. 1973. Calcium, cyclic adenosine $3',5'$-monophosphate, and the control of cell proliferation: a review. In Vitro 8:257−278.

Wilchek, M., T. Oka, and Y. J. Topper. 1975. Structure of a soluble super-active insulin is revealed by the nature of the complex between cyanogen-bromide-activated sepharose and amines. Proc. Natl. Acad. Sci. U.S.A. 72:1055−1058.

Wolf, S., R. Temple, and G. H. Cook. 1973. Stimulation of steroid secretion in adrenal tumor cells by choleragen. Proc. Natl. Acad. Sci. U.S.A. 70: 2741−2744.

Wolfsen, A. R., U. B. McIntyre, and W. D. Odell. 1972. Adrenocorticotropin measurement by competitive binding receptor assay. J. Clin. Endocrinol. Metab. 34:684−689.

Wright, N. A. 1971. Cell proliferation in the prepubertal male rat adrenal cortex: an autoradiographic study. J. Endocrinol. 49:599−609.

Yalow, R. S. 1974. Heterogeneity of peptide hormones. Recent Prog. Horm. Res. 30:597−633.

Anti-Müllerian Hormone

Nathalie Josso, Jean-Yves Picard, and Dien Tran

Although the events and hormonal mechanisms governing postnatal sex maturation have been receiving an increasing amount of attention, knowledge of fetal reproductive physiology has not advanced at a similar pace.

Most of the basic data relative to the differentiation of the genital tract were published by Jost in 1947; in particular, his experiments demonstrated the active and dual role played by the fetal testes. Young fetuses, in the so-called "indifferent" or "ambisexual" stage, possess two sets of genital ducts. Wolffian ducts, the excretory canals of the second provisional kidney, the mesonephros, are incorporated into the genital system when renal function has been taken over by the metanephros. In the male fetus, Wolffian ducts develop into vasa deferentia and seminal vesicles, whereas in the female they degenerate. On the other hand, Müllerian ducts growing down toward the urogenital sinus from invaginations of the coelemic epithelium regress in the male fetus, whereas in the female they develop into tubes, uterus, and the upper part of the vagina. Jost (1947) showed that castration of the male rabbit fetus in utero at the ambisexual stage causes its genital tract to differentiate according to the female pattern, but graft of testicular tissue near the ovary of the female fetus results in virilization of the homolateral tract. These experiments prove that organogenesis of male sex structures and regression of Müllerian ducts are testes-dependent, whereas the opposite evolution does not require the presence of the ovary. The human counterpart of the animal experiments is illustrated by the feminine appearance of agonadal patients with Turner's syndrome or pure gonadal dysgenesis.

In another series of experiments, Jost (1947) compared the action of testosterone with that of the fetal testes. Wolffian maintenance and male differentiation of the external genitalia could be produced either by androgens or by the fetal testes, but regression of the Müllerian ducts was achieved only by the latter. This explains why the Müllerian organs of genetic females exposed to high levels of androgen in utero are always normal, whatever the degree of virilization of their external genitalia and urogenital sinus. The discrete nonandrogenic substance thought to be responsible for the Müllerian-inhibiting activity of the fetal testes is known under many different names: X factor, Müllerian-inhibiting factor or substance, Müllerian inhibitor, or antifeminine substance (Jost, Vigier, and Prépin, 1972). In this laboratory it is called the anti-Müllerian hormone (AMH), although, in view of its essentially local range of action, biologically active concentrations are probably not reached in the blood, except in freemartins, and therefore the term "hormone" may not be appropriate.

This nomenclature explosion contrasts with the lack of hard facts concerning the biochemical nature and physiology of AMH. Experimentation is difficult, because the Müllerian duct is sensitive to AMH only during a short period of its development. Hormonal responsiveness is lost at the end of the ambisexual stage, shortly before the onset of degeneration of Müllerian ducts in the male, i.e., at 15 days in the rat (Picon, 1969), 27 days in the guinea pig (Price et al., 1975), 19 days in the rabbit (Jost, 1947; Tran and Josso, unpublished data), and 7–8 weeks in the human (Josso, 1974a). This time-related sensitivity of the genital tract to morphogenetic hormones is an important factor in sex differentiation and also modulates the effect of testosterone on androgen-dependent structures such as Wolffian ducts (Josso, 1970a) and urogenital sinus (Cunha, 1975).

The demonstration by Picon in 1969 that the Müllerian-inhibiting activity of fetal rat testicular tissue can be studied in vitro with the use of the castrated reproductive tract of 14 ½-day-old fetal rats as target organ opened a new area in the experimental investigation of AMH, because organ culture techniques do not require the survival of fetuses operated in vivo at an early age. Briefly, reproductive tracts of 14 ½-day-old fetal rats of both sexes are dissected free of gonadal tissue and explanted on the grid of a commercial organ-culture dish. The tissue whose anti-Müllerian activity is to be studied is placed between the cranial segments of the tract. Medium is added to the level of the grid, and the explants are fixed and serially sectioned after 3 days of culture. It is necessary to obtain a picture of the entire length of the Müllerian system in order to assess its degree of inhibition in a given tract, because there exists a topographical as well as chronological variation in the sensitivity of the Müllerian duct to AMH; for instance, at 14½ days, responsiveness increases from the ostium to the urogenital sinus.

The 14½-day-old rat Müllerian duct can also be used to study the anti-Müllerian activity of testicular tissue of other mammalian species (Figure 1) (Josso, 1970b, 1971, 1973) and of various liquid media (Josso, Forest, and Picard, 1975). Unfortunately, the histological appearance of the Müllerian duct system upon which rests the appreciation of the intensity of anti-Müllerian activity does not lend itself to quantitation. The subjective aspect of the bioassay, however, can be eliminated by adhering to strict, predefined criteria in the histological evaluation of results and by coding the slides (Josso, Forest, and Picard, 1975). Briefly, 1 section out of 10, representing a total of 25–35 sections of each explant, is mounted and histologically examined. The correspondence between slide number and experimental procedure is not known to the observer at this time. The degree of Müllerian duct regression is scored on each section of the slides, according to the following criteria (Figure 2):

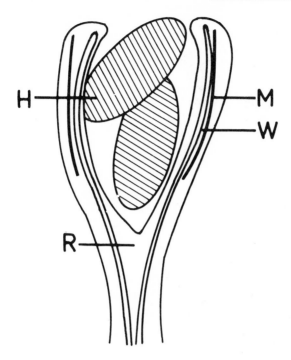

Figure 1. Bioassay of anti-Müllerian activity of human fetal testicular tissue using the Müllerian duct of the 14½-day-old fetal rat. *H,* human testicular tissue; *R,* rat reproductive tract; *M,* rat Müllerian duct; *W,* rat Wolffian duct.

a. No regression: Müllerian and Wolffian ducts have approximately the same width, and Müllerian epithelium is normal, showing frequent mitotic figures. Cell density is increased around the duct, but the cells do not have the elongated morphology characteristic of fibroblasts.

b. Partial regression: duct epithelium is still visible, but its height is decreased and it rarely contains dividing cells. The lumen is narrow, surrounded by a fibroblastic ring.

c. Complete regression: the duct epithelium is replaced by a fibrous whorl.

The scores attributed to the Müllerian duct in each section are used to draw a reconstruction of the Müllerian system of a given reproductive tract. This reconstruction serves to assess the degree of Müllerian inhibition in the reproductive tract as a whole (Figure 2).

A. Tracts showing no alteration of the Müllerian duct on either side are considered normal. *B.* Incomplete inhibition is said to occur when Müllerian regres-

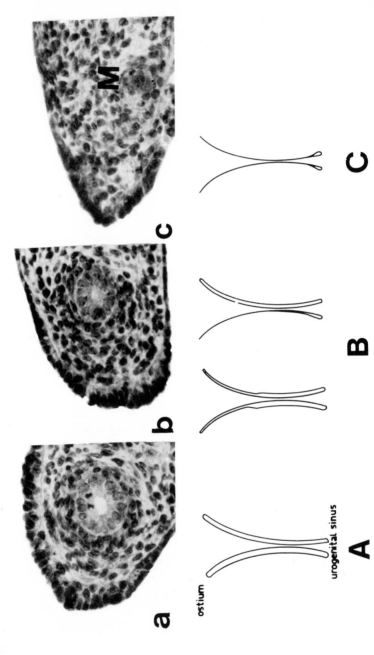

Figure 2. Morphological and topographical criteria of Müllerian duct regression. *Top*, evaluation of regression of Müllerian duct (*M*) on a given section. *a*, no regression; *b*, incomplete regression; *c*, complete regression. *Bottom*, evaluation of inhibition of Müllerian duct of a given rat reproductive tract. *A*, no inhibition; *B*, incomplete inhibition; *C*, complete inhibition.

sion is heterogeneous, asymmetrical, or limited to the anterior segment of the ducts, which is more sensitive to AMH at this stage of development. Because the same concentration of AMH does not always evoke an identical response in individual fetal rat reproductive tracts (Josso, 1972a), an attempt is not made to recognize degrees in the incomplete type of inhibition of the Müllerian duct system. Therefore, small variations of anti-Müllerian activity cannot be measured.

C. Total inhibition is defined as complete regression of the Müllerian duct on both sides and on the entire length of the tract, except in the immediate vicinity of the urogenital sinus.

Efforts to devise a quantitative assay for AMH have been thwarted by the difficulty of obtaining the physiological target organ in pure form. Obviously, the effect of AMH on, for instance, amino acid or thymidine incorporation cannot be studied if the epithelial cells of the Müllerian duct at the responsive stage are admixed with an unknown number of Wolffian and mesonephric cells. Because dissection of Müllerian ducts from 14½-day-old rat fetuses appeared unfeasible, an attempt was made to use fetuses from larger animals such as rabbits, but no great difference was found in size at the early stage of pregnancy in which we were interested. In early rabbit embryos, for instance, Wilson (1973) was unable to separate Wolffian from Müllerian ducts.

In the chick fetus, the large Müllerian duct is easily separated from the rest of the reproductive tract at 8 days of incubation. At that age, chick Müllerian ducts are totally inhibited by chick fetal testes after 4 days in culture. Unfortunately, chick Müllerian ducts are not affected by mammalian fetal testicular tissue, whereas chick testes do inhibit the 14½-day-old rat Müllerian duct (Tran and Josso, in press). These results rule out the possibility of using the chick Müllerian duct as a target organ for mammalian AMH, although the reverse would theoretically be possible, while offering no practical advantage.

Demonstration of other physiological functions for AMH might eventually lead to another type of bioassay. Jost, Vigier, and Prépin (1972) suggest that the same factor could be responsible for the regression of Müllerian ducts and for the inhibition of growth of presumptive ovaries in freemartins, as both events are synchronized. A Sertoli cell-produced hormone, for instance AMH, could also play a role in spermatogenesis by preventing male germ cells from entering meiosis (Jost, 1970). As pointed out by Picon (1970), rat testicular tissue loses its Müllerian-inhibiting activity soon after birth, at the time of initiation of meiotic changes in the testes. However, this correlation does not hold true for other species.

The chronological evolution of the anti-Müllerian activity of the human testes was studied by Josso (1972a). Testicular tissue from human fetuses up to the age of 28 weeks completely inhibited the Müllerian ducts of all 14½-day-old rat reproductive tracts associated to it in organ culture. Müllerian-inhibiting activity waned in the neonatal period and completely disappeared thereafter. AMH production was not resumed at puberty (Figure 3).

Some experimental evidence even suggests depression of testicular anti-Müllerian activity by the pituitary. In the chick, Maraud, Coulaud, and Stoll (1969) showed that decapitation of chick fetuses allowed their testes to retain anti-Müllerian activity until hatching, whereas it normally decreases in the last days of incubation. Growth hormone, thyroid-stimulating hormone, and follicle-stimulating hormone, but not luteinizing hormone, adrenocorticotropic hormone, and prolactin, abolished the effect of decapitation. In the rat, Donahoe et al. (1975), in a preliminary communication, indicated that hypophysectomy of weanling rats extended the range of testicular production of AMH well into postnatal life. However, since hypophysectomy in the first days of life is followed by severe growth and maturation retardation, these, rather than a specific pituitary factor, might be involved in this process. Neither in the human fetus (Gitlin and Biasucci, 1969) nor in the rat fetus (Jost, 1966) does a negative correlation exist between the initiation of pituitary hormonal activity and anti-Müllerian activity of the testes.

The cellular site of secretion of AMH was investigated by Josso (1973), who applied to fetal calf testicular tissue the microdissection procedure described by Christensen and Mason (1965) for adult rats. Whole testicular tissue, isolated interstitial tissue, and seminiferous tubules were obtained from 17 fetal calves, less than 50 cm in crown-rump length, and associated in organ culture with 14-½-day-old fetal rat reproductive tracts. Anti-Müllerian activity was found in whole testicular tissue and in isolated seminiferous tubules, but not in interstitial tissue, except in cases of contamination by tubular remnants (Figure 4).

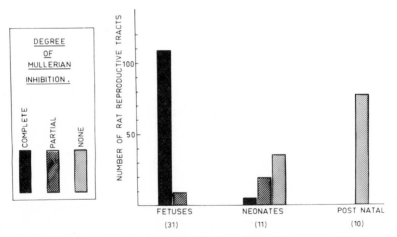

Figure 3. Chronological evolution of anti-Müllerian activity of human testicular tissue. The figures in parentheses indicate the number of cases studied.

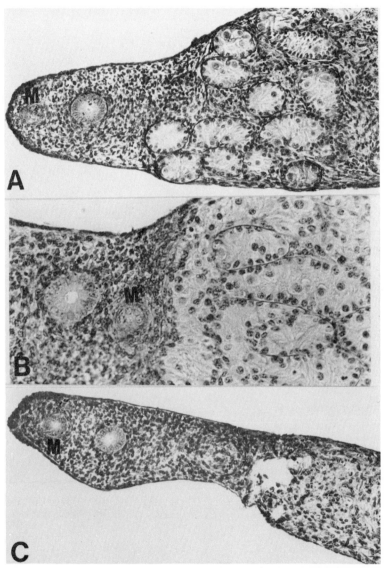

Figure 4. Comparative ability of (A) fetal calf whole testicular tissue, (B) isolated semi-niferous tubules, and (C) isolated interstitial tissue to inhibit the rat fetal Müllerian duct (M). Whole testicular tissue and isolated seminiferous tubules exhibit anti-Müllerian activity, whereas interstitial tissue does not.

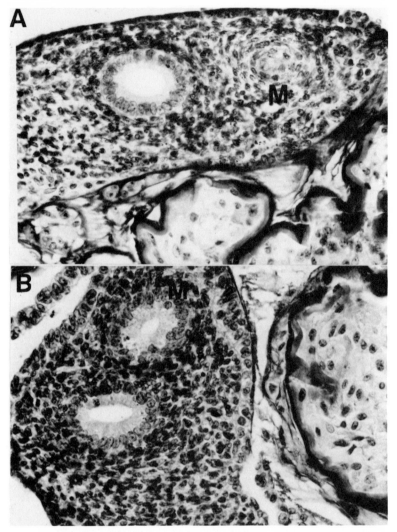

Figure 5. Comparative ability of (*A*) Sertoli cells and (*B*) interstitial cells from calf testes to inhibit the fetal rat Müllerian duct (*M*). Only Sertoli cells exhibit anti-Müllerian activity.

In order to determine which tubular cells are engaged in the synthesis of AMH, advantage was taken of differences which have been demonstrated between biological characteristics of germ and Sertoli cells, such as radiosensitivity and behavior in tissue culture. Human fetal testicular explants were submitted to 500 and 700 rads of ^{60}Co rays; at least 6 days were allowed to elapse between irradiation and AMH bioassay in order to permit irreversibly damaged cells to disappear or exhibit degenerative changes recognizable under the light micro-scope (Josso, 1974b).

The germ cell population in the control and irradiated explants was evaluated by comparing the number of germ cells counted per 50 circular cross-sections of seminiferous tubules to the number present in the same tissue before culture. The average percentage of surviving germ cells was 12.9% in control explants, 7.03% in those exposed to 500 rads, and 3.04% in those exposed to 700 rads ($p < 10^{-5}$). The nearly total destruction of germ cells observed in the irradiated explants did not affect their anti-Müllerian activity, which was similar to that of control testicular explants.

The incapacity of germ cells to attach to the walls of culture vessels was also used to obtain a pure preparation of fetal Sertoli cells (Blanchard and Josso, 1974). Tissue-culture flasks were plated with cellular suspensions from either whole fetal calf testicular tissue, isolated interstitial tissue, or isolated tubules. With the latter, germ cells were eliminated by changing the culture medium, and the cellular monolayer attached to the vessel wall was formed of Sertoli cells only. After 1 week the monolayers were stripped from the flasks by 0.25% trypsin, collected by centrifugation, and placed on the grid of an organ-culture dish, wrapped in the vitelline membrane of a hen's egg. One week after the transfer, anti-Müllerian activity of the cell colonies was tested by placing 14½-day-old fetal rat reproductive tracts on the surface of the vitelline membrane. No anti-Müllerian activity was found in the 9 interstitial cell colonies studied, whereas Müllerian ducts of rat reproductive tracts associated with 15 out of 16 colonies of mixed testicular cells and 10 out of 13 tubular cell colonies were totally inhibited (Figure 5).

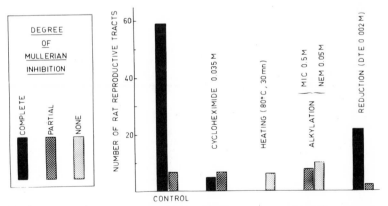

Figure 6. Effect of various treatments on anti-Müllerian activity of incubation media of calf fetal testes. Cycloheximide was added to the medium during incubation. Other treatments, such as heating, monoiodoacetic acid (*MIC*), *N*-ethylmaleimide (*NEM*), and dithioerythritol (*DTE*) were applied to the medium after the completion of incubation.

In summary, it has been shown that AMH is produced by fetal Sertoli cells and that zoological specificity can be demonstrated in certain cases between remotely related species. These experimental data fit with the hypothesis that AMH is a testicular fetoprotein. The macromolecular nature of AMH was already suggested by the inability of fetal testicular tissue to inhibit its target organ when separated from it by the experimental conditions used to this date, in which hormone secretion and bioassay take place simultaneously. The demonstration by Josso, Forest, and Picard (1975) that anti-Müllerian activity can be detected in incubation media of calf fetal testes allowed them to confirm the nondialyzable nature of AMH and also to show that biological activity is thermolabile and partially sulfhydryl-dependent (Figure 6). Furthermore, Picard and Josso (1976) submitted biologically active medium to gel filtration and by studying the Müllerian-inhibiting activity of the effluents estimated the molecular weight of AMH to be in the range of 200,000 to 295,000. Although these biochemical investigations are hampered by the absence of a quantitative test of anti-Müllerian activity, it is hoped that they will eventually lead to the elucidation of one of the last mysterious aspects of modern sex research.

REFERENCES

Blanchard, M. G., and N. Josso. 1974. Source of the anti-müllerian hormone synthesized by the fetal testis: Müllerian inhibiting activity of fetal bovine Sertoli cells in tissue culture. Pediatr. Res. 8:968–972.

Christensen, A. M., and N. R. Mason. 1965. Comparative ability of seminiferous tubules and interstitial tissue of rat testes to synthesize androgens from progesterone-4-C^{14} in vitro. Endocrinology 76:646–656.

Cunha, G. R. 1975. Age-dependent loss of sensitivity of female uro-genital sinus to androgenic conditions as a function of the epithelial stromal interaction in mice. Endocrinology 97:665–673.

Donahoe, P. K., Y. Ito, S. R. Marlatia, and W. H. Hendren. 1975. The range of activity of müllerian-inhibiting substance. Pediatr. Res. 9:289 (Abstr.).

Gitlin, D., and A. Biasucci. 1969. Ontogenesis of immunoreactive growth hormone, follicle-stimulating hormone, thyroid-stimulating hormone, luteinizing hormone, chorionic prolactin and chorionic gonadotropin in the human conceptus. J. Clin. Endocrinol. 29:926–935.

Josso, N. 1970a. Action de la testosterone sur le canal de Wolff du foetus de rat en culture organotypique. Arch. Anat. Microsc. Morphol. Exp. 59:37–50.

Josso, N. 1970b. Action du testicule humain sur le canal de Müller de foetus de rat, en culture organotypique. C. R. Acad. Sci. (Paris) 271:2149–2152.

Josso, N. 1971. Interspecific character of the müllerian-inhibiting substance: action of the human fetal testis, ovary and adrenal on the fetal müllerian duct in organ culture. J. Clin. Endocrinol. 33:404–409.

Josso, N. 1972a. Evolution of the müllerian-inhibiting activity of the human testis. Effect of fetal, peri-natal and post-natal human testicular tissue on the müllerian duct of the fetal rat in organ culture. Biol. Neonat. 20:368–379.

Josso, N. 1972b. Permeability of membranes to the müllerian-inhibiting substance synthesized by the human fetal testis in vitro: a clue to its biochemical nature. J. Clin. Endocrinol. 34:265–270.

Josso, N. 1973. In vitro synthesis of müllerian-inhibiting hormone by seminiferous tubules isolated from the calf fetal testis. Endocrinology 93:829–834.

Josso, N. 1974a. Fetal sexual differentiation in mammals. Ann. Pediatr. (Paris) 3:67–74.

Josso, N. 1974b. Müllerian-inhibiting activity of human fetal testicular cells deprived of germ cells by in vitro irradiation. Pediatr. Res. 8:755–758.

Josso, N., M. G. Forest, and J. Y. Picard. 1975. Müllerian-inhibiting activity of calf fetal testis: relationship to testosterone and protein synthesis. Biol. Reprod. 13:163–167.

Jost, A. 1947. Recherches sur la differentiation sexuelle de l'embryon de lapin. III. Rôle des gonades foetales dans la differentiation sexuel le somatique. Arch. Anat. Microsc. Morphol. Exp. 36:271–315.

Jost, A. 1966. Anterior pituitary function in foetal life. In G. W. Harris and B. T. Donovan (eds.), The Pituitary Gland, pp. 299–323. Butterworths, London.

Jost, A. 1970. Hormonal factors in the sex differentiation of the mammalian foetus. Philos. Trans. R. Soc. Lond. (Biol. Sci.) 259:119–132.

Jost, A., B. Vigier, and J. Prépin. 1972. Free-martins in cattle: the first steps of sexual organogenesis. J. Reprod. Fertil. 29:349–379.

Maraud, R., H. Coulaud, and R. Stoll. 1969. Recherches sur le mécanisme d'inhibition par l'hypophyse de l'inducteur de la répression müllerienne chez l'embryon de poulet. C. R. Soc. Biol. (Paris) 163:2557–2558.

Picard, J. Y., and N. Josso. 1976. Anti-müllerian hormone: estimation of molecular weight by gel filtration. Biomedicine Express 25:147–150.

Picon, R. 1969. Action du testicule foetal sur le développement in vitro des canaux de Müller chez le rat. Arch. Anat. Microsc. Morphol. Exp. 58:1–19.

Picon, R. 1970. Modifications, chez le rat, au cours du développement du testicule, de son action inhibitrice sur les canaux de Müller in vitro. C. R. Acad. Sci. (Paris) 271:2370–2372.

Price, D., J. J. P. Zaaijer, E. Ortiz, and A. O. Brinkmann. 1975. Current views on embryonic sex differentiation in reptiles, birds and mammals. Am. Zool. (Suppl. 1) 15:173–195.

Tran, D., and N. Josso. Zoological specificity of anti-müllerian hormone: relationship between avian and mammalian hormones. Biol. Repr. In press.

Wilson, J. D. 1973. Testosterone uptake by the urogenital tract of the rabbit embryo. Endocrinology 92:1192–1199.

Androgen Receptor Studies in Androgen Insensitivity Syndrome of Man

James A. Amrhein,[1] *Walter J. Meyer, III,*
Bruce S. Keenan, and Claude J. Migeon[2]

Until recently, the classification of male pseudohermaphroditism has been primarily descriptive, based on anatomical characteristics of the genitalia plus the orientation of sexual maturation, if any, occurring at puberty. The difficulty with such classifications is that patients with different biochemical defects may have identical phenotypes; and, conversely, the same biochemical defect may cause diverse clinical characteristics. Therefore, it is now preferable to classify male pseudohermaphroditism into three broad etiological categories: abnormalities in fetal production of androgens; defects in Müllerian-inhibiting factor; and peripheral insensitivity to androgen. In addition, genital abnormalities in the male may be associated with a variety of developmental disorders and dysmorphic syndromes, in this case the defect being considered as a form of congenital malformation.

Examples of the first two types of defects have been adequately discussed by Grumbach and Van Wyk (1974). The ill-defined group with congenital malformations will also be ignored in this discussion. Peripheral insensitivity to androgens may be due to either defective 5α-reductase activity or to a problem in any one of the steps involved in the mode of action of androgens at the cellular level. Several groups (Imperato-McGinley et al., 1974; Walsh et al., 1974) have recently reviewed the pattern of male pseudohermaphroditism which results from a deficiency of 5α-reductase activity in androgen target tissues. Therefore, this chapter will deal exclusively with end organ defects in androgen action subsequent to reductive metabolism of testosterone to dihydrotestosterone (DHT).

This study was supported in part by Research Grant AM-00180-24, and by Traineeship Grant AM-05219-15 from the United States Public Health Service. Portions of this manuscript have been accepted for publication elsewhere: Amrhein, J. A., W. J. Meyer, III, H. W. Jones, Jr., and C. J. Migeon. Androgen insensitivity in man: evidence for genetic heterogeneity. Proc. Nat. Acad. Sci., in press.

[1] Recipient of Postdoctoral Fellowships 5-F22-AM-01224-02 from the National Institute of Arthritis and Metabolic Diseases, United States Public Health Service.

[2] Recipient of Research Career Award 5-K06-AM-21855-12 from the United States Public Health Service.

In recent years, the mechanism of androgen action in responsive tissues has been actively investigated (King and Mainwaring, 1974). In most tissues, reductive metabolism of testosterone to DHT is followed by binding of DHT to a specific cytoplasmic receptor protein. This steroid-receptor complex subsequently translocates to the nuclear compartment, where it binds to specific acceptor sites on the chromatin. Little is known about the exact mechanism by which DHT-receptor complex interacts with chromatin to initiate gene transcription resulting in specific messenger ribonucleic acid (mRNA) synthesis. An alteration at any step in this process could result in defective androgen action.

Over the past few years, attempts have been made to apply this knowledge of the mode of androgen action to the study of patients with male pseudohermaphroditism. To accomplish this, a method has been developed for measuring specific DHT binding in cultured human skin fibroblasts (Keenan et al., 1974; Keenan et al., 1975).

METHODS

Fibroblast cultures were established from skin specimens obtained at the time of surgery or by biopsy. Whole cell DHT binding was measured as previously reported (Keenan et al., 1974; Keenan et al., 1975). Confluent monolayers of fibroblasts were incubated for 30 min at 37°C with [^{3}H]DHT ($0.2-1.5 \times 10^{-9}$ M) dissolved in minimal essential medium without fetal calf serum. Following incubation, the cells were harvested with the use of 0.25% trypsin. All subsequent procedures were carried out at 4°C. After centrifugation at $800 \times g$ for 15 min, the cells were suspended in 1.0 ml of Tris-KCl buffer (0.02 M Tris-HCl, pH 7.5; 0.5 M KCl; 1.5 mM EDTA) and lysed in an ultrasonic cleaner. The sonicate was centrifuged at $1,600 \times g$ for 20 min, and 0.25 ml of the supernatant was taken for DNA measurement (Burton, 1956). Another 0.7 ml was chromatographed on a Sephadex G-25 column (6×0.9 cm) in Tris-KCl buffer. The void volume was collected and counted by liquid scintillation to determine the total protein-bound radioactivity. To quantitatively determine specific DHT binding, a cell aliquot was incubated with [^{3}H]DHT plus an amount of nonradioactive DHT corresponding to 100 times that of [^{3}H]DHT. Bound radioactivity measured in this way was considered nonspecific and was subtracted from the total protein-bound counts to give an estimate of specific binding. By increasing [^{3}H]DHT concentrations in the incubation media a saturation curve was produced. The binding capacity (B_{max}) and apparent dissociation constant (K_d) were determined by linear regression analysis of a double reciprocal plot (Westphal, 1971).

To study the retention of DHT by purified nuclei, confluent monolayer cultures of fibroblasts were incubated with 2×10^{-9} M [^{3}H]DHT for 30 min at 37°C. Similar cultures were incubated in parallel with 2×10^{-9} M [^{3}H]DHT plus a 100-fold excess of nonradioactive DHT. The cells were harvested at 37°C in a 0.25% trypsin–0.05% versene solution. Subsequent isolation procedures were carried out at 4°C. The cells were collected by centrifugation at 800 X g for 15 min, washed with Tris-sucrose buffer, and resuspended in 1 volume of hypotonic buffer (0.02 M Tris-HCl, pH 7.5; 0.5 mM $MgCl_2$; 1.0 mM $CaCl_2$). After 10 min the cells were ruptured by passing them back and forth 10 times through a 25-gauge needle. Exactly one-seventh volume of hypertonic buffer (0.02 M Tris-HCl, pH 7.5; 2.2 M sucrose; 0.5 mM $MgCl_2$; 1.0 mM $CaCl_2$) was added to return the suspension to isotonicity. After centrifugation at 1,600 X g for 20 min, the crude nuclear pellet was washed with Tris-sucrose buffer and purified by centrifuging at 100,000 X g for 1 hr through a 1.8 M sucrose solution. Nuclei prepared in this manner were intact and free from cytoplasmic tage by light microscopy. The purified nuclei were washed once with Tris-sucrose buffer, resuspended in 1 ml of Tris-KCl buffer, lysed by ultrasound, and assayed for bound radioactivity and DNA.

Plasma testosterone and dihydrotestosterone concentrations were determined by a competitive protein-binding method (Tremblay et al., 1970). Serum-luteinizing hormone and follicle-stimulating hormone were evaluated by a double antibody radioimmunoassay (Penny et al., 1970).

RESULTS AND DISCUSSION

The receptor protein for DHT in skin fibroblasts was initially demonstrated by sucrose gradient centrifugation and gel filtration chromatography (Keenan et al., 1974; Keenan et al., 1975). This receptor has a high affinity (K_d of 10^{-9} M) and a high degree of specificity for DHT. Receptor activity is distributed equally between cytoplasmic and nuclear components.

Specific DHT binding in fibroblasts from a number of different anatomical sites, including foreskin, labia, abdomen, and wrist, was measured (Keenan et al., 1974; Keenan et al., 1975). All skin fibroblasts from normal males and females had easily detectable binding activity. Although there was a wide variation in the amount of DHT binding among individuals, binding activity was generally higher in fibroblasts from genital skin as compared to skin from nongenital areas.

Having shown that a receptor protein for DHT is easily detectable in skin fibroblasts from males and females of all ages, studies were performed on patients with complete androgen insensitivity or testicular feminization syndrome. This syndrome is a form of male pseudohermaphroditism characterized by completely female external genitalia, absent Müllerian structures, a 46 XY karyotype, and intra-abdominal or inguinal testes. Spontaneous breast development occurs at puberty if the testes are left in situ. Dr. Lawson Wilkins (1950) suggested many years ago that this disorder represented end organ insensitivity to androgens. Other investigators (Hamilton and Kliman, 1971; Morris and Mahesh, 1963; Strickland and French, 1969) have confirmed the relative unresponsiveness of these patients to exogenous testosterone and dihydrotestoster-

Table 1. DHT binding characteristics of skin fibroblasts from patients with androgen insensitivity

Subjects	Age (years)	Origin of fibroblasts	Apparent K_d (M $\times$ 10^{-9})	B_{max} (mol $\times$ 10^{-18}/μg of DNA)
1[a]	19	Wrist	Unmeasurable	<10
		Pubis	Unmeasurable	0
2[a]	19	Wrist	Unmeasurable	<20
		Labia	Unmeasurable	<10
3	18	Abdomen	Unmeasurable	<20
4	0.1	Arm	Unmeasurable	<10
5	15	Inguinal	Unmeasurable	<20
6 (IV-2)[b]	25	Wrist	1.03	146
7 (IV-4)[b]	39	Wrist	0.92	303
8 (IV-10)[b]	19	Labia	1.01	394
9	22	Pubis	0.60	321
Normal range		Genital	0.20–1.50	170–2,400
		Nongenital	0.10–1.00	60–675

[a]Siblings whose values were reported previously (Keenan et al., 1974).
[b]Refers to Figure 1.

one. Therefore, studies to determine the androgen receptor status of these individuals were conducted.

Initially, five patients with complete androgen insensitivity, ranging in age from 6 weeks to 19 years (Table 1, *subjects 1–5*), were studied. Two of these were siblings. The other three were unrelated patients with no family history of similar disorder. Skin fibroblasts from a variety of sites were investigated, and in all cases there was no detectable specific DHT binding, all of the values being below the sensitivity of the assay. Because of the lack of binding, the K_d could not be determined. These findings were not totally unexpected, because several groups had recently reported a similar defect in androgen binding in the androgen-insensitive mouse kidney and rat preputial gland (Attardi and Ohno, 1974; Bardin et al., 1973; Gehring, Tompkins, and Ohno, 1971).

The identification of the androgen binding deficiency in fibroblasts of affected males provided the means to determine whether or not the condition is X-linked, because the pattern of transmission of this disorder is compatible with either X-linked or sex-linked autosomal dominant inheritance. If the DHT binding deficiency were attributable to a single dose of a mutant autosomal gene, then it could be predicted that both affected males and obligate hetero-zygote females should have a similar lack of androgen binding. X-linked recessive inheritance, on the other hand, would present no binding in affected males but normal or slightly low binding activity in the heterozygote female. The mother of the two siblings with androgen insensitivity (Table 1, *subjects 1 and 2*) was studied and it was found that her fibroblasts of wrist and pubic origin had binding activity within the normal range (Meyer, Migeon, and Migeon, 1975). These results indicate that the mutation is X-linked in man and is, therefore, homologous to the testicular feminization locus in the mouse (Lyon and Hawkes, 1970). In addition, deficient receptor activity in a significant number of clonal populations of maternal fibroblasts was demonstrated, a finding compatible with inactivation of one X-linked allele at this locus.

At the conclusion of these studies, it was believed that the cause of androgen insensitivity syndrome in man had been explained. It apparently resulted from a mutation of the X-linked gene controlling the DHT receptor, causing loss of androgen binding in these individuals. The deficient binding could be due to either the absence of the DHT receptor or to alteration of the receptor, resulting in loss of affinity for the steroid.

In order to confirm and extend our observations, another family with androgen insensitivity was studied. This family was one of the original families with this syndrome seen by Dr. Wilkins (1965). The pedigree of this family (Figure 1) was rather striking in that there were four sisters, all of whom had one or more affected male children. The pattern of transmission was again compatible with either X-linked or sex-linked autosomal dominant inheritance.

We obtained skin specimens from three members of this pedigree (Figure 1, *individuals IV-2, IV-4, and IV-10*). Surprisingly, fibroblasts from these three individuals had levels of DHT binding well within the normal range (Table 1, *subjects 6–8*), regardless of whether fibroblasts were from wrist or genital skin.

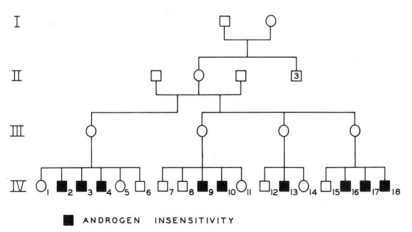

Figure 1. Pedigree showing transmission of androgen insensitivity.

In addition, another unrelated patient with androgen insensitivity was found (Table 1, *subject 9*) whose fibroblasts also showed normal DHT binding.

Therefore, these data indicate that patients with complete androgen insensitivity can be divided into two distinct groups on the basis of the DHT binding characteristics of their fibroblasts—those with undetectable androgen binding and those with normal androgen binding activity. It is important to emphasize that there were no clinical differences between these two groups. All of the patients had phenotypes characteristic of complete androgen insensitivity. In addition, all seven of the postpubertal subjects tested (Table 2) had plasma testosterone levels within or above the normal adult male range, as is characteristic of this syndrome (Rivarola et al., 1967; Tremblay et al., 1972). There was no difference in plasma testosterone between patients with undetectable DHT binding and those with normal DHT binding. Likewise, serum-luteinizing hormone was abnormally high in both groups, whereas follicle-stimulating hormone was normal or only slightly elevated.

Because it is apparent that the four subjects with normal whole cell androgen binding exhibit the characteristic features of androgen insensitivity, it must be assumed that they have a cellular defect at some site other than the initial binding site of the steroid to its cytoplasmic receptor. To investigate this possibility, the nuclear retention of DHT was measured to determine whether cytoplasmic DHT-receptor complex was effectively translocated to the nucleus. As shown in Table 3, there was no difference in specific nuclear retention of labeled DHT between androgen-insensitive subjects and neonatal foreskin controls. In all cases, nuclear-bound DHT accounted for approximately 50% of the whole cell binding. This agrees with previously published data on nuclear binding in normal cells (Keenan et al., 1974; Keenan et al., 1975). The wide range in binding values among individuals in Table 3 is mainly attributable to the site of origin of the skin fibroblasts, wrist skin having generally lower androgen binding capacity than genital or pubic skin. These data indicate that there is no

Table 2. Concentration of testosterone and gonadotrophins in blood of patients with androgen insensitivity

	Plasma testosterone (ng/100 ml)	Gonadotrophins (mI.U./ml)	
		Luteinizing hormone	Follicle-stimulating hormone
Undetectable DHT binding (n = 4)	637–1,090	36.4–62.2	10.0–38.8
Normal DHT binding (n = 3)	640–2,370	31.5–109.6	19.4–21.7
Normal adult male range	300–900	8.8–18	5.5–18

Table 3. Nuclear retention of DHT by fibroblasts from androgen-insensitive subjects with normal whole cell binding

		Specific DHT binding (mol $\times$ 10^{-18}/μg of DNA)	
Subjects	Origin of fibroblasts	Whole cell	Nuclei
Control	Neonatal Foreskin	577	262
Control	Neonatal Foreskin	353	192
7	Wrist	160	109
8	Wrist	106	58
9	Labia	779	269
10	Pubis	497	269

abnormality in nuclear uptake or retention of DHT-receptor complex in these individuals.

At least two basic mechanisms can be invoked to explain the androgen unresponsiveness of the subjects with normal cytoplasmic and nuclear DHT binding. Because the DHT receptor has two primary functions—that of binding to the steroid in the cytoplasm and, following nuclear translocation, binding to specific acceptor sites on the chromatin—it is possible that this variant results from an alteration of the receptor at the site which interacts with chromatin. Or, alternatively, the DHT receptor may be entirely normal, with the mutation involving an alteration of some other protein or proteins essential for androgen-mediated transcription. The exact nature and role of such proteins are unknown, but it has been shown that certain nonhistone proteins are important in determining the specificity of steroid-receptor complex interaction with chromatin (Liao et al., 1973; Mainwaring and Peterken, 1971; O'Malley et al., 1972). Whatever the final answer, the study of cells from androgen-insensitive individuals is certain to lead to a better understanding of the cellular mechanism of androgen action.

SUMMARY

Within the clinical phenotype of complete androgen insensitivity, it has been demonstrated that there are at least two distinct genetic variants.

The first variant is characterized by undetectable DHT binding due to either absence of the receptor protein or alteration of the receptor, resulting in loss of affinity for the steroid. This condition results from a mutation of the X-linked gene specifying the DHT receptor. A similar defect has been observed in androgen-insensitive rodents.

The second variant demonstrates normal cytoplasmic binding and nuclear retention of DHT. The cause of the androgen insensitivity in this variant may be an allelic mutation of the same X-linked gene specifying the DHT receptor, in this case affecting the site on the receptor which interacts with chromatin; or, alternatively, the mutation may involve a separate gene, possibly also on the X chromosome, which codes for other protein or proteins essential for androgen-mediated gene transcription.

It is important for the clinician to recognize these two variants. An XY individual with testes and completely female external genitalia who is found to have undetectable androgen binding clearly has androgen insensitivity and may be expected to feminize spontaneously at puberty. However, a similar prepubertal patient exhibiting normal androgen binding may or may not have androgen insensitivity, and the direction of sexual maturation at puberty remains in doubt. Unfortunately, at the present time there is no way of differentiating between normal androgen-responsive cells and androgen-insensitive cells with normal levels of androgen binding.

Finally, this chapter has dealt only with complete defects resulting in total androgen unresponsiveness. It is highly likely, as with most genetic disorders, that patients will be found with partial androgen insensitivity representing each of these variants. They would be expected to have varying degrees of undervirilization of the external genitalia plus mixed virilization and feminization at puberty.

ACKNOWLEDGMENTS

We are indebted to Mrs. Jacquelyn Kolb for expert technical assistance.

REFERENCES

Attardi, B., and S. Ohno. 1974. Cytosol androgen receptor from kidney of normal and testicular feminized (Tfm) mice. Cell 2:205–212.
Bardin, C. W., L. P. Bullock, R. J. Sherins, I. Mowszowicz, and W. R. Blackburn. 1973. Androgen metabolism and mechanism of action of male pseudohermaphroditism: a study of testicular feminization. Recent Prog. Horm. Res. 29:65–105.
Burton, K. 1956. A study of the conditions and mechanism of the diphenylamine reaction for the colorimetric estimation of deoxyribonucleic acid. Biochem. J. 62:315–323.
Gehring, U., G. M. Tompkins, and S. Ohno. 1971. Effect of the androgen-insensitivity mutation on a cytoplasmic receptor for dihydrotestosterone. Nature (New Biol.) 232:106–107.
Grumbach, M., and J. Van Wyk. 1974. Disorders of sex differentiation. In R.

Williams (ed.), Textbook of Endocrinology, Ed. 5, pp. 480–489. W. B. Saunders Company, Philadelphia.

Hamilton, C. R., Jr., and B. Kliman. 1971. Anabolic effect of dihydrotestosterone in testicular feminization syndrome. Metabolism 20:870–877.

Imperato-McGinley, J., L. Guerrero, T. Gautier, and R. Peterson. 1974. Steroid 5α-reductase deficiency in man: an inherited form of male pseudohermaphroditism. Science 186:1213–1215.

Keenan, B. S., W. J. Meyer, III, A. J. Hadjian, H. W. Jones, and C. J. Migeon. 1974. Syndrome of androgen insensitivity in man: absence of 5α-dihydrotestosterone binding protein in skin fibroblasts. J. Clin. Endocrinol. Metab. 38:1143–1146.

Keenan, B. S., W. J. Meyer, III, A. J. Hadjian, and C. J. Migeon. 1975. Androgen receptor in human skin fibroblasts: characterization of a specific 17β-hydroxy-5α-androstan-3-one-protein complex in cell sonicates and nuclei. Steroids 25:535–552.

King, R., and W. Mainwaring. 1974. Steroid-cell Interactions, pp. 41–101. University Park Press, Baltimore.

Liao, S., T. Liang, T. C. Shao, and J. L. Tymoczko. 1973. Androgen-receptor cycling in prostate cells. In B. W. O'Malley and A. R. Means (eds.), Receptors for Reproductive Hormones, pp. 232–240. Plenum Press, New York.

Lyon, M. F., and S. Hawkes. 1970. X-linked gene for testicular feminization in the mouse. Nature 227:1217–1219.

Mainwaring, W., and B. Peterken. 1971. A reconstituted cell-free system for the specific transfer of steroid-receptor complexes into nuclear chromatin isolated from rat ventral prostate gland. Biochem. J. 125:285–295.

Meyer, W. J., III, B. R. Migeon, and C. J. Migeon. 1975. Locus on the X chromosome for dihydrotestosterone receptor and androgen insensitivity. Proc. Nat. Acad. Sci. U.S.A. 72:1469–1472.

Morris, J., and V. B. Mahesh. 1963. Further observations on the syndrome, "testicular feminization." Am. J. Obstet. Gynecol. 87:731–748.

O'Malley, B., T. Spelsberg, W. Schrader, F. Chytil, and A. Steggles. 1972. Mechanisms of interaction of a hormone-receptor complex with the genome of a eukaryotic target cell. Nature 235:141–144.

Penny, R., H. J. Guyda, A. Baghdassarian, A. J. Johanson, and R. M. Blizzard. 1970. Correlation of serum follicular stimulating hormone (FSH) and luteinizing hormone (LH) as measured by radioimmunoassay in disorders of sexual development. J. Clin. Invest. 49:1847–1852.

Rivarola, M. A., J. M. Saez, W. J. Meyer, F. M. Kenny, and C. J. Migeon. 1967. Studies of androgens in the syndrome of male pseudohermaphroditism with testicular feminization. J. Clin. Endocrinol. Metab. 27:371–378.

Strickland, A. L., and F. S. French. 1969. Absence of response to dihydrotestosterone in the syndrome of testicular feminization. J. Clin. Endocrinol. Metab. 29:1284–1286.

Tremblay, R. R., I. Z. Beitins, A. Kowarski, and C. J. Migeon. 1970. Measurement of plasma dihydrotestosterone by competitive protein-binding analysis. Steroids 16:29–40.

Tremblay, R. R., T. P. Foley, Jr., P. Corvol, I. Park, A. Kowarski, R. M. Blizzard, H. W. Jones, Jr., and C. J. Migeon. 1972. Plasma concentration of testosterone, dihydrotestosterone, testosterone-estradiol binding globulin, and pituitary gonadotrophins in the syndrome of male pseudohermaphroditism with testicular feminization. Acta Endocrinol. (Kbh) 70:331–341.

Walsh, P., J. Madden, M. Harrod, J. Goldstein, P. MacDonald, and J. Wilson. 1974. Familial incomplete male pseudohermaphroditism, type 2: decreased dihydrotestosterone formation in pseudovaginal perineoscrotal hypospadias. N. Engl. J. Med. 291:944—949.

Westphal, U. 1971. Steroid-protein Interactions, pp. 66—83. Springer-Verlag, New York.

Wilkins, L. 1950. The Diagnosis and Treatment of Endocrine Disorders in Childhood and Adolescence, Ed. 1, p. 271. Charles C. Thomas, Springfield, Illinois.

Wilkins, L. 1965. The Diagnosis and Treatment of Endocrine Disorders in Childhood and Adolescence, Ed. 3, pp. 321—322. Charles C. Thomas, Springfield, Illinois.

Naturally Occurring Adrenal Steroids with Salt-losing Properties
Relationship to Congenital Adrenal Hyperplasia

Alfonso H. Janoski

The provocative concept that a naturally occurring steroid with natriuretic properties exerting a physiological or pathophysiological effect on the human organism may exist has been entertained for many years. The likelihood that adrenal steroids evoke the unexplained natriuretic response to extravascular volume expansion has been virtually eliminated, according to publications in this field. There is, however, considerable evidence stemming from both clinical observations and research supporting the role of certain adrenal steroids in sodium balance. Although such steroidal compounds do not fulfill the criteria to be designated natriuretic hormones and are not potent mineralocorticoid antagonists when compared to commercially available spironolactone-like agents, their concerted actions may be significant in their effect on patients with salt-losing congenital adrenal hyperplasia. This chapter discusses specific adrenal steroids with respect to natriuretic activity—namely, progesterone, 17α-hydroxyprogesterone, and 16α-hydroxyprogesterone. Documentation of the natriuretic effects of these steroids in man is reviewed; animal or in vitro studies are excluded to avoid conflicting interpretations, because experience has dictated that natriuretic effects in animals are not consistently reproduced in humans.

Work on the radioimmunoassay of 16α-hydroxyprogesterone was supported by Research Grant AM-15809 from the U.S. Public Health Service. Balance studies on the effects of infusion of 16α-hydroxyprogesterone were supported in part by the Bressler Research Fund from the University of Maryland School of Medicine and the United States Army.

The following trivial names are used in this report:
16α-hydroxyprogesterone, 16α-hydroxy-pregn-4-ene-3,20-dione; 17α-hydroxyprogesterone, 17α-hydroxy-pregn-4-ene-3,20-dione; progesterone, pregn-4-ene-3,20-dione; desoxycorticosterone acetate, pregn-4-ene-21-acetate-3,20-dione; tetrahydrocortisone, 5β-pregnan-3α,17α,21-triol-11,20-dione; 16α-hydroxypregnenolone, 3β,16α-dihydroxypregn-5-ene-20-one; pregnanetriol, 5β-pregnane-3α,17,20-triol; 9α-fluorohydrocortisone, 9α-fluoro-11β,17,21,-trihydroxypregn-4-ene-3,20-dione.

EARLY CLINICAL OBSERVATIONS

The increased urinary sodium excretion that results from the administration of adrenocorticotropic hormone (ACTH) to patients with virilizing congenital adrenal hyperplasia (CAH) was first reported by Lewis and Wilkins (1949). The following year these clinicians observed similar effects in patients with the salt-losing form of CAH. Both physicians suggested a novel hypothesis—the adrenals of patients with salt-losing CAH possibly secrete steroids capable of producing urinary sodium excretion (Wilkins, Klein, and Lewis, 1950). The sodium diuretic effect of ACTH was reviewed by Jailer (1951) and confirmed by other investigators, including the separate efforts of Blizzard et al. (1959), Lieberman and Luetscher (1960), and Prader, Spahr, and Neher (1955).

Adrenal research during this era supported the possible existence of a sodium-excreting steroid or steroids. Eberlein and Bongiovanni (1955) correlated the quantity of tetrahydrocortisone excreted and the sodium-losing tendency. The patients with simple virilizing or non-salt-losing CAH secondary to adrenal 21-hydroxylase deficiency, who had salt loss under stress, excreted less than normal quantities of tetrahydrocortisone but more than that excreted by consistent sodium losers. These studies imply that the adrenals of salt losers produce less cortisol and probably less aldosterone. An additional possible interpretation of these findings is that stress, releasing pituitary ACTH, results in enhanced secretion of salt-losing steroids by adrenal glands having a 21-hydroxylase deficiency.

The relative resistance of patients with the salt-losing form of CAH to the pharmacological action of 11-deoxycorticosterone acetate (DOCA) has been well documented. Crigler, Silverman, and Wilkins (1952) noted that relatively greater dosages of DOCA were required to control such children, but after the pituitary-adrenal axis was suppressed secondary to glucocorticoid therapy the amount of DOCA required to achieve the desired sodium balance was decreased. Others reporting a high degree of resistance to DOCA were Bartter et al. (1951), Lewis and Wilkins (1949), Luetscher and Curtin (1955), and Prader, Spahr, and Neher (1955).

ROLE OF ALDOSTERONE IN
SALT-LOSING FORM OF CONGENITAL ADRENAL HYPERPLASIA

Evidence for the secretion of steroids with sodium-losing properties in patients with 21-hydroxylase block is substantially supported by clinical studies on the role of aldosterone in this disorder. Earlier investigations involved crude bioassays and poor extraction techniques. Despite controversies they caused, certain publications were correct in their initial findings. Blizzard et al. (1959), employing a bioassay technique in which adrenalectomized dogs were used for aldosterone determinations, were the first to report a lack of increased aldosterone excretion in children with virilizing CAH. Lieberman and Luetscher (1960) were the first to document low aldosterone excretion in children with the salt-losing form of CAH by means of a bioassay method. Other contemporary investigators reported data conflicting with those of the previous two groups, stating that aldosterone excretion was normal or elevated. Subsequently, refinement of the double isotope dilution method for measuring aldosterone excretion and production rates was instrumental in settling the dilemma. Quite understandably, publications in this field appeared infrequently: the patients were children who were difficult to study because of age and clinical status, and manipulation of sodium intake or glucocorticoid therapy could result in an Addisonian type of crisis. Despite these serious obstacles, remarkable feats were performed by patients and their clinicians and the controversy was eventually settled. Mattox et al. (1964) and New, Miller, and Peterson (1964) reported low urinary aldosterone excretion in patients with salt-losing CAH and the lack of increase in excretion of this hormone during sodium restriction. The non-salt-losers had "normal" aldosterone excretion on a regular diet, with an increase occurring during a low sodium intake (Mattox et al., 1964).

In Table 1, from the data of New, Miller, and Peterson (1966), three subtypes of patients with 21-hydroxylase deficiency based on sodium balance are suggested. The simple virilizing type has a normal urinary aldosterone level and can increase the urinary aldosterone substantially during sodium restriction. Of the seven patients with the salt-losing form of CAH, four were clinically classified as severe and three as moderate. Of interest is the difference in aldosterone excretion in these two subtypes—both groups of patients lost urinary sodium inappropriately. The severe sodium losers had no compensatory mechanism with baseline levels low and remaining low despite a state of sodium deprivation. The moderate salt losers had "normal" levels of aldosterone in the baseline status, but, on closer scrutiny of the data, some of the levels of urinary aldosterone were inappropriately low for the concomitant urinary excretion of sodium. Because these patients are not sodium-restricted in their everyday life, the disorder is generally mild, and the patients remain free of crisis. During situations in which unusual sodium loss ensues, a crisis is inevitable because there is no increase in aldosterone production (New, Miller, and Peterson, 1966). Data

Table 1. Aldosterone excretion in CAH

	Baseline	After low sodium intake
Severe salt-losing ($n = 4$)	Low	No increase
Moderate salt-losing ($n = 3$)	Normal	No increase
Simple ($n = 3$)	Normal	3-Fold increase

New, Miller, and Peterson (1966).

obtained from the severe salt losers support impaired, low aldosterone production. Interpretation is difficult, however, because these patients require both glucocorticoid and mineralocorticoid therapy even during the studies, and suppression of the renin-angiotensin-aldosterone system can result.

Production rates of aldosterone in salt-losing and simple virilizing CAH were reported from three different sources in 1965. Degenhart et al. (1965), using the double isotope dilution technique, determined aldosterone secretion rates in nine children with CAH, three of whom were salt losers. In the six non-salt-losers, aldosterone secretion rates were normal (60–125 μg/24 hr) and rose after salt deprivation (100–380 μg/24 hr). Extremely low values were obtained for the three children with the salt-losing type (10 μg/24 hr), and there was no increment in secretion rate following restriction of sodium. Table 2 summarizes the findings of Kowarski et al. (1965), Bryan, Kliman, and Bartter (1965) and Bartter, Henkin, and Bryan (1968), who independently determined low aldosterone production rates in patients with salt-losing CAH. Kowarski's group classified 17 children with CAH as salt losers or non-salt-losers, according to clinical symptoms. One patient did not fit this classification and was designated as an intermediate type; this patient lost moderate amounts of urinary sodium only

Table 2. Production rates of aldosterone in CAH

	Sodium intake (mEq/day)	Treatment	Production rates (μg/day)
A. Salt-losing ($n = 6$)	Ad lib	None	4.0–22
Intermediate ($n = 1$)	Ad lib	None	64
Simple ($n = 10$)	Ad lib	None	113–345
Case 1	85	None	184
	9	None	628
Case 2	119	None	350
	9	None	600
Case 3	100	None	269
	100	Gluc[a]	47
Normal	Ad lib	None	29–95
B. Salt-losing ($n = 7$)	Ad lib	Gluc	2.0–27
	Depletion	Gluc	2.0–78
Control ($n = 6$)	Ad lib	None	26–198
	Depletion	None	110–460
C. Simple			
($n = 8$)	83–133	None	112–1,697
($n = 9$)	9	None	254–3,244
($n = 5$)	61–182	Gluc	26–121
	9–14	Gluc	116–361

Modified from A, Kowarski et al. (1965); B, Bryan, Kliman, and Bartter (1965), and C, Bartter, Henkin, and Bryan (1968).
[a]Gluc, glucocorticoid suppressive therapy.

when put on a low sodium diet, but maintained a greater aldosterone production rate than the salt losers. Patients with untreated simple virilizing CAH were found to secrete aldosterone in amounts greater than normal for their sodium intake when compared to normal controls of comparable ages. On suppressive glucocorticoid therapy, these patients, as typified by case 3 (see Table 2), reduced the aldosterone production rates to normal. Non-salt-losers could increase aldosterone production with sodium restriction, whereas salt losers continued to have a fixed, low rate of production. Bartter, Henkin, and Bryan (1968) confirmed the observations that patients with the simple non-salt-losing form of CAH have elevated aldosterone production rates when not treated with appropriate doses of glucocorticoids. As shown in Table 2, such patients have abnormally increased aldosterone production during periods of normal sodium intake, but aldosterone secretion can increase still further during salt restriction. During suppressive glucocorticoid therapy, the production rates return to the normal baseline. Quite recently, the abnormally elevated secretion of aldosterone in non-salt-losers was substantiated by Loras, Haour, and Bertrand (1970).

The conclusions which can be drawn from these investigations have been summarized by Bartter, Henkin, and Bryan (1968) and Kowarski et al. (1965). The biosynthetic pathways for aldosterone production are defective in salt-losing CAH, but are intact in the non-salt-losing form (Bartter, Henkin, and Bryan, 1968). Of significance is the clinical observation that untreated patients with simple CAH, while maintaining hyperproduction of aldosterone during normal sodium intakes, were normotensive and did not develop hypertension or alkalosis (Bartter, Henkin, and Bryan, 1968; Kowarski et al., 1965). Two hypotheses concerning the overproduction of aldosterone in the non-salt-losing adrenogenital syndrome were suggested by these investigators. According to the "biogenetic" sequence, increased ACTH secretion causes an overproduction of aldosterone precursors, resulting in enhanced aldosterone production. With a "physiological hypothesis," the overproduction of aldosterone can be considered an attempt of physiological compensation to counteract the sodium loss secondary to increased release of the sodium-losing steroids by the adrenal (Kowarski et al., 1965). This latter hypothesis is more attractive because, according to the biogenetic sequence, a direct hypersecretion of aldosterone should eventually result in hypokalemic alkalosis, hypertension, and a fixed aldosterone secretion. During sodium loading of untreated patients with simple CAH, aldosterone production decreased according to Kowarski et al. (1965), and this effect would not occur if overproduction of precursor steroids were responsible for the hyperproduction of aldosterone. Evidence supporting an antagonism by natriuretic adrenal steroids to aldosterone is gained from these observations, because such steroids can block sodium for potassium exchange and sodium for hydrogen exchange, preventing hypokalemic alkalosis and hypertension (Bartter, Henkin, and Bryan, 1968).

ROLE OF PROGESTERONE

Studies on the effect of progesterone in five volunteers on a constant diet were reported by Landau and Lugibihl (1958). There was an increase in urinary sodium excretion and a decline in urinary potassium excretion within the first few days of progesterone administration. The progesterone was given intramuscularly in a buffered medium with an oil vehicle. As little as 12.5 mg of progesterone/day reportedly elicited urinary sodium loss. The total quantity of sodium excreted was dependent on the dose and duration of administration. In one subject, 300 mg of progesterone intramuscularly for 8 days evoked a cumulative loss of 336 mEq; in a second subject, 200 mg/day for a 6-day comparable period resulted in a loss of 396 mEq of sodium in the urine. The investigators believed that the administration of 12.5 mg of progesterone/day was consistent with the quantity of this steroid produced during the luteal phase of the menstrual cycle and that doses of 200 mg/day were consistent with levels found in pregnancy near term, suggesting a physiological effect on sodium balance under these conditions. Landau and Lugibihl (1958) furnished evidence that progesterone in doses of 50 mg/day given to an Addisonian patient could antagonize the sodium-retaining effects of d,l-aldosterone in doses of 300 mg/day. In other studies, these researchers were the first to demonstrate a lack of natriuretic response to progesterone in patients with adrenal insufficiency who were deficient in mineralocorticoids either naturally or therapeutically. These findings implied a peripheral antagonism of aldosterone at the site of action in the kidney.

Additional confirmation of the antialdosterone effect of progesterone in humans was attained by Laidlaw, Ruse, and Gornall (1962), who evaluated the effect of progesterone administration on sodium balance and aldosterone excretion in volunteers on constant diet and sodium intake. All eight subjects responded to 100 mg of progesterone/day with a rise in aldosterone excretion during the entire time the progesterone was administered. Quite recently, Sundsfjord (1971) has shown that progesterone in doses of 100 mg/day given to four male normal volunteers, resulting in plasma concentrations varying from 4.5–29 ng/ml, produced a sodium diuresis on the 1st day, but aldosterone excretion did not rise appreciably until the 3rd day of the study. In the patients with the untreated non-salt-losing form of CAH, Strott, Yoshimi, and Lipsett (1969) reported plasma progesterone levels 6–10 times greater than those of normal males. Simopoulos et al. (1971) verified this observation, but also noted comparably high levels in untreated salt losers.

ROLE OF 17α-HYDROXYPROGESTERONE

The natriuretic effects of 17α-hydroxyprogesterone (17-OHP) in five normal volunteers and two patients with adrenal insufficiency were published by Jacobs et al. (1961). A constant diet and electrolyte intake were imposed during the studies. Each subject took 500 mg of 17α-hydroxyprogesterone/day by mouth while receiving 5 mg of DOCA/day. After a 10-day control or equilibration period for electrolyte balance, the study was initiated with 17-OHP and continued for 10–20 days. Urinary sodium rose by day 6, reaching a peak excretion by the 6th to 9th day of 17-OHP administration for all normal volunteers. The negative sodium balance persisted for 72 hr after the steroid was discontinued. In one case of adrenal insufficiency maintained on cortisone and DOCA, the response to 17-OHP was similar to that of normal volunteers. In the second patient with adrenal insufficiency, maintained on cortisone and adequate salt but not DOCA, there was no response to 17-OHP. These studies established the natriuretic action of 17α-hydroxyprogesterone in humans, and, as with progesterone, the sodium-excreting effect is the result of antagonism to the sodium-retaining activity of mineralocorticoids. In the non-sodium-losing adrenogenital syndrome, Strott, Yoshimi, and Lipsett (1969) measured plasma levels of 17-OHP that were 50–200 times greater than those in normal males. Studies by Simopoulos et al. (1971) found equally high levels in salt-losing CAH.

ROLE OF 16α-HYDROXYPROGESTERONE

Interest in 16α-hydroxyprogesterone (16-OHP) as a naturally occurring natriuretic steroid was aroused by the isolation of large quantities of metabolically reduced 16α-hydroxylated C-21 steroids from the urine of patients with the salt-losing adrenogenital syndrome (Neher, Meystre, and Wettstein, 1959). These were later established by Ruse and Solomon (1966) as urinary metabolites of 16-OHP. Two of these metabolites—3β,16α-dihydroxy-5α-pregnane-20-one and its isomer 3β,16α-dihydroxy-5β-pregnane-20-one—have not demonstrated any evidence of natriuretic activity in man (Coppage and Liddle, 1960; George, Saucier, and Bartter, 1965). As early as 1965, however, there was evidence that 16-OHP in intramuscular doses of 200 mg/day evoked a natriuretic response on the day following withdrawal of the steroid (George, Saucier, and Bartter, 1965). This effect may represent the lag period of 3–4 days reported by others with substances possessing antialdosterone- or spironolactone-like activity. In all the aforementioned clinical experiments in which the steroids were administered intramuscularly, by rectal suppository, or orally, there is no information available about rate of absorption or blood levels produced. A delay in achieving optimal levels is conceivable.

Janoski and fellow workers, using the double isotope dilution technique, found enhanced production rates of 16-OHP in two salt losers who did not have glucocorticoid suppression of the pituitary-adrenal axis (Janoski et al. 1969b) (Table 3). When both patients had urinary excretion of pregnanetriol greater than 35 mg/day, the production rates of 16-OHP were 24 and 28 mg/day, compared to a normal subject who had less than 1 mg/day. In an earlier

Table 3. Production rates of 16α-hydroxyprogesterone

Subject	Clinical state[a]	Production rate (mg/day)
Male salt loser, age 15 years	Suppressed	0.6
	Unsuppressed	2.8
Female salt loser, age 10 years	Partially suppressed	7.9
	Unsuppressed	2.4

[a]State of suppression determined by excretion of urinary pregnanetriol.

experiment using the same subjects, when both had partial to almost complete suppression of the adrenal secretion during glucocorticoid therapy, the 16-OHP production rates were lower, correlating adrenal release of 16-OHP with ACTH levels.

In the same year, Jacobs (1969) described the effects of administration of 16-OHP on electrolyte balance in three normal subjects and a patient with adrenal insufficiency. After a control period, on a constant balance diet for 6 days, each volunteer received 250 mg of 16-OHP orally every 12 hr. The total urinary electrolyte concentrations were averaged over consecutive periods of 2–3 days for comparison of control to experimental periods. In brief, these studies verified the natriuretic effect of 16-OHP in man. Furthermore, in a patient with adrenal insufficiency, maintained on DOCA (15 mg/day) and cortisone acetate (37.5 mg/day), 16-OHP in a dose similar to that used in the controls produced increased urinary sodium excretion.

Preliminary studies of intravenous infusions of 16-OHP were reported by Janoski et al. (1969a). Two normal volunteers were selected and placed on a constant fluid and electrolyte balance diet with high sodium and normal potassium intake (Figure 1). 16-OHP (30 mg/day) was infused in 5% dextrose and water containing 1.8% absolute ethanol by volume. The dose was based on earlier estimates of the daily production rates of 16-OHP in two patients with salt-losing CAH (Janoski et al. 1969b). Following an equilibration period of 7 days, the volunteers were infused with control solutions for 2 consecutive days. The control infusions were devoid of 16-OHP. During the study period, 16-OHP was added to the intravenous fluids, and the volunteers were infused for 6–10 days (Figure 1). Prior to these studies, the investigators had established that the infusate was pyrogen-free in rabbits. There were no untoward effects or febrile reactions produced in these human volunteers. The results show a significant rise in urinary aldosterone excretion in both subjects (Figure 1), indicating that infusion of 16-OHP in doses comparable to adrenal production in untreated patients with salt-losing CAH will antagonize the action of aldosterone and evoke a compensatory increase in the secretion of this hormone.

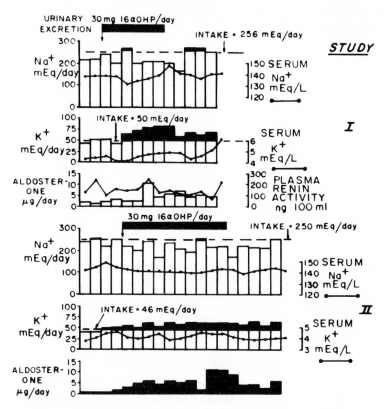

Figure 1. Effect of infusion of 16α-hydroxyprogesterone on urinary sodium, potassium, and aldosterone excretion in two normal adult male volunteers (*I* and *II*).

Quite recently, an infusion study was concluded by this investigator with the aid of a bilaterally adrenalectomized volunteer housed in a metabolic unit on a constant balance diet. This patient was maintained on cortisone acetate and 9α-fluorohydrocortisone with sodium intake adjusted to provide the least intake necessary to maintain well being. On this regimen, the patient required 90 mEq of sodium/day (Table 4). On days 6 and 7 of the study period, there was a substantial increase in the urinary sodium to potassium ratio. This occurred when the infusion rate was changed from 30 mg/24 hr or approximately 2 μg/min to 35 μg/min for the first 12 hr and 7 μg/min for the remainder of each of 2 days. During *I-6* and *I-7* (Table 4), the total quantity of fluid, dextrose, and alcohol infused and the rate of infusion of these substances were unchanged from *C-1* through *I-5,* the only variable being the rate of 16-OHP infused. Further studies are required to confirm these preliminary findings and determine the log-dose response.

108   Janoski

Table 4. Infusion of 16-OHP in adrenalectomized volunteer[a] on constant fluid and electrolyte intake[b]

| Day | Urinary | | Rate of steroid infusion (30 mg/day) |
	Sodium (mEq/day)	Na:K ratio	
C[c]-1	70	0.96	
C-2	83	0.97	
C-3	75	1.01	
I-1	76	1.02	15 mg q 12 hr
I-2	72	0.95	15 mg q 12 hr
I-3	75	1.06	15 mg q 12 hr
I-4	97	1.20	15 mg q 12 hr
I-5	92	1.13	15 mg q 12 hr
I-6	98	1.35	25 mg q 12 hr
			5 mg q 12 hr
I-7	100	1.39	25 mg q 12 hr
			5 mg q 12 hr

[a]White male adult.
[b]Intake, 100 mEq of sodium and 80 mEq of potassium per day.
[c]The following abbreviations are used: C, control infusion; I, 16-OHP infusion.

To date, there is no information available on blood levels of 16-OHP in the simple or salt-losing types of CAH. Quite recently, the daily urine specimens of some patients with CAH have been obtained in collaboration with Drs. Salvatore Raiti and Noel Maclaren of the Department of Pediatrics, University of Maryland School of Medicine. The daily urinary concentration of 16-OHP in two patients with documented CAH secondary to 21-hydroxylase deficiency and one child with 11-hydroxylase deficiency is presented in Table 5.

The free 16-OHP corresponds to unconjugated 16-OHP in the urine and is measured following extraction of an aliquot of the 24-hr urine. Prior to extraction, labeled 16-OHP is added for recovery. Total 16-OHP represents all urinary 16-OHP determined following the addition of labeled 16-OHP, enzymatic hydrolysis, and extraction. The steroid concentration is measured by a highly specific radioimmunoassay following chromatography of the extract on thin layer plates (Janoski, Schultz, and Connor, 1974). The normal values for urinary excretion of this steroid are obtained from the adult population. Currently, attempts are being made to match age and sex in these and other patients to controls. The preliminary data show that the untreated salt loser, age 3 weeks, had a 10-fold elevation of free 16-OHP and a 25-fold increase in total 16-OHP compared to normal adults and a child of the same age. The untreated 6-year-old with simple virilizing CAH had higher free 16-OHP levels, but reduced total

Table 5. Urinary excretion of 16α-hydroxyprogesterone

	Free (μg/day)	Total[a] (μg/day)
Adults		
Normal males (n = 40)	0.22 ± 0.20 (S.D.)	11.0 ± 7.6 (S.D.)
Normal females (n = 75)	0.31 ± 0.22 (S.D.)	12.2 ± 7.6 (S.D.)
Children		
T. W. (age 3 weeks, salt-losing CAH)	2.02	308
	2.03[b]	310[b]
M. B. (age 6 years, 21-CAH)[c]	4.74	80.7
P. M. (age 1 year, 11-CAH)	1.7	.4.24

[a]Following enzymatic hydrolysis.
[b]Determined on a different day.
[c]Simple virilizing CAH.

levels compared to the salt loser. The untreated child with 11-hydroxylase deficiency had still lower urinary levels for both free and conjugated 16-OHP. Of interest is that the 24-hr urinary excretion of 16-OHP during infusion studies with 30 mg of this steroid is approximately 290–300 μg (total 16-OHP). Further studies are underway to determine the relationship of 16-OHP to aldosterone excretion in patients with 21-hydroxylase block in order to determine whether a correlation exists in sodium balance.

INDIRECT EVIDENCE OF NATRIURETIC STEROID ACTIVITY: MENSTRUAL CYCLE AND PREGNANCY

There is additional provocative indirect evidence supporting the concept of naturally occurring natriuretic steroids. Documented reports of significant increases in the blood concentrations of 17α-hydroxyprogesterone and progesterone in normal menstruating women during the luteal phase of the cycle and in maternal blood during the latter part of pregnancy are to be considered (Craft, Whyman, and Sommerville, 1969; Holmdahl and Johansson, 1972a, 1972b). Janoski and others have recently reported enhanced maternal plasma levels of 16-OHP beginning at week 31 of pregnancy and rising at term to levels 40-fold above the nonpregnant state (Janoski and Schultz, 1975a). A significant rise in plasma and urinary 16-OHP also has been established during the luteal phase of the cycle (Janoski and Schultz, 1975b). Knowledge that production rates of aldosterone increase during these times—the postovulatory phase of the cycle and late in pregnancy—strongly suggests a compensatory adjustment to the effects of these natriuretic steroids acting in concert to evoke urinary sodium loss. Whether or not their role is purely a negative one awaits further investigation.

SUMMARY

Abundant evidence exists that progesterone, 17α-hydroxyprogesterone, and 16α-hydroxyprogesterone have natriuretic activity in humans. From the data available, the sodium-losing effect is best explained as a spironolactone-like pharmacological action anatagonizing aldosterone at its site of activity in the distal tubule of the kidney. When each steroid is considered separately, this antialdosterone, natriuretic effect is weak. From the literature reviewed, it is obvious that simple or salt-losing CAH permits overproduction of all three steroids, creating an additive effect. The concerted action of such steroids can explain the compensatory rise in aldosterone production in the non-salt-losing form of CAH, in late pregnancy, and in the luteal phase of the menstrual cycle. In the salt-losing form of CAH, these three steroids probably act collectively and antagonize the action of the reduced quantities of aldosterone secreted secondary to impaired adrenal production, thereby contributing significantly to the urinary sodium loss.

ACKNOWLEDGMENTS

Gratitude is extended to Karen Schultz for her excellent technical assistance, Myra Barlow for dietary consultations, and all the volunteers and patients for their enthusiastic cooperation.

REFERENCES

Bartter, F. C., F. Albright, A. P. Forbes, A. Leaf, E. Dempsey, and E. Carroll. 1951. Effects of adrenocorticotropic hormone and cortisol in the adrenogenital syndrome associated with congenital adrenal hyperplasia: an attempt to explain and correct its disordered pattern. J. Clin. Invest. 30:237.

Bartter, F. C., R. I. Henkin, and G. T. Bryan. 1968. Aldosterone hypersecretion in "non-salt-losing" congenital adrenal hyperplasia. J. Clin. Invest. 47:1742.

Blizzard, R. M., G. W. Liddle, C. Migeon, and L. Wilkins. 1959. Aldosterone secretion in virilizing adrenal hyperplasia. J. Clin. Invest. 38:1442.

Bryan, G. T., B. Kliman, and F. C. Bartter. 1965. Impaired aldosterone production in "salt-losing" congenital adrenal hyperplasia. J. Clin. Invest. 44:957.

Coppage, W. S., and G. W. Liddle. 1960. Metabolic studies with a steroid isolated from the urine of patients with "salt-losing" congenital adrenal hyperplasia. J. Clin. Endocrinol. 20:729.

Craft, I., H. Whyman, and I. F. Sommerville. 1969. Serial analyses of plasma progesterone and pregnandiol in human pregnancy. J. Obstet. Gynaecol. Br. Commonw. 76:1080.

Crigler, J. F., S. H. Silverman, and L. Wilkins. 1952. Further studies on the treatment of congenital adrenal hyperplasia with cortisone. IV. Effect of cortisone and compound B in patients with disturbances of electrolyte metabolism. Pediatrics 10:397.

Degenhart, H. J., H. K. Visser, R. Wilmink, and W. Croughs. 1965. Aldosterone and cortisol secretion rates in infants and children with congenital adrenal hyperplasia suggesting different 21-hydroxylation defects in salt-losers and non-salt-losers. Acta Endocrinol. 48:587.

Eberlein, W. R., and A. M. Bongiovanni. 1955. Partial characterization of urinary adrenocortical steroids in adrenal hyperplasia. J. Clin. Invest. 34:1337.

George, J. M., G. Saucier, and F. C. Bartter. 1965. Is there a potent naturally occurring sodium-losing steroid hormone? J. Clin. Endocrinol. 25:621.

Holmdahl, T. H., and E. Johansson. 1972a. Peripheral plasma levels of 17α-hydroxyprogesterone, progesterone and oestradiol during normal menstrual cycles in women. Acta Endocrinol. 71:743.

Holmdahl, T. H., and E. Johansson, 1972b. Peripheral plasma levels of 17α-hydroxyprogesterone during human pregnancy. Acta Endocrinol. 71:765.

Jacobs, D. R. 1969. Natriuretic activity of 16α-hydroxyprogesterone in man. Acta Endocrinol. 61:275.

Jacobs, D. R., J. van der Poll, J. L. Gabrilove, and L. J. Soffer. 1961. 17α-hydroxyprogesterone—a salt-losing steroid: relation to congenital adrenal hyperplasia. J. Clin. Endocrinol. 21:909.

Jailer, J. W. 1951. Evidence for a salt-losing adrenal hormone in congenital adrenal virilism associated with Addisonian-like symptoms. J. Clin. Endocrinol. (Abstr.) 11:798.

Janoski, A. H., R. H. Herman, J. G. Hilton, and W. G. Kelly. 1969a. Natriuretic activity of 16α-OH-progesterone. Clin. Res. (Abstr.) 17:589.

Janoski, A. H., M. S. Roginsky, N. P. Christy, and W. G. Kelly. 1969b. On the metabolism of 16α-hydroxy-C_{21} steroids. III. Evidence for high rates of production of 16α-hydroxyprogesterone and 16α-hydroxypregnenolone in the salt-losing form of congenital adrenal hyperplasia. J. Clin. Endocrinol. 29:1301.

Janoski, A. H., and K. E. Schultz. 1975a. 16α-hydroxyprogesterone in human pregnancy: maternal plasma and umbilical cord blood concentrations by radioimmunoassay. Clin. Res. 23:238A.

Janoski, A. H., and K. E. Schultz. 1975b. Plasma and urinary concentrations of unconjugated 16α-hydroxyprogesterone during the human menstrual cycle. In Program of the Fifty-seventh Annual Meeting of the Endocrine Society, Suppl. Endocrinol. (Abstr.) 96:256.

Janoski, A. H., K. E. Schultz, and T. B. Connor. 1974. Radioimmunoassay of plasma 16α-hydroxyprogesterone in man. J. Steroid Biochem. (Abstr.) 5:306.

Kowarski, A., J. W. Finklestein, J. S. Spaulding, G. H. Holman, and C. J. Migeon. 1965. Aldosterone secretion rate in congenital adrenal hyperplasia. A discussion of the theories on the pathogenesis of the salt-losing form of the syndrome. J. Clin. Invest. 44:1505.

Laidlaw, J. C., J. L. Ruse, and A. G. Gornall. 1962. The influence of estrogen and progesterone on aldosterone excretion. J. Clin. Endocrinol. 22:161.

Landau, R. L., and K. Lugibihl. 1958. Inhibition of the sodium-retaining influence of aldosterone by progesterone. J. Clin. Endocrinol. 18:1237—1245.

Lewis, R. A., and L. Wilkins. 1949. The effect of adrenocorticotropic hormone in congenital adrenal hyperplasia with virilism and in Cushing's syndrome treated with methyl testosterone. J. Clin. Invest. 28:394.

Lieberman, H. H., and J. A. Luetscher. 1960. Some effects of abnormalities of pituitary, adrenal or thyroid function on excretion of aldosterone and the response to corticotropin or sodium deprivation. J. Clin. Endocrinol. 20:1004.

Loras, B., F. Haour, and J. Bertrand. 1970. Exchangeable sodium and aldosterone secretion in children with congenital adrenal hyperplasia due to 21-hydroxylase deficiency. Pediatr. Res. 4:145.

Luetscher, J. A., and R. H. Curtin. 1955. Relation of aldosterone in urine to sodium balance and to some other endocrine functions. J. Clin. Invest. 34:951.

Mattox, V. R., A. B. Hayles, R. M. Salassa, and F. R. Dion. 1964. Urinary steroid patterns and loss of salt in congenital adrenal hyperplasia. J. Clin. Endocrinol. 24:517.

Neher, R., C. H. Meystre, and A. Wettstein. 1959. Neue 16α-hydroxysteroide aus menschlichen urin und aus schweinenebennieren isolierung, konstitution, synthesen. Helv. Chim. Acta. 42:132.

New, M. I., B. Miller, and R. E. Peterson. 1964. Excretion of aldosterone metabolites in normal children and in children with congenital adrenal hyperplasia. In The Society for Pediatric Research Program, 34th Annual Meeting, p. 51 (Abstr.).

New, M. I., B. Miller, and R. E. Peterson. 1966. Aldosterone secretion in normal children and children with adrenal hyperplasia. J. Clin. Invest. 45:412.

Prader, A., A. Spahr, and R. Neher. 1955. Erhote aldosteronausschedung beim kongenitalen adrenogenitalen syndrom. Schweiz Med. Wochenschr. 85:1085.

Ruse, J. L., and S. Solomon. 1966. The in vivo metabolism of 16α-hydroxyprogesterone. Biochemistry 5:1065.

Simopoulos, A. P., J. R. Marshall, C. S. Delea, and F. C. Bartter. 1971. Studies on the deficiency of 21-hydroxylation in patients with congenital adrenal hyperplasia. J. Clin. Endocrinol. 32:438.

Strott, C. A., T. Yoshimi, and M. B. Lipsett. 1969. Plasma progesterone and 17α-hydroxyprogesterone in normal man and children with congenital adrenal hyperplasia. J. Clin. Invest. 48:930.

Sundsfjord, J. A. 1971. Plasma renin activity and aldosterone excretion during prolonged progesterone administration. Acta Endocrinol. 67:483.

Wilkins, L., R. Klein, and R. A. Lewis. 1950. The response to ACTH in various types of adrenal hyperplasia. In Proceedings of the First Clinical ACTH Conference, p. 184. Blakiston Co., Philadelphia.

Mechanism of Salt Loss in Congenital Virilizing Adrenal Hyperplasia

A. Avinoam Kowarski

ANALYSIS OF CLINICAL DATA BY COMPUTER

Detailed information on a large number of patients suffering from endocrinological disorders has been accumulated for over 30 years at the Division of Pediatric Endocrinology of The Johns Hopkins Hospital. This wealth of data has been of great value to many investigators in the past. However, the retrieval of data was time-consuming and subject to human error. A rapid and accurate retrieval system, as well as a method for the analysis of accumulated information, was needed. The Division of Pediatric Endocrinology has used a computer program for this purpose, hoping that the convenience and speed of the computer would

00052	AL,CAMERON 581157/48/B/49/S/CVAH/21-OH/FEMALE PSEUDO/GENDER CHANGE/GONADECTOMY/CLITOROMEGALY/M/$
00057	AL,ANITA 4427876/63/B/71/S/CVAH/21-OH/FEMALE PSEUDO/CLITORIDECTOMY/F/$
00076	AN,VICKY 754337/58/B/59/S/CVAH/21-OH/DELAYED B.A./SHORT STATURE/FEMALE PSEUDO/CLITORIDECTOMY/F/$
00112	AS,JANE 457834/48/B/49/S/CVAH/ADRENALECTOMY/FEMALE PSEUDO/F/$
00122	AU,ANN 237890/11/B/58/S/CVAH/HYPERTENSION/11-OH/F/$
00170	BA,BETTY 433675/31/B/54/S/CVAH/21-OH/MARRIED/F/$
00201	BA,JOETTE 222536/57/B/57/S/CVAH/FEMALE PSEUDO/HYPOSPADIAS/CRYPTORCHIDISM/DEAD/F/$
00240	BE,MARCIA 365974/41/B/46/S/CVAH/21-OH/MARRIED/F/$
00264	BE,SHARON 878806/43/B/53/S/CVAH/FEMALE PSEUDO/CLITORIDECTOMY/F/$
00306	BL,STEPHEN 1288875/64/B/68/S/CVAH/21-OH/ADVANCED B.A./M/$
00440	BR,DELORES 783825/47/B/60/S/CVAH/21-OH/MARRIED/F/$
00465	BR,ALAN 781940/48/B/52/S/CVAH/M/$
00474	BR,DAVID 976234/43/B/48/S/CVAH/M/$
00558	BU,BONNIE 1061432/39/B/62/S/CVAH/21-OH/MARRIED/DEAD/F/$
00559	BU,BRENDA 2018384/47/B/62/S/CVAH/21-OH/FEMALE PSEUDO/CLITORIDECTOMY/F/$
00655	CH,RHONDA 222896/61/B/64/S/CVAH/FEMALE PSEUDO/CLITORIDECTOMY/SHORT STATURE/F/$

Figure 1. Partial list of patients with congenital virilizing adrenal hyperplasia. The numerical descriptor preceding /B/ represents the last two digits of the year of birth. The numerical descriptor preceding /S/ represents the last two digits of the year in which the patient was first seen at the clinic.

113

encourage frequent and better use of our clinical data. The use of a similar computer system by other pediatric endocrine clinics could help in combining data from many centers, particularly when dealing with relatively rare diseases.

Figure 1 gives an example of an alphabetical list of patients with congenital virilizing adrenal hyperplasia generated by the computer. One hundred and ninety-nine such patients were listed, representing 4.7% of the 4,250 patients presently entered on our computer tapes. The list consists of the name and history number of each patient and a series of descriptors to which additional descriptors can be added at will.

Figure 2 shows an example of a computer analysis of the 77 cases of the salt-losing form of the disease which were retrieved by the computer. These cases represent 39.8% of the total number of patients with congenital virilizing adrenal hyperplasia. The various descriptors stored on the tape are listed by the computer in their order of frequency. The ages at which the patients were first seen in the clinic are also shown. Thirty-nine patients (51%) were below the age of 1 year on their first visit. Forty-nine (64%) were below the age of 2 years.

The same analysis was performed for the non-salt-losing form of the disease. The computer found 122 such patients. Six of them had the hypertensive form of the syndrome. The ages at which the first visit to the clinic occurred had a distribution that was strikingly different from that of the salt-losing form. Only 14% had their first visit before the age of 1 year and 24% before the age of 2 years. Thus, it is possible to use the computer, not only to store and retrieve

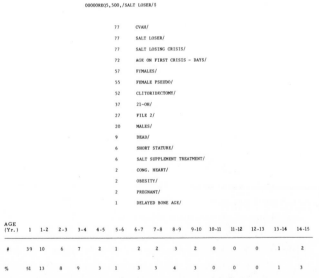

Figure 2. Analysis of 75 cases of the salt-losing form of congenital adrenal hyperplasia (see "Analysis of Clinical Data by Computer").

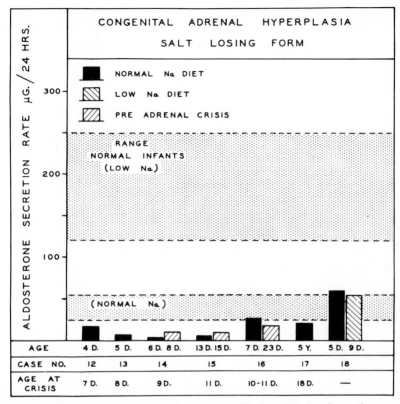

Figure 3. Aldosterone secretion rate in patients with the salt-losing form of congenital adrenal hyperplasia. The seven patients presented in this figure had no therapy and were receiving a normal sodium diet at the time of the study. A second study was performed on *patients 14, 15,* and *16* just before an adrenal crisis and on *patient 18* when on a low sodium diet. The patients are listed according to the severity of their salt-losing tendency as determined by their age at the time of the first spontaneous adrenal crisis; *patient 18* did not go into crisis even when put on a low sodium diet for 4 days. (J. Clin. Invest. 1965. 44:1505.)

data, but also to carry out mathematical calculations with the numerical descriptors.

This program can be used for 1) storage of unlimited amounts of data, 2) selective retrieval of the stored data, and 3) analysis of the stored data.

TIME OF FIRST ADRENAL CRISIS

The secretion rate of aldosterone in untreated babies with the salt-losing form of the syndrome (Figure 3) (Kowarski et al., 1965) varied from very low to normal values, being lower in patients with the greater salt-losing tendency and increasing toward normal in those with the milder form of the disease. The salt-losing patients differed from the non-salt-losing patients in their inability to increase their aldosterone secretion rate when depleted of sodium. Indeed, this inability was probably the cause of their salt-losing tendency. Infant salt losers, who were unable to secrete enough aldosterone to maintain sodium balance on a normal diet, had their first crisis at an early age. Infants who were secreting somewhat more aldosterone were able to maintain sodium homeostasis for a period of time. Only at a later age, when their need for an increased amount of aldosterone was not met, did sodium loss become apparent. Thus, the age at which the first crisis occurred was directly related to the ability to secrete aldosterone.

MECHANISM FOR DELAY IN ADRENAL CRISIS

Figure 4 shows the age at which 70 of our salt-losing patients had their first crisis. Thirty-four of the 70 patients had their initial crisis during the first 2 weeks of life—one on the 3rd day and all the others on or after 6 days of age. The 36 other salt losers had their first crisis at later ages—16 during the 3rd week of life, 3 during the 4th and 5th weeks, and the remaining patients only during specific stressful conditions which led to decreased salt intake or increased sodium loss.

  The data highlight the fact that the first adrenal crisis very rarely occurs during the 1st week of life. An explanation for this delay was suggested by the following observations. As shown in Figure 5 (Kowarski, Weldon, and Migeon, 1968; Weldon, Kowarski, and Migeon, 1967), the secretion rate of aldosterone in normal newborn babies during the first days of life was surprisingly low (9–38 μg/24 hr). The aldosterone secretion rate of these children had doubled when

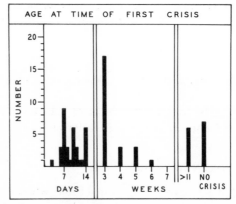

Figure 4. Age at which the first salt-losing crisis occurred in the 70 salt-losing patients for whom this information was available.

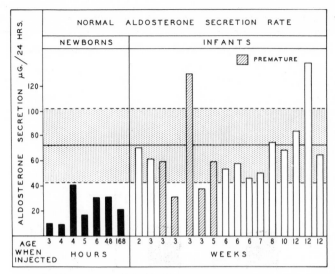

Figure 5. Aldosterone secretion rates in normal infants under 1 week of age, compared to infants 2–12 weeks of age. The *horizontal shaded area* represents the mean ± 1 S.D. for the 8-day to 12-month age group. (Pediatrics. 1967. 39:713.)

they were retested after 2 weeks of age, suggesting a dramatic rise in aldosterone requirement after the age of 3–7 days.

It should be noted that even the most severely affected salt-losing children secreted small amounts of aldosterone. This small amount was in the range of the normal secretion rate during the 1st week of life. Thus, it may have met their requirements at that age. The sudden increase in physiological requirement for aldosterone during the 2nd week of life may explain the prevalence of crisis during that period.

Our explanation for the surprisingly low requirement for aldosterone during the first days of life is based on the relationship between the secretion rate and the metabolic clearance rate of aldosterone. The concentration of aldosterone in plasma is a function of its secretion rate as well as of its metabolic clearance rate.

SECRETION RATE = METABOLIC
CLEARANCE RATE × PLASMA CONCENTRATION

Figure 6 (Beitins et al., 1972b) contains the findings of this study on the plasma level of aldosterone during the first 3 days of life, compared with the level in cord blood and in supine adult subjects. The concentration of aldosterone in the plasma was found to be high during the period of low secretion rate. This indicated a low metabolic clearance rate during that period. It could, therefore,

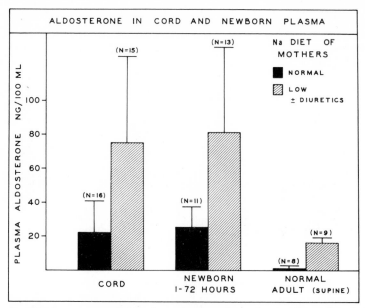

Figure 6. Aldosterone concentration in cord and newborn plasma. The mothers had been on normal or low sodium intake or diuretics before delivery. These values are compared to values obtained on normal, nonpregnant adults in supine position on similar dietary conditions. (J. Clin. Invest. 1972. 51:386.)

be concluded that the increased concentration of aldosterone during the first 3 days of life was mainly due to a decreased metabolic clearance rate, whereas during the latter part of infancy the increased plasma concentration was mainly due to an increased secretion rate. It can be speculated that an immaturity of the liver, the main organ clearing aldosterone, was the cause for the low secretion of aldosterone during the first few days of life.

The salt-losing crisis was delayed in affected newborn babies because of the very low requirement for aldosterone at this age. The maturation of the liver brought about an increase in the amount of aldosterone required for the maintenance of an adequate plasma level. Adrenal crisis occurred when the requirement for aldosterone could no longer be met. Infants with a partial salt-losing tendency had a salt-losing crisis at an older age, because they were able to secrete enough aldosterone to maintain sodium homeostasis and delay the appearance of crisis until circumstances requiring more aldosterone were encountered.

SALT-LOSING HORMONES

Deficiency in aldosterone is not the only cause for salt loss in congenital virilizing adrenal hyperplasia. Figure 7 (Beitins et al., 1972a) illustrates an

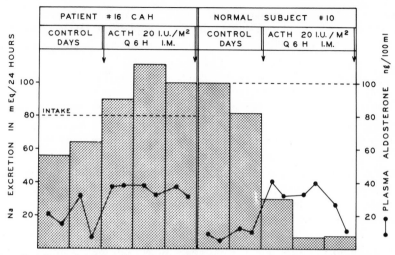

Figure 7. Effect of ACTH administration on urinary excretion of sodium in a patient with congenital adrenal hyperplasia receiving glucocorticoid therapy and in a normal subject. The response of aldosterone in the patient was inappropriate in view of the sodium loss produced by ACTH administration. (J. Clin. Endocrinol. Metab. 1972. 35:595.)

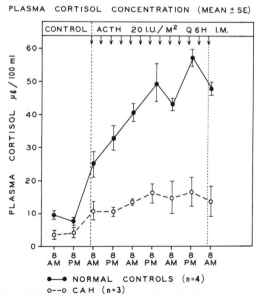

Figure 8. Cortisol concentration in plasma of normal subjects and patients with congenital adrenal hyperplasia during I.M. administration of ACTH (20 I.U./M² every 6 hr). (J. Clin. Endocrinol. Metab. 1972. 35:595.)

experiment which proves this point. An adequately treated patient with the non-salt-losing form of congenital adrenal hyperplasia (CAH) was put on a constant sodium intake for 5 days. After demonstrating adequate sodium balance, the patient was treated with adrenocorticotropic hormone (ACTH) (20 I.U./M^2 every 6 hr for 3 days). A negative sodium balance resulted. A normal control subject demonstrated sodium retention under the same circumstances.

What was the mechanism of the sodium loss in the patient? A sodium-retaining effect was expected in normal control subjects, because ACTH increased the plasma level of cortisol and aldosterone (Figures 8 and 9) (Beitins et al., 1972a). In contrast, the plasma levels of cortisol did not change in the CAH patients. Their plasma concentrations of aldosterone, which started at a higher level than normal, showed a further increase under ACTH treatment. In addition, the concentration of aldosterone remained high in the patients on the 3rd day of ACTH, whereas they came back to baseline levels in the normal subjects. Despite these high concentrations of aldosterone, the patients exhibited a negative sodium balance. The obvious conclusions from these studies were that

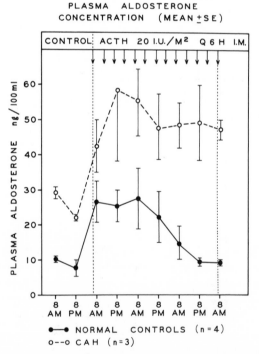

Figure 9. Aldosterone concentration in plasma of normal subjects and patients with congenital adrenal hyperplasia during I.M. administration of ACTH (20 I.U./M^2 every 6 hr). (J. Clin. Endocrinol. Metab. 1972. 35:595.)

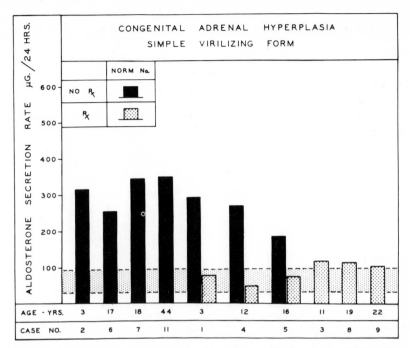

Figure 10. Aldosterone secretion rate in 10 patients with the simple virilizing form of congenital adrenal hyperplasia. All patients were on a normal sodium diet and were either untreated or treated for at least 7 days. The *horizontal shaded area* represents the range of variation of aldosterone secretion rate in six normal adults on a normal sodium diet. When patients were untreated, the secretion rates were greater than normal, whereas they fell to or near the normal range after 1 week of treatment. (J. Clin. Invest. 1965. 44:1505.)

the effect of aldosterone was inhibited in these patients and that the inhibiting effect was augmented by ACTH administration.

Figure 10 (Kowarski et al., 1965) demonstrates the effect of treatment on aldosterone secretion. The secretion rate of untreated non-salt-losers was significantly higher than that of normal subjects and was often in the range found in patients suffering from hyperaldosteronism. Treatment with glucocorticoids consistently lowered the aldosterone secretion rate of these patients to normal levels.

It is felt that the presence of high concentrations of steroids such as 17-hydroxyprogesterone and progesterone, which are competitive inhibitors of aldosterone at the kidney level, caused secondary hyperaldosteronism in the non-salt-losing patients. The salt-losing effect of ACTH could also be attributed to an increased secretion of these steroids. The competitive inhibiting effect of various adrenal steroids on aldosterone was discussed by Dr. A. H. Janoski in the preceding chapter.

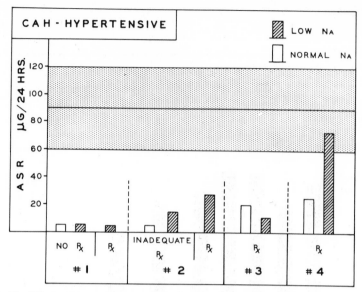

Figure 11. Aldosterone secretion rate in patients with the hypertensive form of congenital adrenal hyperplasia. The *horizontal shaded area* represents the mean ± 1 S.D. for normal subjects on a normal sodium diet. (J. Clin. Endocrinol. Metab. 1968. 28:1445.)

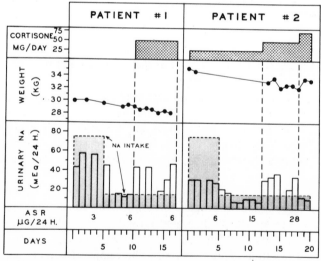

Figure 12. Effect of dietary sodium and of cortisone treatment on sodium balance and aldosterone secretion rate of a patient with the hypertensive form of congenital adrenal hyperplasia. (J. Clin. Endocrinol. Metab. 1968. 28:1445.)

SALT LOSS IN HYPERTENSIVE FORM OF VIRILIZING CAH

The hypertensive form of CAH is due to inefficient 11-hydroxylation by the adrenals. This steroid is necessary for the biosynthesis of aldosterone as well as of cortisol. Figure 11 contains data demonstrating that these patients had a low secretion rate of aldosterone although they were sodium retainers rather than salt losers. Increased secretion of deoxycorticosterone by the fasciculata and reticularis of the adrenal glands more than compensated for their decreased ability to secrete aldosterone.

It should be noted, however, that the compensating effect of deoxycorticosterone may be removed by an adequate replacement therapy. Figure 12 shows a study in a patient suffering from the hypertensive form of CAH. This patient was able to maintain adequate sodium balance when his sodium intake was lowered from 75 mEq/day to 10 mEq/day, as long as he was untreated. When put on replacement glucocorticoid therapy, a paradoxical negative sodium balance was demonstrated.

This observation has practical implications. One patient with 11-hydroxylase defect almost died of a salt-losing crisis when deprived of food (hence on a low salt intake) while still receiving cortisol therapy. By continuing to take his cortisol tablets during a period of starvation, the patient adequately suppressed his oversecretion of deoxycorticosterone and was transformed in effect from a salt retainer to a salt loser.

CONCLUSIONS

Salt loss in CAH is due to an insufficient secretion of aldosterone. This inadequacy is further aggravated by an increased demand for aldosterone because of the presence of other steroids which inhibit the effect of aldosterone on the kidney. Adrenal crisis occurs whenever a need for additional secretion of aldosterone is not met.

Patients with a severe form of the syndrome have their initial crisis at an earlier age than patients with a milder form. Yet, even the most severe cases do not exhibit salt loss during the first days of life. This delay is due to a low metabolic clearance rate of aldosterone at this age.

Patients with the hypertensive form of CAH can become salt losers by treatment. Glucocorticoid therapy lowers their oversecretion of deoxycorticosterone, thus exposing their inability to secrete adequate amounts of aldosterone.

REFERENCES

Beitins, I. Z., F. Bayard, A. Kowarski, and C. J. Migeon. 1972a. The effect of ACTH administration on aldosterone production in non-salt-losing congenital adrenal hyperplasia. J. Clin. Endocrinol. Metab. 35:595–603.

124   Kowarski

Beitins, I. Z., F. Bayard, L. Levitsky, I. G. Ances, A. Kowarski, and C. J. Migeon. 1972b. Plasma aldosterone concentration at delivery and during the newborn period. J. Clin. Invest. 51:386–394.

Kowarski, A., J. W. Finkelstein, J. S. Spaulding, G. H. Holman, and C. J. Migeon. 1965. Aldosterone secretion rate in congenital adrenal hyperplasia: a discussion of the theories on the pathogenesis of the salt-losing form of the syndrome. J. Clin. Invest. 44:1505–1513.

Kowarski, A., A. Russell, and C. J. Migeon. 1968. Salt losing tendency in the hypertensive form of congenital adrenal hyperplasia induced by treatment with glucocorticoids. J. Clin. Endocrinol. Metab. 28:1445–1449.

Kowarski, A., V. V. Weldon, and C. J. Migeon. 1968. Adrenal cortical function in human growth. In D. B. Cheek (ed.), Human Growth, pp. 541–567. Lea and Febiger, Philadelphia.

Kowarski, A., H. Katz, and C. J. Migeon. 1974. Plasma concentration of aldosterone in normal subjects from infancy to adulthood. J. Clin. Endocrinol. Metab. 38:489–491.

Kowarski, A., L. de Lacerda, and C. J. Migeon. 1975. Integrated concentration of plasma aldosterone in normal subjects: correlation with cortisol. J. Clin. Endocrinol. Metab. 40:205–210.

Weldon, V. V., A. Kowarski, and C. J. Migeon. 1967. Aldosterone secretion rate in normal subjects from infancy to adulthood. Pediatrics 39:713–723.

HORMONE MEASUREMENT IN DIAGNOSIS AND MANAGEMENT

Usefulness of Plasma Renin Activity to Monitor Mineralocorticoid Replacement in Salt-losing Congenital Adrenal Hyperplasia

H. Lansing Lipton,[1] *Siang Y. Tan,*
Robert Noth, Patrick J. Mulrow, and Myron Genel

Congenital adrenal hyperplasia, most commonly 21-hydroxylase deficiency, is usually thought to have two forms—a salt-losing and a simple virilizing form—although the difference at times may not be clear cut. Glucocorticoid replacement in both forms can be reliably estimated from the known cortisol secretory rate and approximates 24 mg/m^2/day. Furthermore, glucocorticoid replacement can be monitored by urinary pregnanetriol and 17-ketosteroid excretion, as well as by bone age and other parameters. Assessment of the adequacy of mineralocorticoid replacement, however, has been somewhat problematic. Not only is there some uncertainty as to the requirements of individual patients with the salt-losing form, but the usual signs of sodium depletion, such as orthostatic changes in blood pressure and pulse, may be difficult to assess in children. Other parameters, such as blood urea nitrogen (BUN) and serum electrolytes, may not be sufficiently sensitive. This is potentially a very critical area, because there is some reason to suspect that growth retardation, so frequently seen in the salt-losing form of adrenal hyperplasia, may be related to chronic salt depletion. It is known that experimental animals grow poorly when they are chronically deprived of salt. Furthermore, patients with the rare disorder of selective

This research was conducted in the inpatient and ambulatory facilities of the Yale Children's Clinical Research Center and was supported by Grant RR-00125 from the General Clinical Research Centers Branch, Division of Research Resources, National Institutes of Health, United States Public Health Service.

These studies were initiated by Melvin Firestone, M.D., as part of a doctoral dissertation, "Clinical Therapeutics of the Adrenogenital Syndrome," submitted in April, 1975, to fulfill the requirements for graduation from the Yale University School of Medicine.

[1] Postdoctoral fellow in Endocrinology, Department of Internal Medicine, Yale University School of Medicine.

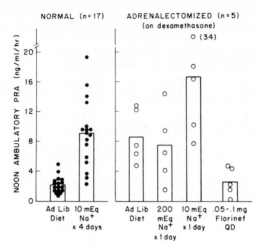

Figure 1. Response of plasma renin activity to acute salt restriction in normal adult volunteers (*left*) and in five adrenalectomized adults (*right*) subjected to various manipulations of salt intake. (See under "Results.")

unresponsiveness to adrenocorticotropic hormone (ACTH), but with normal aldosterone secretion, do not develop growth retardation (Kelch et al., 1972; Kershnar, Roe, and Kogut, 1972); whereas patients with selective aldosterone deficiency (David, Golan, and Drucker, 1968) and renal salt wasting (Raine and Roy, 1962; Rösler et al., 1973) commonly do.

For the past year, plasma renin activity has been studied as a more sensitive measure of sodium balance in children with the salt-losing form of congenital adrenal hyperplasia. Elevated plasma renin activity (PRA) has been reported by others in congenital adrenal hyperplasia (Godard et al., 1968; Imai, Igarashi, and Sokabe, 1968; Strickland and Kotchen, 1972) and has been interpreted as reflecting a state of chronic sodium deprivation.

MATERIALS AND METHODS

For the most part, specimens were drawn in the outpatient clinic and represented ambulatory afternoon plasma renin activity, except as measured in infants. PRAs were measured by a modification of the radioimmunoassay technique of Haber et al. (1969). BUNs and electrolytes were determined by autoanalyzer. Urinary pregnanetriol was determined by Bio-Science Laboratories, Van Nuys, California, and urinary 17-ketosteroids were determined by the Zimmerman reaction.

RESULTS

Figure 1 presents plasma renin responsiveness in five young adult volunteers, all of whom have had bilateral adrenalectomy for Cushing's syndrome. Two days before admission they stopped their mineralocorticoid replacement and went on an ad lib sodium diet. They were maintained on 1 mg of dexamethasone/day as their only replacement. The *right panel* represents noon ambulatory plasma renin activity in adrenalectomized patients, and the *left panel* represents normal volunteers. Even though the adrenalectomized patients were taking in as much sodium as they wished, their mean PRA was more than 3 times the mean PRA of normal patients on ad lib diets. On the next day, the patients were sodium-loaded on a 200-mEq high sodium diet for 1 day, and although plasma renin activity fell slightly it still remained markedly elevated. Following this and 1 day of sodium deprivation on 10 mEq/day, plasma renin activity was clearly elevated into an abnormal range. In contrast, it took 4 days of sodium restriction to elevate PRA in normal volunteers, and at the end of this time the mean PRA for the group was in the same range as for the adrenalectomized patients on an ad lib sodium diet. In Figure 1, the column at the *far right* represents the patients' PRAs when seen in clinic under the usual fluorohydrocortisone replacement of 0.05–0.1 mg/day; they are in the same range as those of the normal volunteers. Thus, it appears to be difficult to achieve normal plasma renin suppression in adrenalectomized patients merely by sodium loading or with ad lib sodium. A similar phenomenon has been reported with Addisonian patients (Linquette et al., 1975). Although it was evident that these patients were salt-depleted during the experimental period, the usual laboratory parameters changed very little, suggesting that they were not sufficiently sensitive. BUN did rise slightly, but not significantly. Serum creatinine, sodium, potassium, and bicarbonate were essentially unchanged. The only significant difference was in serum chloride, which fell a mean of 6 mEq/liter, significant at the 0.05 level, but this phenomenon has not been repeated.

With this information in hand, an attempt to assess plasma renin activity in children was undertaken. One difficulty was the acquisition of a range of normal PRA for children, particularly infants. In these studies it was found that plasma renin activity in children over the age of 2 years was approximately 50% higher than in young adults, placing the mean at about 3.27 ng/ml/hr. Allowing two standards of deviation, the upper limit of normal was 6.0 ng/ml/hr. From 6 months to 2 years of age, there was another 50% increase, and the mean in this age group was approximately 4.5 ng/ml/hr, with the upper limit of normal being estimated at 10 ng/ml/hr. This was in the same range as other published estimations (Kotchen et al., 1972; Sassard et al., 1975).

An attempt was made to see whether plasma renin activity correlated with more easily measured parameters—in particular, to correlate plasma renin activity with BUN, sodium, and potassium (Figure 2). In the scattergrams illustrated,

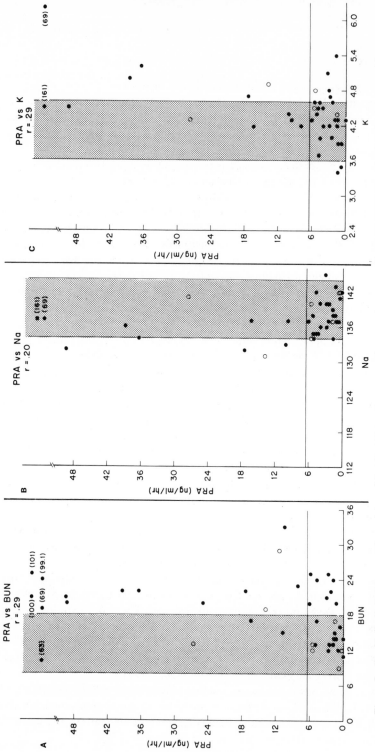

Figure 2. Correlation of plasma renin activity with (A) BUN, (B) serum Na^+, and (C) serum K^+ in infants and children with salt-losing congenital adrenal hyperplasia. *Shading* represents normal range for BUN (8–18 mg%), serum Na^+ (134–144 mEq/liter), and serum K^+ (3.6–4.6 mEq/liter), and the *horizontal line* represents the upper limit of PRA in normal children >2 years. The *r* values are not significant.

the normal range for the respective chemistries is *shaded,* and the upper limits of normal for PRA are represented by a *horizontal line.* The *closed circles* represent children with congenital adrenal hyperplasia and the *open circles* those with idiopathic Addison's disease. The linear correlation was very poor in all of these scattergrams and did not represent a significant relationship. Although a few of the values represented infants, the upper limit of normal PRA was certainly not much higher than 12 ng/ml/hr. Although patients with abnormal plasma renin activities tended to have BUNs of 13 mg/100 ml or higher, there were still several PRAs which were quite high when other chemistries were only minimally abnormal.

CASE STUDIES

Donna S. (Figure 3) is now 16 years old and is the oldest of three sisters, all affected with the salt-losing form of congenital adrenal hyperplasia. At age

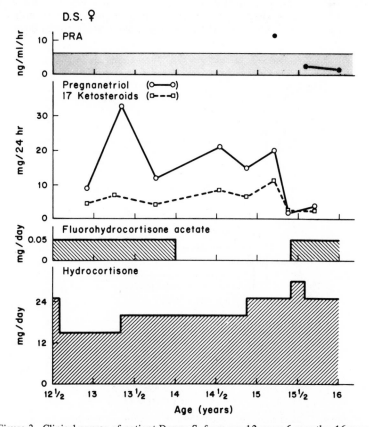

Figure 3. Clinical course of patient Donna S. from age 12 years 6 months–16 years.

14, the patient stopped her fluorohydrocortisone, and because she appeared to be in no difficulty clinically and was able to increase her sodium intake ad lib, it was elected not to insist upon her restarting. Pregnanetriol and 17-ketosteroid excretions were elevated, and glucocorticoid supplemention in the form of hydrocortisone was raised in an attempt to suppress the abnormal steroid precursors. The lag seen in the graph between laboratory values and manipulation of therapy reflects time elapsed between obtaining and reporting of the specimens. Plasma renin activities were originally measured routinely when the patient was about 15 years old, and the first value, at 11 ng/ml/hr, is well above the normal range for a 16-year-old (*shaded*), despite the fact that she was receiving 25 mg of hydrocortisone a day as well. It was felt that glucocorticoid replacement was also probably inadequate; therefore, her hydrocortisone replacement subsequently was raised to 30 mg/day and fluorohydrocortisone was resumed. The drop of PRA into the normal range might be attributed to increased hydrocortisone, but, even when the dose was later attenuated to 25 mg/day, PRA remained in the normal range. This observation is comparable to that made earlier with the adult adrenalectomized patients.

Carmen D. (Figure 4) is a 5-year-old girl with the salt-losing form of congenital adrenal hyperplasia. Plasma renins were initially normal when measured in this patient, at a time when pregnanetriol excretion was elevated. PRA rose acutely when the patient was dehydrated for an intravenous

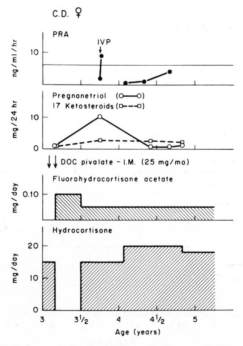

Figure 4. Clinical course of patient Carmen D. from age 3–5 years 3 months.

pyelogram and, when measured again, PRA was normal. Normalization of pregnanetriol excretion by increasing the glucocorticoid therapy did not make much difference in the PRA level.

Ryan A. (Figure 5) is a male with salt-losing CAH. Good suppression of pregnanetriol and 17-ketosteroid excretion and of PRA was initially seen, but at the age of 2 years and 10 months both PRA and pregnanetriol levels rose into the abnormal range. Mineralocorticoid dose was not altered; instead, the hydrocortisone was increased, and both the pregnanetriol and plasma renin activity returned once more to normal. This may be due to some mineralocorticoid effect of hydrocortisone; alternatively, controlling the disease may suppress the production of abnormal steroid precursors which may be natriuretic.

Michael D. (Figure 6) is affected with a partial loss of 3β-ol-dehydrogenase (Schneider et al., 1975) and is now 18 years old. At about the age of 17–17 1/2, there was a rise in his pregnanetriol and 17-ketosteroid excretion, probably not a good measure of suppression in this enzyme deficiency. However, his condition did seem to be out of control, and because he was a postpubertal male it was elected to err on the side of undercontrol rather than to risk oversuppression. It might be speculated that he would not produce as many natriuretic precursors as patients with 21-hydroxylase deficiency; in any event, his plasma renin activity appeared to be normal and stabilized on fluorohydrocortisone, again demonstrating the lack of correlation obtained in most patients between optimal glucocorticoid and mineralocorticoid replacement.

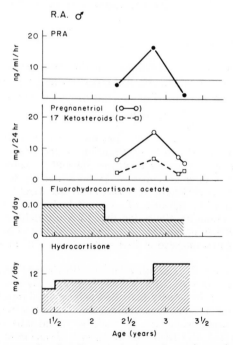

Figure 5. Clinical course of patient Ryan A. from age 1 year 3 months–3 years 4 months.

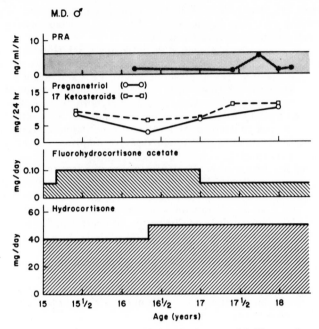

Figure 6. Clinical course of patient Michael D. from age 15–18 years 2 months.

The use of plasma renin determination has been particularly helpful in assessing sodium balance in infants. Although the upper limits of normal for children under 2 years and for infants are not firmly established, they have been estimated at approximately 12 ng/ml/hr.

Patrina M. is an infant recently diagnosed as having the salt-losing form of CAH (Figure 7). On initial presentation to the hospital, PRA was 122 ng/ml/hr, along with elevated pregnanetriol and 17-ketosteroid excretion. She was treated with hydrocortisone by mouth and a deoxycorticosterone acetate (DOCA) pellet (Percorten, CIBA Pharmaceutical Co.). The next PRA was drawn during an episode of acute dehydration and was markedly elevated at 158 ng/ml/hr. Following this, PRA normalized. At 5 months of age, the first DOCA pellet became exhausted, detected by a rise in plasma renin activity. When the second DOCA pellet was implanted, PRA fell into the normal range.

Carol H. (Figure 8) is another infant with the salt-losing form of CAH and was initially treated with a DOCA pellet. As the pellet began to dissipate, plasma renin activity increased and then fell immediately after the institution of oral fluorohydrocortisone. Shortly thereafter, the patient had an Addisonian crisis secondary to acute gastroenteritis and became profoundly dehydrated. Her BUN rose along with plasma renin activity. Fluorohydrocortisone was increased, then decreased again after PRA had fallen into

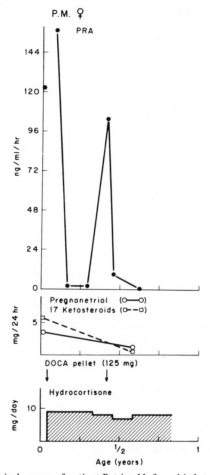

Figure 7. Clinical course of patient Patrina M. from birth to 10 months of age.

the normal range. Because of a persistently elevated BUN, fluorohydrocortisone again was increased, but plasma renin activity, when reported, remained normal. The elevated BUN was unexplained, with no signs of renal disease. In this case, the elevated BUN gave a "false positive" indication of the patient's state of dehydration.

Brian K., a male infant with the salt-losing form of CAH, was initially treated with a DOCA pellet, as well as with added salt (Figure 9). In response to a markedly elevated PRA, the sodium dose was increased. PRA fell to 17 ng/ml/hr, but was still above the normal range, again a situation analogous to that of the adult adrenalectomized patients who could not suppress PRA simply with increased salt intake. When salt was discontinued and the patient

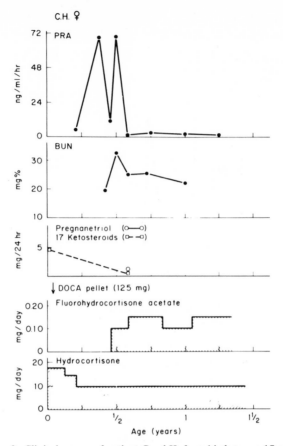

Figure 8. Clinical course of patient Carol H. from birth to age 17 months.

given fluorohydrocortisone, renin activity was immediately suppressed. Throughout the course, urinary pregnanetriol excretion remained normal.

Alexis A., a two-year-old male infant from Venezuela, presented at age 5 months with severe failure to thrive. At that time, length and weight were less than at birth (Figure 10). He initially presented a diagnostic puzzle, because there were no signs of virilization and bone age was retarded. A salt-losing defect was immediately apparent, but it was not until confirmation with elevated serum 17-hydroxyprogesterone levels that the diagnosis of congenital virilizing adrenal hyperplasia was established. After beginning therapy, he caught up to the third percentile for height and paralleled the third percentile since that time. His requirement for mineralocorticoids (approximately 4 mg of 11-deoxycorticosterone/day) seemed extraordinary during the initial hospitalization. This would have converted to 100 mg of

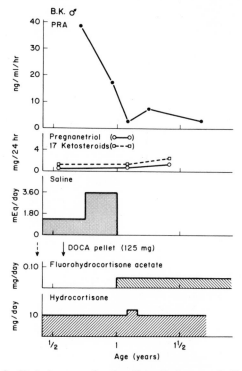

Figure 9. Clinical course of patient Brian K. from age 5–20 months.

11-deoxycorticosterone pivilate/month, but, inasmuch as there was reluctance to discharge him on such a huge dose, he was dismissed on 35 mg/month, with added salt. Subsequently, plasma renin values were very low, implying oversuppression, and the patient became hypertensive (systolic blood pressure was 150 mm/Hg). 11-Deoxycorticosterone pivilate was reduced to 25 mg/month and salt was discontinued; however, hypertension persisted. As the injection dissipated, PRA rose, and the therapy was changed to fluorohydrocortisone, which could be stopped acutely to restudy his actual mineralocorticoid requirements. With the institution of fluorohydrocortisone therapy, plasma renin activity was suppressed, and the patient is presently on 0.1 mg of fluorohydrocortisone daily. The most recent PRAs are now approaching the normal range. After acute cessation of mineralocorticoid therapy (fluorhydrocortisone) at 8 months of age, serum sodium levels became low normal, potassium levels were slightly high, and the pregnanetriol excretion remained normal. Three days after cessation of fluorohydrocortisone, plasma renin activity was measured at 63 ng/ml/hr. After another 3 days, it had risen to 146 ng/ml/hr. The elevated plasma renin activity was the only indication that the patient was becoming volume-depleted.

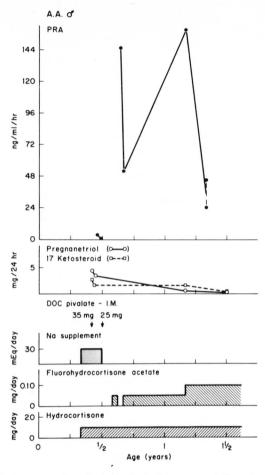

Figure 10. Clinical course of patient Alexis A. from presentation at age 5 months with failure to thrive to age 19 months.

SUMMARY

Plasma renin activity has been used to follow the sodium balance of patients with the salt-losing form of congenital virilizing adrenal hyperplasia. Plasma renin activity seems to more readily reflect salt and volume depletion than BUN or serum electrolytes in mineralocorticoid-deficient patients. It would appear that in congenital virilizing adrenal hyperplasia plasma renin activity can be independent of glucocorticoid suppression, the important exception being that loss of control may result in the excretion of abnormal steroid precursors which may be natriuretic. In these studies, serial measurement of plasma renin activity in congenital virilizing adrenal hyperplasia has permitted rational adjustment of mineralocorticoid treatment.

ACKNOWLEDGMENTS

The assistance of Mrs. Jean Smith, Mrs. Louise Tomaso, Mrs. Sue Richardson, and Mrs. Tatieta Sergievsky in the collection of control PRA specimens is gratefully acknowledged.

REFERENCES

David, R., S. Golan, and W. Drucker. 1968. Familial aldosterone deficiency: enzyme defect, diagnosis and clinical course. Pediatrics 41:403–412.

Godard, C., A. M. Riondel, R. Veyrat, A. Mégevand, and A. F. Muller. 1968. Plasma renin activity and aldosterone secretion in congenital adrenal hyperplasia. Pediatrics 41:883–904.

Haber, E., T. Koerner, L. B. Page, B. Kliman, and A. Purnode. 1969. Application of a radioimmunoassay for Angiotensin I to the physiologic measurements of plasma renin activity in normal human subjects. J. Clin. Endocrinol. Metab. 29:1349–1355.

Imai, M., Y. Igarashi, and H. Sokabe. 1968. Plasma renin activity in congenital virilizing adrenal hyperplasia. Pediatrics 41:897–903.

Kelch, R. P., S. L. Kaplan, E. G. Biglieri, G. H. Daniels, C. J. Epstein, and M. M. Grumbach. 1972. Hereditary adrenocortical unresponsiveness to adrenocorticotropic hormone. J. Pediatr. 81:726–736.

Kershnar, A. K., T. F. Roe, and M. D. Kogut. 1972. Adrenocorticotropic hormone unresponsiveness: report of a girl with excessive growth and review of 16 reported cases. J. Pediatr. 80:610–619.

Kotchen, T. A., A. L. Strickland, T. W. Rice, and D. R. Walters. 1972. A study of the renin-angiotensin system in newborn infants. J. Pediatr. 80:938–946.

Linquette, M., J. Lefebvre, P. Fossati, J. C. Fourlinnie, J. P. Cappoen, and P. Lecieux. 1975. L'activité rénine plasmatique dans la surveillance due traitement de la maladie d'Addison. Ann. Endocrinol. (Paris) 36:103–104.

Raine, D. N., and J. Roy. 1962. A salt-losing syndrome in infancy. Arch. Dis. Child. 37:548–556.

Rösler, A., R. Theodor, E. Gazit, H. Biochis, and D. Rabinowitz. 1973. Salt wastage, raised plasma-renin activity, and normal or high plasma-aldosterone: a form of pseudohypoaldosteronism. Lancet 1:959–961.

Sassard, J., L. Sann, M. Vincent, R. Francois, and J. F. Cier. 1975. Plasma renin activity in normal subjects from infancy to puberty. J. Clin. Endocrinol. Metab. 40:524–525.

Schneider, G., M. Genel, A. M. Bongiovanni, A. S. Goldman, and R. L. Rosenfield. 1975. Persistent testicular Δ^5-isomerase-3β-hydroxysteroid dehydrogenase (Δ^5-3β-HSD) deficiency in the Δ^5-3β-HSD form of congenital adrenal hyperplasia. J. Clin. Invest. 55:681–690.

Strickland, A. L., and T. A. Kotchen. 1972. A study of the renin-aldosterone system in congenital adrenal hyperplasia. J. Pediatr. 81:962–969.

17-Hydroxyprogesterone and Plasma Renin Activity in Congenital Adrenal Hyperplasia

Ieuan A. Hughes[1] *and Jeremy S. D. Winter*[2]

The usual techniques for diagnosis and monitoring of therapy in patients with the C-21-hydroxylase form of congenital adrenal hyperplasia (CAH) include measurement of urinary 17-ketosteroids and pregnanetriol (as indices of glucocorticoid replacement) and serum electrolytes (as an index of mineralocorticoid replacement in salt losers). Despite these aids, children treated for CAH often exhibit poor growth (Bailey and Komrower, 1974; Brook et al., 1974; Rappaport et al., 1973; Rappaport, Cornu, and Royer, 1968; Sperling et al., 1971), delayed menarche (Jones and Verkauf, 1971), and possibly reduced fertility (Kirkland et al., 1974). Possible causes for these complications include inadequate suppression of adrenal androgens, excessive cortisol therapy, or chronic depletion of sodium in the salt-losing patients.

This study investigated the possible value of measuring serum 17-hydroxyprogesterone (17-OHP) in the diagnosis and long-term management of CAH patients. In salt losers, this technique was coupled with assays of plasma renin activity as an index of the effectiveness of mineralocorticoid therapy. The data provide information concerning the range of serum 17-OHP in healthy children and demonstrate the value of this assay both in diagnosis of CAH and in the management of common treatment problems. In addition, the relationship between changes in serum 17-OHP and alterations in serum concentrations of progesterone, androstenedione, and testosterone—steroids which may have more direct implications for reproductive function than 17-OHP—has been explored.

This research was supported by the Medical Research Council of Canada (Grant MT2997) and the Children's Hospital of Winnipeg Research Foundation.

The following trivial names are used: pregnanetriol, 5β-pregnane-3α,17α,20α-triol; progesterone, pregn-4-ene-3,20-dione; 17-hydroxyprogesterone, 17α-hydroxypregn-4-ene-3,20-dione; androstenedione, androst-4-ene-3,17-dione; testosterone, 17β-hydroxyandrost-4-ene-3-one; cortisol (Compound F), pregn-4-ene-11β,17α,21-triol-3,20-dione.

[1] Supported by a Fellowship of the Medical Research Council of Canada.

[2] A Queen Elizabeth II Scientist.

141

Finally, suggestions are made as to how this new assay can be used in a practical way in the management of the CAH patient in the clinic.

MATERIALS AND METHODS

A total of 15 patients with the C-21-hydroxylase form of CAH was studied, all except 2 of whom were salt losers. Their ages ranged from 2 days to 16 years. Five infants and one adolescent patient were studied before the initiation of cortisol therapy. Blood samples were collected every 6 hr for a 30-hr period from the infants and every 2 hr over a similar time period from the adolescent patients. Simultaneous 24-hr urine samples were collected for determination of 17-ketosteroids, pregnanetriol, electrolytes, and creatinine. Blood for measurement of plasma renin activity and serum sodium and potassium concentrations was collected from each patient while resting in the supine position at 0900 hr. Each treated patient continued to receive his pretest amount of cortisol, divided into three doses orally at 0900, 1500, and 2100 hr. In addition, the salt-losing patients received their usual dose of Florinef (9α-fluorohydrocortisone) orally once daily at 0900 hr. All patients were maintained on a standard diet for age without a salt supplement. Mixed cord blood from 42 newborn infants and venous blood from 500 healthy children ranging in age from birth to 16 years and 20 young adults were assayed to establish normal 17-OHP values. These samples were collected between 0800 and 1700 hr.

All of the serum steroids were measured by specific radioimmunoassay following separation from cross-reacting steroids by column chromatography. The extract for analysis of 17-OHP was chromatographed on a column of Sephadex LH-20, and a specific antiserum to the 6-(O-carboxymethyl)-oxime-bovine serum albumin derivative of 17-OHP was used in the assay (Hughes and Winter, 1976). Progesterone, androstenedione, and testosterone were separated from each other by chromatography on a column of Lipidex (hydroxyalkoxypropyl Sephadex). Antisera to the 6-(O-carboxymethyl)-oxime-bovine serum albumin derivatives of androstenedione, testosterone, and progesterone were used in the radioimmunoassay. The specificities of the antisera used have been reported previously (Winter et al., 1976). Plasma renin activity was measured by radioimmunoassay of the angiotensin I generated after standard incubation of plasma (Haber et al., 1969). Urinary pregnanetriol was measured by gas-liquid chromatography (Kinoshita et al., 1968) and 17-ketosteroids by a standard method (Peterson and Pierce, 1960).

VALUES IN HEALTHY CHILDREN

The values for serum 17-OHP (mean ± 1 S.D.) from birth through adolescence are shown in Figure 1. Cord values were extremely high (males, 3,119 ± 1,365

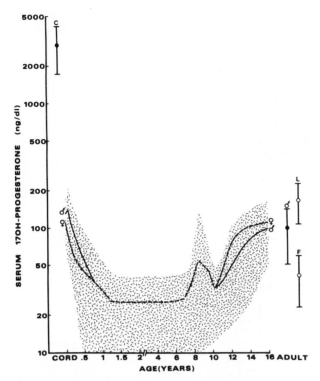

Figure 1. Semilogarithmic plot of serum 17-OHP concentrations in 500 healthy subjects. The *lines* indicate the mean for each sex, as denoted by the symbols. The *shaded area* and the *vertical bars* encompass mean ± 1 S.D. *C* indicates cord sera. The *bars* on the right show mean ± 1 S.D. for adult males (♂) and adult females in the follicular (*F*) and luteal (*L*) phases of the menstrual cycle.

ng/dl; females, 2,591 ± 824 ng/dl), but fell rapidly within hours after birth. During the first 4 months of life, mean levels were higher in male infants than in females, but thereafter levels were similar in both sexes until puberty. A transient rise in mean 17-OHP levels was observed in each sex at about age 8 years, but this may only represent an artifact of the cross-sectional study. Mean values for adult females were 30 ng/dl and 140 ng/dl in the follicular and luteal phases, respectively, of the menstrual cycle. For the purpose of defining a normal serum 17-OHP value in the CAH patients, a level of 200 ng/dl was arbitrarily selected, because this value exceeded the 95% confidence limits for the healthy children. This level may, however, be too low for use with young infants and postmenarchal girls.

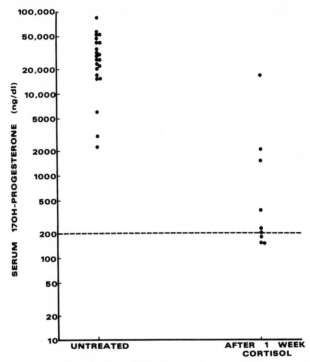

Figure 2. Serum 17-OHP levels in CAH infants (<3 years) before and after 1 week of cortisol therapy. Five infants were sampled repeatedly over 24 hr on each occasion. The *dashed line* indicates the upper limit of normal used in this study.

USE OF 17-HYDROXYPROGESTERONE ASSAYS IN DIAGNOSIS

The serum 17-OHP values obtained in five infants with CAH sampled repeatedly over a 24-hr period before treatment and again following 1 week of cortisol therapy are shown in Figure 2. In all samples from the untreated infants, levels greater than 10 times the upper limit of 200 ng/dl were obtained, which illustrates the diagnostic value of serum 17-OHP. Following treatment, there was a marked fall, but uniformly normal values were not observed after 1 week of cortisol therapy.

APPLICATION OF
17-HYDROXYPROGESTERONE ASSAYS IN MONITORING THERAPY

These methods were then applied to a group of treated CAH infants, including both salt losers and non-salt-losers (Figure 3). Plasma renin activity was normal (<5 ng/ml/hr) in all these infants, whether they were non-salt-losers or salt losers

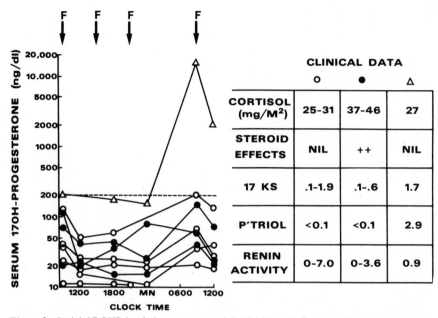

	CLINICAL DATA		
	O	●	Δ
CORTISOL (mg/M²)	25-31	37-46	27
STEROID EFFECTS	NIL	++	NIL
17 KS	.1-1.9	.1-.6	1.7
P'TRIOL	<0.1	<0.1	2.9
RENIN ACTIVITY	0-7.0	0-3.6	0.9

Figure 3. Serial 17-OHP levels in seven treated CAH infants (<3 years). The vertical arrows (F) indicate the time of each cortisol dose. Patients are shown as well controlled (o), overtreated with signs of cortisol excess (●), or poorly controlled (Δ), according to the data in the inset. In the table, urinary 17-ketosteroids (17-KS) and pregnanetriol (p'triol) are expressed in mg/24 hr and plasma renin activity in ng/ml/hr. The *dashed line* indicates the upper limit of normal.

receiving mineralocorticoid replacement therapy. Three types of patients could be defined. Well controlled patients had normal serum 17-OHP values throughout the day and night, normal urinary 17-ketosteroids and pregnanetriol, and no clinical signs of cortisol excess. Their oral cortisol dose ranged from 25–31 mg/m² /day. The second group was receiving larger doses of cortisol (37–46 mg/m² /day), and all infants showed clinical signs of cortisol excess. In this group, serum 17-OHP, like the urinary steroids, was no lower than in the first group. This demonstrates that serum 17-OHP assays cannot be used to identify patients receiving excessive steroid therapy. The third group was exemplified by a single infant with elevated urinary pregnanetriol excretion (2.9 mg/day), suggesting inadequate cortisol replacement. Analyses of serum 17-OHP showed abnormally elevated values only during the morning hours. This patient required a larger dose of cortisol at bedtime to suppress the morning rise of 17-OHP; this could be achieved, however, without any increase in total daily dose of cortisol.

Similar studies were performed on adolescent patients of both sexes (Figure 4). Again, plasma renin activity was normal in all of these patients, who included non-salt-losers and Florinef-treated salt losers. Two patients were well con-

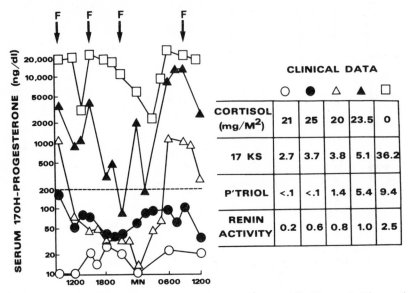

Figure 4. Serial 17-OHP levels in treated CAH adolescents (13–16 years). The vertical arrows (*F*) indicate the time of each cortisol dose. Each symbol identifies a separate patient whose data are summarized in the table. The *dashed line* indicates the upper limit of normal. 17-KS, 17-ketosteroids; p'triol, pregnanetriol.

trolled, with normal serum 17-OHP values throughout the day and night, normal urinary 17-ketosteroids and pregnanetriol, and no clinical signs of cortisol excess. This would seem to be the optimal situation. Their oral cortisol doses were 21 and 25 mg/m² /day, respectively. Another patient had normal urinary 17-ketosteroids and pregnanetriol, but had elevated serum 17-OHP values during the morning hours. This suggested a need for an increase in the evening cortisol dose but not necessarily an increase in the total daily dose. A fourth patient was poorly controlled, with consistently elevated serum 17-OHP levels throughout the day and night and increased urinary pregnanetriol. This patient required an increase in the total daily dose of cortisol. The last patient was untreated at the time of the study. As seen previously in the untreated infants, his serum 17-OHP was markedly elevated at all times.

Because an early morning rise in serum 17-OHP values has been seen in several of these patients, an improvement in control of nocturnal steroid secretion might be obtained by the use of a synthetic steroid such as prednisone, which should have a longer suppressive effect than cortisol. Some preliminary results with this mode of therapy are illustrated in Figure 5. Three patients had normal serum 17-OHP levels throughout the day and night, together with normal urinary ketosteroids and pregnanetriol. However, in order to achieve this con-

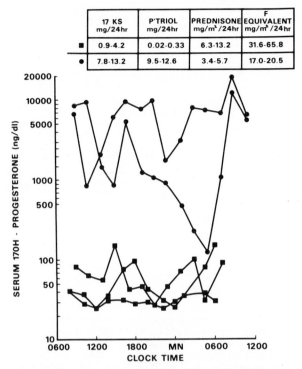

	17 KS mg/24hr	P'TRIOL mg/24hr	PREDNISONE mg/m²/24hr	F EQUIVALENT mg/m²/24hr
■	0.9-4.2	0.02-0.33	6.3-13.2	31.6-65.8
●	7.8-13.2	9.5-12.6	3.4-5.7	17.0-20.5

Figure 5. Serum 17-OHP in prednisone-treated CAH patients. The symbols (■ and ●) indicate the steroid values observed while the patients received two different prednisone doses. A ratio of 5:1 was used in expressing prednisone dose in cortisol equivalents. 17-KS, 17-ketosteroids; p'triol, pregnanetriol.

trol, their prednisone dose, when expressed as cortisol equivalents, was in the range of 31–65.8 mg/m²/day.

This is excessive glucocorticoid therapy and undoubtedly these patients would in time show clinical signs of cortisol excess. A smaller dose, equivalent to 17–20.5 mg/m²/day of cortisol, was tried in two patients. They showed elevated serum 17-OHP and urinary pregnanetriol and clearly were receiving doses that were inadequate for proper control. Although other dosage schedules have not yet been explored, it would seem that prednisone has no obvious advantages over a daily cortisol regimen divided into appropriate doses throughout the day.

COMBINED USE OF SERUM 17-HYDROXYPROGESTERONE AND PLASMA RENIN ACTIVITY IN SALT LOSERS

Figure 6 shows serial serum 17-OHP concentrations on four different occasions in a 2-year-old, treated salt loser who received varying doses of Florinef, but a

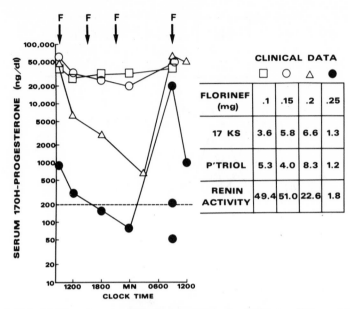

Figure 6. Relationship of serum 17-hydroxyprogesterone (17P) to efficacy of mineralo-corticoid replacement therapy as reflected by plasma renin activity in a single infant with salt-losing CAH. Symbols (□, ○, △, ●) refer to separate studies at 1-week intervals on varying doses of Florinef. The vertical arrows (F) indicate the time of each cortisol dose. The total daily cortisol dose throughout the four study periods remained at 29.4 mg/m²/24 hr. The two *single points* (●) represent serum 17-OHP values obtained 1 and 4 months later while receiving the same dose of cortisol and Florinef (0.25 mg/day). The *dashed line* indicates the upper limit of normal. 17-KS, 17-ketosteroids; p'triol; pregnanetriol.

constant dose of cortisol (29.4 mg/m²/day). Her serum electrolytes were always normal. On a Florinef dose of 0.1 mg/day, serum 17-OHP was elevated, as were urinary 17-ketosteroids and pregnanetriol. Plasma renin activity was extremely high, indicating inadequate mineralocorticoid replacement. Increasing the Florinef dose to 0.15 mg/day had no effect on the elevated steroid levels and plasma renin activity. A further increase to 0.2 mg/day was followed by a reduction in afternoon serum 17-OHP levels, but urinary 17-ketosteroids and pregnanetriol and plasma renin activity were still elevated. When the dose of Florinef was increased to 0.25 mg/day, plasma renin activity became normal and there was a striking reduction in urinary 17-ketosteroids and pregnanetriol; some normal serum 17-OHP values were obtained, but levels were still increased in the morning. Continued treatment with this same dose of Florinef and cortisol subsequently produced normal morning levels of 17-OHP. After several months on this regimen, it was possible to reduce the dose of Florinef to 0.2 mg/day and then to 0.15 mg/day. The patient's serum 17-OHP values and plasma renin activity remained normal, and her cortisol dose remained unchanged.

A possible mechanism for this apparent effect of chronic salt depletion upon serum 17-OHP levels in the presence of apparently adequate cortisol replacement is suggested in Figure 7. The serum sodium and potassium concentrations may be normal (as was the case in the above patient), but the elevated plasma renin activity is the clue to the salt-depleted state. It is postulated that this chronic "stress" can be a stimulus for increased adrenocorticotropic hormone production and consequently increased production of 17-OHP. The treatment in such a situation would be more salt or mineralocorticoid, not necessarily more cortisol.

RELATIONSHIP OF 17-HYDROXYPROGESTERONE TO OTHER STEROIDS

In this initial study, an attempt was made to determine the dose of cortisol for each patient which would keep all serum 17-OHP values below 200 ng/dl. Because this level was selected arbitrarily on the basis of levels seen in healthy children, the possible pathophysiological consequences of elevated 17-OHP levels were studied through an examination of the correlation between 17-OHP levels and serum levels of progesterone, androstenedione, and testosterone. The relationship of progesterone to 17-OHP in CAH infants is seen in Figure 8. There was a high degree of correlation between the levels of these two hormones ($r =$ 0.90), with progesterone levels remaining approximately one-tenth those of 17-OHP. When 17-OHP rose above 500 ng/dl, consistently elevated levels of progesterone were obtained. Figure 9 shows the relationship between progesterone and 17-OHP in adolescent CAH patients. In males, the relationship appeared similar to that obtained for infants, as seen in Figure 8. The initial data available in female patients was from well controlled patients, and no 17-OHP levels above 200 ng/dl were seen. The samples were collected at random throughout the menstrual cycle, and no significant correlation between levels of progesterone and 17-OHP was present. No postovulatory or luteal levels of progesterone were seen in these girls.

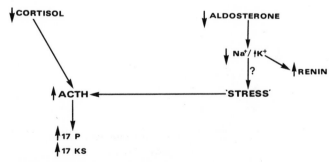

Figure 7. A suggested mechanism for the effect of chronic salt depletion on 17-hydroxyprogesterone (17P) production. 17-KS, 17 ketosteroids.

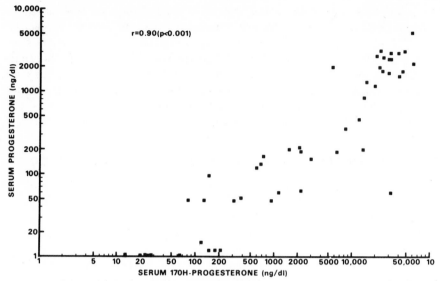

Figure 8. Log-log plot of the relationship of progesterone to 17-OHP in CAH infants. Each point represents values obtained from a single blood sample.

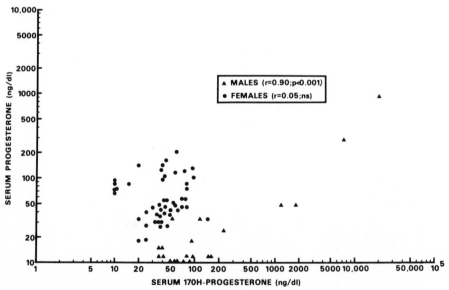

Figure 9. Log-log plot of the relationship of progesterone to 17-OHP in adolescent CAH patients. *ns,* not significant.

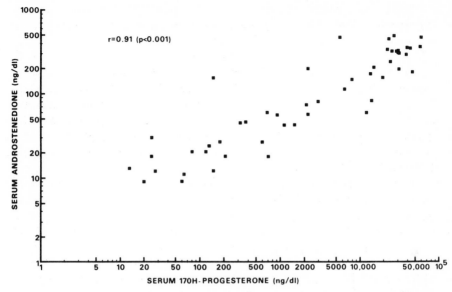

Figure 10. Log-log plot of the relationship of androstenedione to 17-OHP in CAH infants.

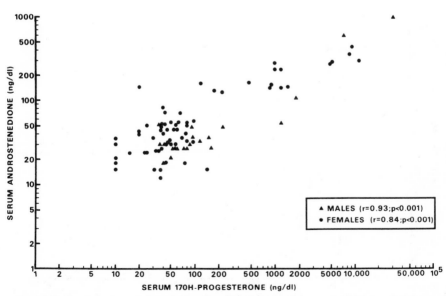

Figure 11. Log-log plot of the relationship of androstenedione to 17-OHP in adolescent CAH patients.

There was a highly significant correlation (r = 0.91) between serum androstenedione and 17-hydroxyprogesterone levels in male and female infants (Figure 10). Androstenedione levels began to rise when serum 17-OHP exceeded 200 ng/dl, but consistently abnormal androstenedione concentrations (above 80 ng/dl) were not observed until 17-OHP levels exceeded 1,000 ng/dl. The same androstenedione-17-OHP relationship in adolescent CAH patients is illustrated in Figure 11. There was a high degree of correlation present in both sexes, with androstenedione levels somewhat higher in the females than in the males. In spite of the linear relationship of androstenedione to 17-OHP, abnormally elevated levels (>200 ng/dl) were not observed until 17-OHP levels exceeded 1,000 ng/dl.

Figure 12 shows that there was a highly significant correlation between serum testosterone and 17-OHP in infants with CAH. An occasional abnormal testosterone value (>30 ng/dl) was seen when 17-OHP reached 300 ng/dl, but many of the testosterone levels were still within the normal range when 17-OHP was 1,000 ng/dl or higher. If a major goal of glucocorticoid therapy in infancy is to prevent virilization and if it is assumed that this will not occur unless serum testosterone levels exceed the normal range, then it is possible that levels of 17-OHP as high as 500 or even 1,000 ng/dl will not be associated with virilization.

The relationship of testosterone to 17-OHP in adolescents with CAH is shown in Figure 13. Adolescent girls showed a high degree of correlation

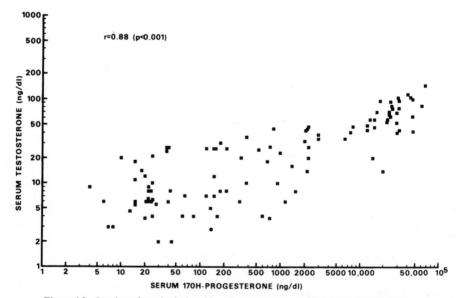

Figure 12. Log-log plot of relationship of testosterone to 17-OHP in CAH infants.

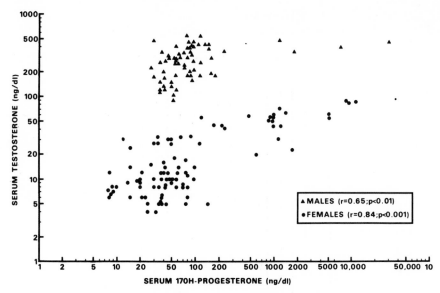

Figure 13. Log-log plot of relationship of testosterone to 17-OHP in adolescent CAH patients.

between these two hormones (r = 0.84), but again abnormal levels of testosterone (>65 ng/dl) did not occur until 17-OHP levels exceeded 1,000 ng/dl. Not surprisingly, the correlation in adolescent boys was less significant (r = 0.65). Presumably, as adrenal androgen secretion increases, there is some suppression of Leydig cell testosterone production, and this tends to obscure the relationship.

PRACTICAL CLINICAL APPLICATIONS

This study has attempted to show how serum 17-OHP levels reflect the degree of adrenal suppression in patients with CAH and to indicate how increases in serum 17-OHP might serve as indicators of excessive adrenal secretion of androgens or progesterone. These preliminary studies, however, involved repeated blood sampling over a 30-hr period, which is obviously not practical for use in the clinic. The data have therefore been reanalyzed to determine which samples provide the most reliable indication of the state of control as compared to the information derived from assay of urinary pregnanetriol. The diagnostic accuracy (in terms of adequacy of adrenal suppression) of serum 17-OHP determinations at four different times in the day was compared in 36 instances with the interpretations derived from simultaneous assays of urinary pregnanetriol, urinary 17-ketosteroids, and serum testosterone (Figure 14). In 14 of the 36 instances, there was increased excretion of pregnanetriol, whereas in only 8 instances was there a

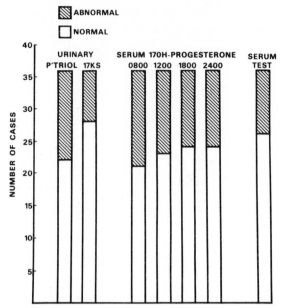

Figure 14. A comparison of the interpretations assigned to each value in 36 patient visits at which simultaneous assays of 24-hr urinary pregnanetriol (p'triol) and total 17-ketosteroids (17-KS), plus serum 17-OHP (at 0800, 1200, 1800 and 2400 hr) and testosterone (at 0800 hr) were available. The *shaded area* of each bar shows the number of abnormal values obtained, while the *clear area* indicates the number of values within the normal range for the patient's age.

concomitant elevation of urinary 17-ketosteroids. Assays of serum 17-OHP in blood collected at 0800 and 1200 hr were abnormal in 15 and 13 cases, respectively, each agreeing with the urinary pregnanetriol result in every instance but one. Sampling for serum 17-OHP at 1800 and 2400 hr did not appear to provide any further diagnostic information in these instances. For comparison, the serum testosterone concentration was elevated in only 10 of the instances in which pregnanetriol was abnormal. It would seem, therefore, from this analysis that a normal serum 17-OHP value from a blood sample collected at 0800 hr from a patient taking three divided oral doses of cortisol can be taken as evidence that adrenal suppression is adequate. It cannot alone, however, indicate whether the cortisol dose is excessive.

From this study, certain conclusions concerning the value of serum 17-hydroxyprogesterone assays can be made.

1. The assay can be used to make a rapid and accurate diagnosis of the C-21-hydroxylase form of CAH, even in circumstances (as in the first few days of life) when urinary pregnanetriol may be normal (Shackleton, Mitchell, and Farquhar, 1972).

2. The serum level of 17-OHP is the most sensitive index of the adequacy of glucocorticoid therapy, provided that accurate information is available concerning the normal level for the age of the patient, the timing of the blood sample in relation to the previous dose of cortisol, and finally the state of sodium balance in a salt loser.
3. Plasma renin activity is the most sensitive index available to determine the adequacy of mineralocorticoid replacement.
4. Serum 17-OHP is of no value in the detection of excessive steroid therapy, which must be expected in any patient receiving more than 30 mg of cortisol/ m^2/day (Migeon, 1968).

For routine use in the management of CAH patients in the clinic, regular estimations of plasma renin activity at 0900 hr and serum 17-OHP at 0800 and 1200 hr would appear to provide as much or more information regarding control as the usual assay of urinary 17-ketosteroids or pregnanetriol. If these serum values are normal, then the patient can be considered to be adequately controlled. If the levels are elevated, then consideration should be given to obtaining serial serum 17-OHP values to determine exactly how the steroid therapy should be altered. It is hoped that these new techniques will permit continued suppression of adrenal androgen levels to normal levels without causing hypercortisolism, with the use of doses of cortisol in the range of 15–25 mg/m²/day. This more exact control of CAH therapy should maximize each patient's chance for normal growth and reproductive potential.

ACKNOWLEDGMENTS

The authors acknowledge the excellent assistance of Miss D. Dzydz, Mr. D. Grant, Mr. D. Powell, Mr. I. Riyaz, and Miss E. Gulbis.

REFERENCES

Bailey, C. C., and G. M. Komrower. 1974. Growth and skeletal maturation in congenital adrenal hyperplasia. Arch. Dis. Child. 49:4–7.
Brook, C. G. D., M. Zachmann, A. Prader, and G. Mürset. 1974. Experience with long-term therapy in congenital adrenal hyperplasia. J. Pediatr. 85:12–19.
Haber, E., T. Koerner, L. B. Page, B. Kliman, and A. Purnode. 1969. Application of a radioimmunoassay for angiotensin I to the physiologic measurements of plasma renin activity in normal healthy subjects. J. Clin. Endocrinol. Metab. 29:1349–1355.
Hughes, I. A., and J. S. D. Winter. 1976. The application of a serum 17OH-progesterone radioimmunoassay to the diagnosis and management of congenital adrenal hyperplasia. J. Pediatr. 88:766–773.
Jones, H. W., and B. S. Verkauf. 1971. Congenital adrenal hyperplasia: age at menarche and related events at puberty. Am. J. Obstet. Gynecol. 109:292–298.
Kinoshita, K., K. Isurugi, Y. Matsumoto, and H. Takayasu. 1968. Gas chromatographic estimation of urinary Δ^5-pregnene-3β,17α,20α-triol. Steroids 11:1–11.

Kirkland, J., R. Kirkland, L. Librik, and G. Clayton. 1974. Serum gonadotropin levels in female adolescents with congenital adrenal hyperplasia. J. Pediatr. 84:411–414.

Migeon, C. J. 1968. Updating of the treatment of congenital adrenal hyperplasia. J. Pediatr. 73:805–806.

Peterson, R. E., and C. E. Pierce. 1960. Methodology of urinary 17-ketosteroids. *In* F. W. Sunderman and F. W. Sunderman, Jr. (eds.), Lipids and the Steroid Hormones in Clinical Medicine, pp. 147–161. Lippincott, Philadelphia.

Rappaport, R., E. Bouthreuil, C. Marti-Hennenberg, and A. Basmaciogullari. 1973. Linear growth rate, bone maturation and growth hormone secretion in prepubertal children with congenital adrenal hyperplasia. Acta Paediatr. Scand. 62:513–519.

Rappaport, R., G. Cornu, and P. Royer. 1968. Statural growth in congenital adrenal hyperplasia treated with hydrocortisone. J. Pediatr. 73:760–766.

Shackleton, C. H., F. L. Mitchell, and J. W. Farquhar. 1972. Difficulties in the diagnosis of the adrenogenital syndrome in infancy. Pediatrics 49:198–205.

Sperling, M. A., F. M. Kenny, J. C. Schutt-Aine, and A. L. Drash. 1971. Linear growth and growth hormonal responsiveness in treated congenital adrenal hyperplasia. Am. J. Dis. Child. 122:408–413.

Winter, J. S. D., I. A. Hughes, F. I. Reyes, and C. Faiman. 1976. Pituitary-gonadal relations in infancy. II. Patterns of serum gonadal steroid concentrations in man from birth to two years of age. J. Clin. Endocrinol. Metab. 42:679–686.

17-Hydroxyprogesterone, Progesterone, Estradiol, and Testosterone in Congenital Adrenal Hyperplasia

Solomon A. Kaplan, Barbara M. Lippe,
Stephen H. LaFranchi, and Albert Parlow

The serum concentrations of 17-hydroxyprogesterone (17-OHP) in patients with adrenal hyperplasia have been studied in this laboratory over the past 3 or 4 years to determine whether this measurement would be of help in the diagnosis and treatment of this disorder. Simultaneous assessments of 17-OHP and 24-hr urinary excretion of 17-ketosteroids and pregnanetriol were made. In addition, serum levels of progesterone, estradiol, and testosterone were measured and correlated with other measurements of plasma steroids. Methods used have been published previously (Lippe et al., 1974).

Mean values for serum 17-OHP, progesterone, estradiol, and testosterone in cord blood, infants 1–6 weeks old, prepubertal boys, and prepubertal girls are listed in Table 1.

Figure 1 depicts results of simultaneous measurements of serum 17-OHP and 24-hr urinary pregnanetriol. A general lack of correlation is seen between random blood samples and simultaneous 24-hr urine measurements. A similar plot of 24-hr 17-ketosteroids and serum 17-OHP demonstrates an equivalent lack of good correlation. If the data are grouped according to degree of control (Figure 2), it is found that mean serum 17-OHP concentrations in patients judged to be in good control were 4.2 ng/ml. The mean value in patients not considered to be in good control was 30.7 ng/ml. Similar plots for serum progesterone and urinary pregnanetriol or 17-ketosteroids also indicated a general lack of correlation. The mean value for serum progesterone for patients considered in good control was 1.1 ng/ml, whereas those in poor control had a mean level of 2.7 ng/ml.

In an effort to determine the reasons for lack of better correlations between serum 17-OHP and urinary steroids, the variation of serum 17-OHP over the day

This work was supported in part by Grants RR865 and AM11214 from the United States Public Health Service.

Table 1. Serum steroid concentrations in normal prepubertal children (mean ± S.E.M.)

	Number of patients	17-OHP (ng/ml)	Progesterone (ng/ml)	Estradiol (pg/ml)	Testosterone (ng/dl)
Cord blood	6	26.7 ± 4.10	838 ± 269	11,400 ± 900	
Infants (1 day–6 weeks)	6	2.1 ± 0.36	2.12 ± 1.25	22 ± 2.5	51 ± 18.6
Prepubertal boys	15	0.28 ± 0.11	0.13 ± 0.01	14.2 ± 1.4	20 ± 3.4
Prepubertal girls	14	0.35 ± 0.08	0.22 ± 0.02	23.2 ± 3.4	

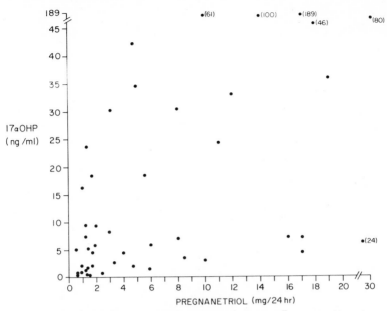

Figure 1. Correlation of serum 17-OHP with pregnanetriol excretion in 20 patients with congenital adrenal hyperplasia.

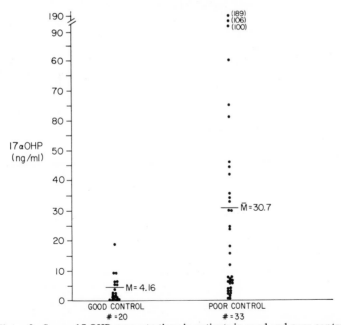

Figure 2. Serum 17-OHP concentrations in patients in good and poor control.

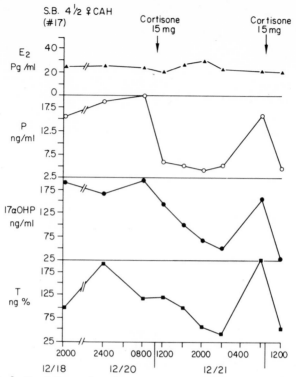

Figure 3. Effects of oral doses of cortisone on serum estradiol, progesterone, 17-OHP, and testosterone in a newly diagnosed patient with congenital adrenal hyperplasia.

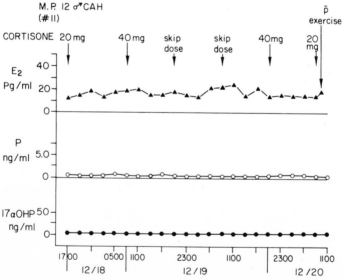

Figure 4. Effects of oral doses of cortisone on serum estradiol, progesterone, and 17-OHP in a well controlled patient with congenital adrenal hyperplasia.

Table 2. Laboratory values at time of initial diagnosis

Patient	Sex	Salt loss	Age	17-Ketosteroids (mg/24 hr)	Pregnanetriol (mg/24 hr)	17-OHP (ng/ml)	Progesterone (ng/ml)
1	F	+	10 days	5.0	5.5	718	
2	M	+	16 days	4.7	0.1	60	
3	M	+	21 days	4.0	3.4	157	
4	F	+	25 days	3.1	3.8	130	
5	M	+	30 days	9.2	2.4	277	7.2
6	F	–	3 months	6.3	3.6	312	24
7	F	–	4 years	16	17	189	16
8	F	–	6 years	15	14	100	7.0

with and without oral cortisone treatment was studied. Figure 3 shows the variation in serum 17-OHP, progesterone, estradiol, and testosterone in a newly diagnosed 4 1/2 year-old female with congenital adrenal hyperplasia. Marked fluctuation in the plasma steroids is seen over the day, both before and after treatment. By contrast, Figure 4 depicts similar observations made in a 12-year-old male with congenital adrenal hyperplasia. This patient was considered to be in good control; serum levels of 17-OHP, progesterone, and estradiol underwent very little fluctuation during the day.

Measurement of 17-OHP is of particular value in the diagnosis of congenital adrenal hyperplasia. Table 2 lists initial values for serum 17-OHP, progesterone, estradiol, testosterone, and urine 17-ketosteroids and pregnanetriol in eight patients at the time of initial diagnosis of the disorder, and demonstrates that plasma 17-OHP measurement is of considerable value in the diagnosis of congenital adrenal hyperplasia, especially in those patients with the 21-hydroxylase deficiency.

REFERENCES

Lippe, B. M., S. H. LaFranchi, N. Lavin, A. Parlow, J. Coyotupa, and S. A. Kaplan. 1974. Serum 17-hydroxyprogersterone, progesterone, estradiol, and testosterone in the diagnosis and management of congenital adrenal hyperplasia. J. Pediatr. 85:782–787.

Blood Testosterone Values in Patients with Congenital Virilizing Adrenal Hyperplasia

Irene L. Solomon and Edgar J. Schoen

Earlier work with the use of blood testosterone measurements in the evaluation of the chemical course of congenital virilizing adrenal hyperplasia (CVAH) has been reported (Solomon and Schoen, 1975). This investigation has continued to follow testosterone levels in patients with CVAH and to compare blood testosterone with urinary steroid values. This presentation will review and update these studies of the use of blood testosterone values in the treatment of CVAH.

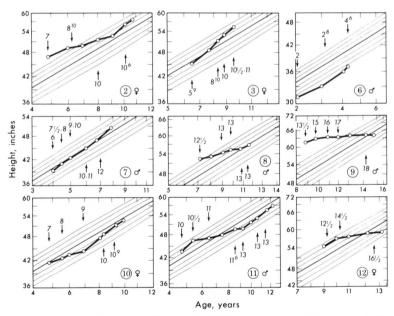

Figure 1. Growth charts of nine patients with CVAH studied sequentially during childhood. The *arrows* indicate the age at which bone age was assessed. The *numerals* associated with the arrows indicate the bone age level. The *circled numbers* in each growth chart are case numbers, corresponding to the text and Tables 1 and 2. Reproduced by permission from J. Clin. Endocrinol. Metab. 40:355 (1975).

Table 1. Comparison of 17-KS, pregnanetriol, and testosterone levels in six females and six prepubertal males

| Case | Sex | Age (Years^{month}) | Urinary | | Blood testosterone (ng/100 ml) | Oral glucocorticoid (mg/m^2/day) |
			17-KS (mg/24 hr)	Pregnanetriol (mg/24 hr)		
1	F	3^3	1.6	1.5	20	31 Cortisone acetate
		6^2	7.0	1.0	7	25 Cortisone acetate
2	F	4^{10}	7.5	6.5	72	Pretreatment
		8^5	2.0	2.5	0	7 Prednisone
		10$^{2-3}$	4.0	2.3	18	6.8 Prednisone
		10$^{9-10}$	3.2	2.6	13	6.8 Prednisone
		11^3	4.1	3.2	16	6.8 Prednisone
		12^4	7.0	4.6	14	5.8 Prednisone
3	F	7^8	6.2	6.4	29	16 Cortisone acetate
		9^7	10.6	5.7	36	17 Cortisone acetate
		10^6	12.2		66	24 Cortisone acetate
		10^{10}	11	10	106	24 Cortisone acetate
		11^2	8.5	11	74	27 Cortisone acetate
4	F	19^5	24	61	115	Off therapy 1 month
		20$^{6-7}$	32	62	74	8.4 Prednisone
		20^{10}	5.5	4.5	16	8.4 Prednisone
		21^1	11	10	81	8.4 Prednisone
		21$^{9-10}$	4.4	2.1	16	8.4 Prednisone
		22$^{4-5}$	8.2	7.0	16	8.4 Prednisone

Patient	Sex	Age				Treatment
5	M	0^{6}	0.3	1.4	2	10 Cortisone acetate[a]
6	M	2^{1}	2.0	3.7	1	18.5 Hydrocortisone
		2^{8}	6.6	15	8	15 Hydrocortisone
		4^{4}	7.4	9.6	44	16 Hydrocortisone
		5^{1}	5.4	14	42	22 Hydrocortisone
		5^{4}	2.0	2.2	5	29.5 Hydrocortisone
		5^{8}				28 Hydrocortisone
7	M	5	9.7	33	73	12.5 Prednisone
		6	3.0		2	17 Prednisone
		7	11.5	1.62	48	16.5 Prednisone
		7^{9}			5	9.5 Prednisone
8	M	9^{6}	9.2	4.8	24	18 Cortisone acetate
		9^{10}	10.5	4.7	26	18 Cortisone acetate
9	M	8^{10}	16.2	15	105	Pretreatment
		12^{5}	9.1		587	6.4 Prednisone
		13^{9}	2.2	2.4	356	6 Prednisone
14	M	7^{3-4}	11	5.2	20	61 Prednisone
		8^{2}	6.7	6.0	17	41 Prednisone
		8^{7}	12	21	17	40 Prednisone
		8^{9}	9	16	28	40 Prednisone
15	F	4^{6-7}	2.4	0.5	3	20 Hydrocortisone
16	F	1^{6-7}	<1.0	0.5	3	40 Hydrocortisone

[a]Administered intramuscularly.

Eighteen patients with CVAH who were followed by pediatricians of The Permanente Medical Group in Northern California have been studied. Cases 10, 11, and 12 (siblings) and case 17 have an 11-hydroxylase defect. Of the 14 patients with 21-hydroxylase deficiency, cases 2, 4, 8, and 9 have simple virilization; the rest are salt losers.

Blood testosterone in these studies was drawn, in most instances, between 2 and 4 p.m. Testosterone in serum or plasma was measured by a modification of the radioimmunoassay method of Furuyama, Mayes, and Nugent (1970). Laboratory normals for testosterone in adult females were 20–50 ng/100 ml; in the adult male, >300 ng/100 ml; in prepubertal children, <20 ng/100 ml. Urinary 17-ketosteroid (17-KS) and pregnanetriol levels were measured at Bioscience Laboratory, Van Nuys, California.

Patients with CVAH in whom testosterone was measured were evaluated according to the following criteria: growth, periodic assessment of bone age by comparison with the Greulich and Pyle standards (1959), measurements of urinary 17-KS and pregnanetriol, treatment prescribed, and compliance with therapy.

These studies have been divided into two parts. In the first group were patients for whom there were available values of urinary steroids from reliable 24-hr urine collections to compare with blood testosterone levels. This group comprised patients 1–8 and 14–16. In a second group of patients, it was not possible to obtain reliable urinary steroid values for comparison with blood testosterone levels. In this latter group of patients, cases 10–13, 17, and 18, sequential testosterone values were compared with the clinical assessment of the patient's control.

Normal urinary steroid values in treated patients with CVAH, based on those of Wilkins (1965) and Bongiovanni and Root (1963), include a 17-KS value of less than 1.5 mg/24 hr before age 2, from 2–4 mg/24 hr from ages 2–6, and 4–6 mg/24 hr from below age 6 until puberty. Urinary pregnanetriol levels should be less than 1 mg/24 hr until age 6 and less than 2 mg/24 hr thereafter. A summary of the growth and bone age data from nine patients studied during childhood is presented in Figure 1. Table 1 lists the 17-KS, pregnanetriol, and testosterone values from patients with CVAH whose blood testosterone and urinary assays were available for comparison.

Cases 5, 15, and 16 each were studied on a single occasion while their disease was satisfactorily controlled. Testosterone values in all three were in the prepubertal range, and urinary steroids were suppressed. Growth in cases 5 and 16 was normal; the height of case 15 was below the third percentile for age. In case 1, both testosterone values were 20 ng/100 ml or below; urinary pregnanetriol values at 3 years 3 months of age were minimally elevated, whereas at 6 years 2 months they were suppressed.

Case 2, whose control on therapy was excellent (Figure 1), showed elevated urinary steroids and testosterone above the normal level of adult women prior to the initiation of therapy at 4 years 10 months. All testosterone values on treatment were below 20 ng/100 ml, 17-KS were suppressed, and pregnanetriol levels remained minimally elevated. At age 12, 7 months after menarche, height was 61.2 inches and bone age was 12 years 6 months.

In case 3, whose cortisone dose was inadequate, all testosterone values were above the prepubertal range, and all 17-KS and pregnanetriol levels were elevated. Growth was excessive and the bone age advanced (Figure 1). Similarly, all urinary 17-KS and pregnanetriol values obtained in case 8 were elevated, and testosterone levels were slightly above the prepubertal range. However, in spite of this, growth was poor (Figure 1) in this patient. Therefore, a low steroid dose was maintained.

At age 19 years 5 months, after therapy had been stopped for 4 weeks for investigation, case 4 showed elevated urinary 17-KS and pregnanetriol and a blood testosterone level above the upper limit for normal adult women. Treatment was resumed, but compliance was poor. At 20 years 6–7 months, when

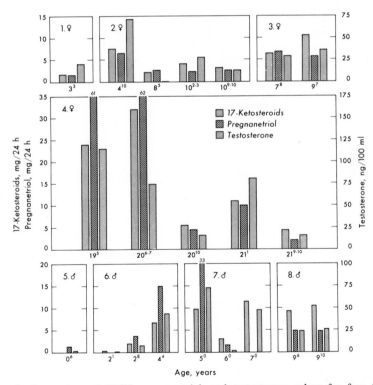

Figure 2. Comparison of 17-KS, pregnanetriol, and testosterone values for four female patients and four prepubertal males with CVAH; case numbers are as in Table 1. Reproduced by permission from J. Clin. Endocrinol. Metab. 40:355 (1975).

Table 2. Testosterone values in five patients with CVAH correlated with clinical control

Case	Sex	Age (Years^{month})	Blood testosterone (ng/100 ml)	Oral glucocorticoid (mg/m^2/day)	Clinical course
10	F	7^7	100		Off steroid 1 month
		9	129	6.8 Prednisone	Uncertain compliance
		9^4	32	6.2 Prednisone	Uncertain compliance
		9^{10}	123	5.8 Prednisone	Uncertain compliance
		10^5	103	7.4 Prednisone	Uncertain compliance
		10^7	41	7.4 Prednisone	Parental supervision encouraged
		10^{11}	124	7.4 Prednisone	Uncertain compliance
		11^3	184	7.4 Prednisone	Uncertain compliance
		11^4	<10	7.4 Prednisone	Parental supervision encouraged
11	M	7^{11}	14	11 Prednisone	
		9^{10}	3	9 Prednisone	
		9^{11}	51		Off treatment 4 weeks
			66		Off treatment 6 weeks
12	F	10	10		Off steroid 1 month
		10^{10}	94	7.8 Prednisone	
		11^{11}	250		
		12^5	13	8 Prednisone	
		12^9	87		
		13^3	186		
		13^{10}	13		
		14	<10	9.3 Prednisone	Not taking prescribed steroid
		14^5	<10	8.8 Prednisone	Not taking prescribed steroid
		14^8		8.9 Prednisone	Not taking prescribed steroid

13	M	20^{11}	4		Prednisone	Dosage uncertain
		23^{8}	200		Prednisone	Dosage uncertain; erratic administration
		26	183		Prednisone	Dosage uncertain; erratic administration
		26^{1}	54	100^{a}	Cortisone acetate	
		27^{10}	168		Prednisone	Dosage uncertain; erratic administration
		28^{8}	298		Prednisone	Dosage uncertain; questionable compliance
17	F	$0^{1\,1/2}$	48			Pretreatment
		0^{4}	8	25	Cortisone acetate	
18	F	2 days	580		Cortisone acetate[b]	Pretreatment
		2 weeks	250	20	Cortisone acetate[c]	
		3 weeks	27			

[a] Administered intramuscularly the preceding day.
[b] After two doses intramuscularly.
[c] Administered intramuscularly.

seen with amenorrhea, she admitted failing to take her prescribed therapy. Blood and urinary steroid values were again elevated. At 20 years 10 months, again on treatment, menses resumed and testosterone fell below 20 ng/100 ml. The same pattern of elevated testosterone values was repeated at age 21 years 1 month, when the patient took steroid irregularly. On resumption of therapy at 21 years 9–10 months, urinary steroids fell and testosterone dropped below 20 ng/100 ml.

Case 6 was thought to have growth suppression, despite a low dose of hydrocortisone (Figure 1). Corresponding testosterone levels were below 20 ng/100 ml. When steroid therapy was further reduced in an attempt to correct growth retardation, urinary 17-KS rose above normal and testosterone became elevated above 20 ng/100 ml. At age 5 years 4 months, after his steroid dosage had been increased, testosterone fell below 20 ng/100 ml, although urinary steroids remained elevated. Subsequently, urinary 17-KS fell to normal.

In case 7, compliance with treatment was poor. At age 5, treatment was taken irregularly. Urinary steroids were elevated and testosterone was above the prepubertal range. When adequate treatment had been resumed at age 6, urinary steroids were suppressed and testosterone fell within the prepubertal range. At age 7, again with erratic therapy, urinary 17-KS were elevated and testosterone rose above 20 ng/100 ml. With resumption of therapy, testosterone fell below 20 ng/100 ml.

In contrast to the previously discussed cases, case 14 showed consistently elevated urinary steroid levels when three of four corresponding blood testosterone values were 20 ng/100 ml or below. Despite the high urinary steroid values, the child's growth was inadequate. On a lowered dose of cortisone, his growth rate began to accelerate.

Following institution of steroid therapy in a pubertal boy with CVAH (case 9), although 17-KS and pregnanetriol levels fell, testosterone rose concomitantly with progressive testicular enlargement as puberty advanced.

In Figure 2, the correspondence between urinary 17-KS, pregnanetriol, and blood testosterone in cases 1–8 is shown diagrammatically. The correlation coefficients calculated for all the data from Table 1 are 0.88 for 17-KS and pregnanetriol, 0.69 for 17-KS and testosterone, and 0.66 for pregnanetriol and testosterone. In most instances, the urinary steroids and the blood testosterone yielded the same interpretation of the adequacy of a patient's control. Where there is a discrepancy between interpretation of the blood and urinary levels, the urinary steroids usually were elevated, while the blood testosterone remained within the prepubertal range.

The blood testosterone data from cases 10–13, 17, and 18 are shown in Table 2. In cases 10–12, compliance with therapy was poor and urine collections probably incomplete. Case 10, at 7 years 6 months, showed marked elevation of testosterone 1 month after treatment was stopped for investigation. Subsequently, testosterone levels dropped when it appeared that medication was taken regularly.

Case 11 showed a low testosterone level at age 9 years 10 months on treatment, but 4 and 6 weeks after treatment was stopped for investigation testosterone rose above 20 ng/100 ml. Case 12 at 10 years 10 months showed a testosterone value in the prepubertal range, which rose above 20 ng/100 ml 4 weeks after treatment was stopped for investigation. Like her younger sister, case 12 complied poorly with instructions to take medicine. At 12 years 5 months, 13 years 3 months, and 13 years 10 months, when treatment was not taken, menses stopped, acne increased, and testosterone rose above 20 ng/100 ml. At 12 years 9 months and from age 14 on, menses were regular and testosterone values below 20 ng/100 ml.

Case 13, reported previously (Schoen, di Raimondo, and Dominguez, 1961), had bilateral orchiectomies. His cooperation with medical management was poor; his history of medication, inaccurate. His testosterone values, which reflect only adrenal androgen output, range from 4–298 ng/100 ml. The high values presumably reflect failure to take prescribed steroid. The testosterone level recorded at age 26 years 1 month followed intramuscular steroid administration during hospitalization for a salt-losing crisis.

In case 17, testosterone prior to treatment at age 6 weeks was 48 ng/100 ml. The value fell below 20 ng/100 ml following suppressive therapy. In case 18, the testosterone value at 2 days of age was 580 ng/100 ml. After several doses of parenteral therapy at age 2 weeks, testosterone was 250 ng/100 ml, still greatly elevated. After intramuscular suppression on maintenance therapy, testosterone at age 3 weeks was 27 ng/100 ml, minimally above the prepubertal range.

Although testosterone levels in untreated patients with CVAH vary, a testosterone value of 20 ng/100 ml appears to be critical in treated patients. Lower values indicate at least adequate adrenal gland suppression and higher values suggest inadequate adrenal gland suppression in children and adult females with CVAH. The serial measurement of blood testosterone is a useful adjunct to the chemical monitoring of patients with CVAH. When urine collections are inaccurate or impossible to obtain, measurement of the blood testosterone offers a satisfactory alternative to the chemical evaluation of the patient with CVAH.

ACKNOWLEDGMENTS

We gratefully acknowledge the technical assistance of Larry Donelan and David Brandt-Erichsen.

REFERENCES

Bongiovanni, A. M., and A. W. Root. 1963. The adrenogenital syndrome. N. Engl. J. Med., 268:1342–1351.
Furuyama, S., D. M. Mayes, and C. A. Nugent. 1970. A radioimmunoassay for plasma testosterone. Steroids 16:415–428.
Greulich, W. W., and S. I. Pyle. 1959. Radiographic Atlas of Skeletal Develop-

ment of the Hand and Wrist, Ed. 2. Stanford University Press, Stanford, California.

Schoen, E. J., V. di Raimondo, and O. V. Dominguez. 1961. Bilateral testicular tumors complicating congenital adrenocortical hyperplasia. J. Clin. Endocrinol. Metab. 21:518–532.

Solomon, I. L., and E. J. Schoen. 1975. Blood testosterone values in patients with congenital virilizing adrenal hyperplasia. J. Clin. Endocrinol. Metab. 40:355–362.

Wilkins, L. 1965. The Diagnosis and Treatment of Endocrine Disorders in Childhood and Adolescence, Ed. 3, pp. 67, 360, 416. Charles C Thomas, Springfield, Illinois.

Congenital Adrenal Hyperplasia
A New Index of Adrenal Activity and Evidence for Adrenal Suppression in the Undertreated and Well Treated Patient

Terence J. McKenna, Anthony S. Jennings,
Grant W. Liddle, and Ian M. Burr[1]

The methods presently used for monitoring the adequacy of therapy in adreno-genital syndrome rely heavily on measurement of urinary 17-ketosteroid and pregnanetriol excretion. These methods have some disadvantages. First, considerable difficulty is often encountered in obtaining 24-hr urine collections in infants. Second, there is difficulty in interpreting urinary 17-ketosteroid and pregnanetriol values obtained around puberty due to the variability in the gonadal contribution to these steroids. Third, a lower limit for steroid excretion has not been established for young children. Recently it has been demonstrated that there are significant increases in plasma testosterone (Baulieu, Peillon, and Migeon, 1967) and in plasma progesterone and 17-hydroxyprogesterone (Strott, Yoshimi, and Lipsett, 1969) in patients with 21-hydroxylase deficiency, a finding that provides possible solutions to the first disadvantage noted above. However, some difficulty has been reported in distinguishing between under-treated and optimally treated patients on the basis of plasma concentrations of these steroids (Lippe et al., 1974).

The adrenal glands are a major source of both plasma pregnenolone and plasma 17-hydroxypregnenolone, and both upper and lower limits for plasma

This study was supported in part by Grants AMO-5318, HDO-5797, AMO-5092, MOI-RR-95, and AM-15269 from the National Institutes of Health and by International Fellowship 1-FO5-TWO1805-02 from the United States Public Health Service.

[1] An investigator of the Howard Hughes Medical Institute.

concentrations have been defined (Abraham and Chakmakjian, 1973; McKenna and Brown, 1974; McKenna et al., 1974; Strott, Bermudez, and Lipsett, 1970). However, the gonadal contribution to plasma 17-hydroxypregnenolone is minimal (McKenna et al., 1974). Therefore, measurement of plasma 17-hydroxypregnenolone theoretically should avoid the major disadvantages associated with urinary steroid determinations.

In the present study, the efficacy of assays of plasma pregnenolone and 17-hydroxypregnenolone for assessing the status of patients with adrenogenital syndrome has been determined. In addition, these assays have been used to determine the responsiveness of the adrenal cortex and the pituitary-adrenal axis in treated patients by measuring the changes in the plasma concentrations of these steroids in response to adrenocorticotropic hormone (ACTH) administration and to a reduction in glucocorticoid dosage.

METHODS

Pregnenolone, 17-hydroxypregnenolone, and testosterone were measured by previously described techniques (Coyotupa, Parlow, and Abraham, 1972; DiPietro, Brown, and Strott, 1972; McKenna et al., 1974). Urinary 17-ketosteroids were measured by colorimetry (Allen, 1950; Callow, Callow, and Emmens, 1938) following extraction (Drekter et al., 1952). Pregnanetriol was measured by the method of Bongiovanni and Eberlein (1958).

Plasma steroid concentrations used for the calculation of correlation coefficients were those found in blood drawn between 7 and 9 a.m. prior to administration of exogenous steroid on that day. Plasma testosterone values from pubescent and mature males were excluded when making correlations. All plasma values of <0.1 ng/ml were arbitrarily assigned a value of 0.1 ng/ml for statistical purposes.

STUDY PROTOCOL

A total of 22 patients, 21 with 21-hydroxylase deficiency and 1 with 3β-ol-dehydrogenase deficiency (all but one of whom were currently under treatment), were studied after informed consent had been obtained and after approval by the Clinical Investigation Committee. Patients were admitted to the clinical research center. The following day, blood was drawn prior to the administration of the usual morning steroid dose for estimation of plasma pregnenolone, 17-hydroxypregnenolone, and testosterone. Urine collections commenced and continued as sequential 24-hr samples for the duration of the hospital stay for measurement of 17-ketosteroids, pregnanetriol, creatinine, and volume. ACTH (α1-24 ACTH, 25 U. I.M.) was given to 14 patients on the morning of the 3rd day 1 hr prior to administration of the usual glucocorticoid dose. Blood was drawn before and 1 hr after the administration of ACTH. Sixteen patients were given 20–40 U. (according to size) of repository ACTH (Acthar Gel, Armour) I.M. q. 12 hr for 36–48 hr, starting on the morning of day 3. Blood was drawn at least twice a day. Six patients were followed at home for 1 week on half their previous glucocorticoid dose after baseline measurements had been made. These measurements (24-hr urinary 17-ketosteroids and pregnanetriol and plasma steroids) were repeated in the hospital on day 7.

RESULTS

The normal ranges of pregnenolone and 17-hydroxypregnenolone in this laboratory were 0.3–2 ng/ml and 0.3–4.4 ng/ml, respectively. The range observed in patients with adrenogenital syndrome (7–9 a.m. samples) were 0.1–20.3 ng/ml and 0.1–25.0 ng/ml, respectively. As indicated in Figure 1, there was good correlation between both plasma pregnenolone and plasma 17-hydroxypregnenolone with urinary pregnanetriol excretion ($r = 0.85, p < 0.001$ and $r = 0.87, p < 0.001$, respectively). Similar correlations were observed with these plasma steroids and both plasma testosterone ($r = 0.82, p < 0.001$ and $r = 0.87, p < 0.001$) and urinary 17-ketosteroids ($r = 0.91, p < 0.001$ and $r = 0.79, p < 0.001$). These correlations illustrated that all patients with plasma pregnenolone and 17-hy-

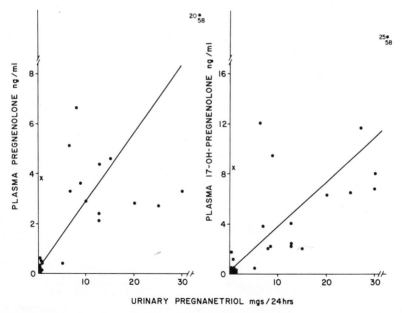

Figure 1. Plasma pregnenolone (*left*) and 17-hydroxypregnenolone (*right*) plotted on a vertical axis against urinary pregnanetriol on the horizontal axis. ●, patients with 21-hydroxylase deficiency; X, patient with 3β-ol-dehydrogenase deficiency.

droxypregnenolone concentrations above the normal range had high urinary steroids and plasma testosterone; conversely, all patients with plasma pregnenolones <0.1 ng/ml had low urinary steroid concentrations. Correlations were less significant for pregnenolone when the patient with the highest values was excluded from analysis and when ketosteroids were corrected for the patient's age and simultaneous creatinine excretion.

Figure 2 demonstrates the effect of glucocorticoid administration on plasma pregnenolone and 17-hydroxypregnenolone concentrations over a 5-hr period. Patients with normal or elevated plasma pregnenolone and 17-hydroxypregnenolone exhibited marked falls in the concentration of these steroids following glucocorticoid administration. No significant changes were observed over this time period when glucocorticoid was not given.

Administration of ACTH ($\alpha 1-24$ ACTH) had no acute effect on the plasma levels of pregnenolone and 17-hydroxypregnenolone in most patients; cf. normal subjects, Figure 3. After 36–48 hr of ACTH, a small but consistent increase in the plasma concentrations of these steroids was observed in all patients, those with higher baselines having the greater responses (Figure 4).

Reduction of glucocorticoid dosage by 50% for a period of 1 week had no significant effect on basal (7–9 a.m.) plasma steroid concentrations (Figure 5) or on urinary 24-hr 17-ketosteroid or pregnanetriol excretions.

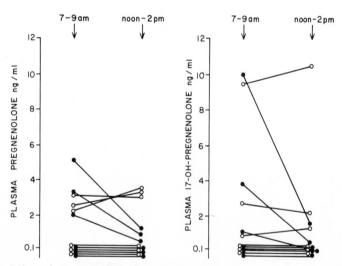

Figure 2. Effect of glucocorticoid administration (•) on plasma pregnenolone (*left*) and 17-hydroxypregnenolone (*right*) and a comparison of changes observed when glucocorticoid was not given (o).

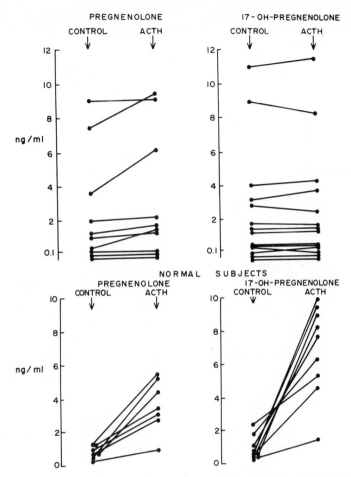

Figure 3. Plasma pregnenolone and 17-hydroxypregnenolone before and 1 hr after ACTH administration in patients with adrenogenital syndrome (*upper panels*) and in normal individuals (*lower panels*).

DISCUSSION

These results indicate that plasma concentrations of pregnenolone and 17-hydroxypregnenolone can be used to assess the status of patients with adrenogenital syndrome secondary to 21-hydroxylase deficiency. Plasma concentrations of 17-hydroxypregnenolone consistently correlated well with the degree of control as assessed clinically and by urinary 17-ketosteroid and pregnanetriol excretion. The correlations of the other steroids with plasma pregnenolone

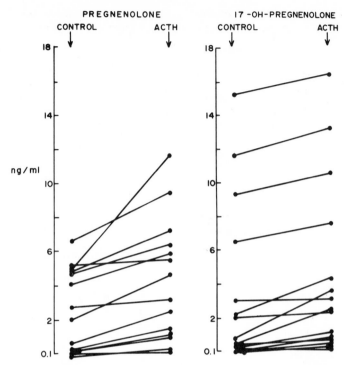

Figure 4. Plasma pregnenolone and 17-hydroxypregnenolone before and after 36–48 hr of ACTH administration.

tended to lose significance when values from overly suppressed patients were excluded. In addition, plasma pregnenolone (McKenna and Brown, 1974), 17-hydroxyprogesterone (Strott, Yoshimi, and Lipsett, 1969), and testosterone vary markedly with gonadal activity, and plasma 17-hydroxypregnenolone concentrations do not (McKenna et al., 1974). Therefore, measurement of 17-hydroxypregnenolone as a monitor of adrenal activity in patients treated with glucocorticoids for adrenogenital syndrome would circumvent the disadvantages of measuring urinary 17-ketosteroids and pregnanetriol, including the difficulty in collection of urine in infants and in interpretation at puberty. For these reasons, it would appear that assay of 17-hydroxypregnenolone is the measurement of choice in assessing the adrenal activity of patients under treatment for congenital adrenal hyperplasia.

It is worthy of note that while plasma concentrations of pregnenolone and 17-hydroxypregnenolone were markedly reduced within 5 hr of administration of the morning dose of oral glucocorticoids, they remained relatively constant over this period of time when the morning dose was omitted. That is, despite evidence for diurnal variation in the plasma concentration of these steroids in

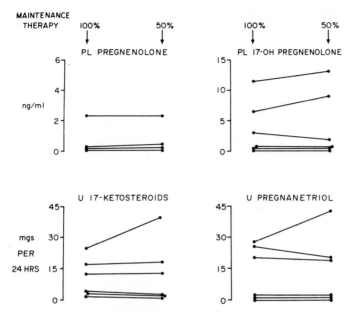

Figure 5. Effect of a 50% reduction in glucocorticoid dosage for 1 week on plasma pregnenolones and urinary 17-ketosteroids and pregnanetriol in patients with adrenogenital syndrome.

normal subjects (McKenna et al., 1974) and in untreated patients (McKenna et al., unpublished observation), moderate variation in the time of sampling in the morning will not affect the validity of the result in treated patients, provided sampling occurs prior to glucocorticoid administration.

Two further observations deserve comment. First, stimulation with exogenous ACTH produced sluggish and modest increases in plasma pregnenolone and 17-hydroxypregnenolone in treated patients with adrenogenital syndrome when compared with the acute, marked increase observed in normal subjects (Bermudez and Lipsett, 1972; McKenna and Brown, 1974; McKenna et al., 1974). Second, reduction of the administered glucocorticoid dose to 50% did not alter either plasma (7–9 a.m. sample drawn some 12 hr after the therapeutic glucocorticoid dose administered the night before) or urinary steroid concentrations after 1 week, whether the patient had been previously well or poorly controlled. These data suggest that the steroid doses needed to produce "normal" pregnanetriol and 17-ketosteroid excretion are such as to produce suppression of the pituitary-adrenal axis and that such suppression can be demonstrated even in patients with plasma and urinary steroid concentrations higher than desired. The potential clinical significance lies in the fact that excess steroids can contribute to growth retardation. Thus, the disturbing possibility is raised that it may not be possible to obtain suppression of pregnanetriol and 17-ketosteroid production to the normal range with "physiological" doses of exogenous glucocorticoid. It is theoretically reasonable that the amount of ACTH required to drive the adrenal to produce excess ketosteroids and pregnanetriol in the presence of enzyme deficiency is less than that amount required for appropriate cortisol production and the associated normal 17-ketosteroids and pregnanetriol excretion in the absence of enzyme deficiency.

On a more optimistic and less speculative note, it has been a general experience that significant reductions in total glucocorticoid replacement dosage can be achieved by using a dual or multiple dose regime while retaining the same degree of control as achieved by higher doses on a single dose regime (as assessed by clinical and urinary steroid criteria). Thus, the present daily dose range used in this laboratory is $10-15$ mg/m^2/day. The data presented in this paper provide experimental support for this approach. Acute (within 5 hr) reductions in plasma pregnenolone and 17-hydroxypregnenolone were observed following small doses of glucocorticoid in both appropriately treated and undertreated patients. However, plasma concentrations of the pregnenolones had risen markedly 12 hr after glucocorticoid administered the previous evening. The challenge remains to define the optimal frequency and dosage level for administering exogenous glucocorticoid. Measurement of plasma 17-hydroxypregnenolone may facilitate this endeavor.

ACKNOWLEDGMENTS

The expert technical assistance of Becky Miller and the secretarial assistance of Laura Drury are gratefully acknowledged.

REFERENCES

Abraham, G. E., and Z. H. Chakmakjian. 1973. Serum steroid levels during the menstrual cycle in a bilaterally adrenalectomized woman. J. Clin. Endocrinol. Metab. 37:581–587.

Allen, W. M. 1950. A simple method for analyzing complicated absorption curves of use in the colorimetric determination of urinary steroids. J. Clin. Endocrinol. Metab. 10:71–83.

Baulieu, E. E., F. Peillon, and C. J. Migeon. 1967. Adrenogenital syndrome. In A. B. Eisenstein (ed.), The Adrenal Cortex, pp. 553–637. Little, Brown and Company, Boston.

Bermudez, J. A., and M. B. Lipsett. 1972. Early adrenal response to ACTH: plasma concentrations of pregnenolone, 17-hydroxypregnenolone, progesterone and 17-hydroxyprogesterone. J. Clin. Endocrinol. Metab. 34:241–243.

Bongiovanni, A. M., and W. R. Eberlein. 1958. Critical analysis of methods for measurement of pregnane-3-alpha,17-alpha,20-alpha-triol in human urine. Anal. Chem. 30:388–393.

Callow. N. H., R. K. Callow, and C. W. Emmens. 1938. Colorimetric determinations of substances containing the grouping–CH_2CO–in urine extracts as an indication of androgen content. Biochem. J. 32:1312–1331.

Coyotupa, J., A. F. Parlow, and G. E. Abraham. 1972. Simultaneous assay of plasma testosterone and dihydrotestosterone. Analyt. Lett. 5:329–332.

DiPietro, D. L., R. D. Brown, and C. A. Strott. 1972. A pregnenolone radio-immunoassay utilizing a new fractionation technique for sheep antiserum. J. Clin. Endocrinol. Metab. 35:729–755.

Drekter, I. J., A. Heisler, G. R. Scism, S. Stern, S. Pearson, and T. H. Mac-Gavock. 1952. The determination of urinary steroids. 1. The preparation of pigment free extracts and a simplified procedure for the estimation of total 17-ketosteroids. J. Clin. Endocrinol. Metab. 12:55–65.

Lippe, B. M., S. H. LaFranchi, N. Lavin, A. Parlow, J. Coyotupa, and S. A. Kaplan. 1974. Serum 17α-hydroxyprogesterone, progesterone, estradiol and testosterone in the diagnosis and management of congenital adrenal hyperplasia. J. Pediatr. 85:782–787.

McKenna, T. J., and R. D. Brown. 1974. Pregnenolone in man: plasma levels in states of normal and abnormal steroidogenesis. J. Clin. Endocrinol. Metab. 38:480–485.

McKenna, T. J., D. L. DiPietro, R. D. Brown, C. A. Strott, and G. W. Liddle. 1974. Plasma 17-OH-pregnenolone in normal subjects. J. Clin. Endocrinol. Metab. 39:833–841.

Strott, C. A., J. A. Bermudez, and M. B. Lipsett. 1970. Blood levels and production rate of 17-hydroxypregnenolone in man. J. Clin. Invest. 49:1999–2007.

Strott, C. A., T. Yoshimi, and M. B. Lipsett. 1969. Plasma progesterone and 17-hydroxyprogesterone in normal men and children with congenital adrenal hyperplasia. J. Clin. Invest. 48:930–939.

Management of Congenital Adrenal Hyperplasia by Determinations of Plasma Testosterone, 17-Hydroxyprogesterone, and Adrenocorticotropic Hormone Levels and Plasma Renin Activity
A Comparison with the Classic Method Based on Urinary Steroids Determination

M. David, I. Ghali, P. Gillet, Louis David, Jean Bertrand, R. Francois, and M. Jeune

Wilkins et al. (1950) first reported on the successful treatment of patients with congenital adrenal hyperplasia (CAH) by the administration of cortisone. Since then the prognosis for life has been markedly improved, and many patients now attain adult life. However, the long-term follow-up of the patients is sometimes difficult. The aim of this work is to report the experience in this laboratory in the last 24 yr with the management of patients with CAH and to compare two different methods of control. These two methods are the classic one used before 1972, based mainly upon 24-hr urinary steroid determinations, and a new one introduced in January, 1972, based upon plasma determinations of renin activity (PRA), testosterone, 17-hydroxyprogesterone (17-OHP), and adrenocorticotropic hormone (ACTH).

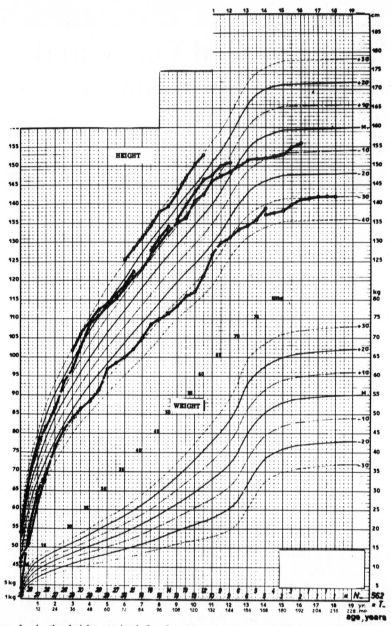

Figure 1, *A*, the height attained for female patients with CAH due to 21-hydroxylase deficiency. A general growth pattern was constructed by plotting the extreme upper and lower individual segments of curves from 46 of the 50 girls. Four individual curves lie above

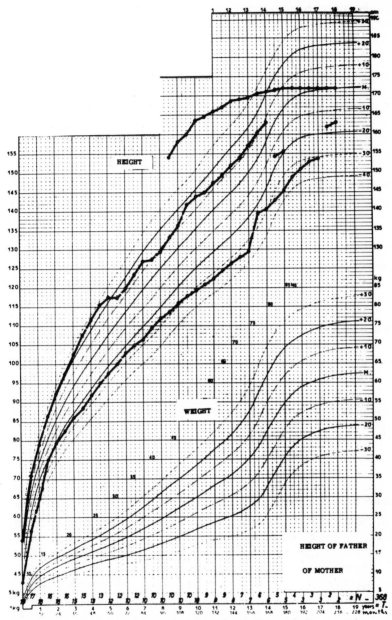

this upper segment. Figure 1, *B,* the height attained by 25 male patients with congenital adrenal hyperplasia due to 21-hydroxylase deficiency. With one exception, the extreme upper and lower individual segments of curves are plotted.

MATERIALS AND METHODS

Patients

Thirty-three males and 52 females with 21-hydroxylase deficiency were diagnosed and treated. Among these patients were two women raised as boys, who were virilized at puberty; their growth patterns were eliminated from this study. Seventeen patients died (14 before 1966 and 3 between 1966 and 1970). Growth data of some of them were included in the study if the period of observations was 1 year or longer. Seventeen other cases had achieved their final adult height at the time of the onset of the new method of evaluation.

Clinical Investigations

Height, weight, and roentgenograms of the left hand were obtained at intervals of approximately 6 months. Growth curves were plotted for each sex and were compared with standard charts of the centre d'Etude de la Croissance et du Dévelopement (Sempe and Masse, 1965). Deviations from normal mean were expressed as standard deviation (S.D.). Because of the extreme variability of the shape of the different individual curves and because several segments of individual curves were lacking, the general growth pattern was constructed by plotting the extreme upper or lower individual segment of curves. All the individual growth curves from the 50 girls lay inside the area limited by the extreme curves, except for the four individual segments of curves lying above (Figure 1A). The general growth pattern for the boys was studied in a similar manner (Figure 1B). The effect of under- or overtreatment was assessed on individual distance and velocity curves. Annual height velocity curves were determined by the increase in height in cm/year every 6 months. Skeletal maturation was determined at 6-month intervals with the use of the maturity scoring system of Sempe (1972). The curve for osseous maturation was plotted for each patient and was compared to the standard distance curve and velocity bone curve available for the normal French population.

Laboratory Investigations

From 1950 to 1971, estimates of urinary corticosteroids—17-ketosteroids (17-KS) and ketogenic steroids(KGS)—were used for diagnosis and for control of the disease. The treatment regimen was adjusted to keep 17-KS and KGS levels within normal, according to chronological age. Since 1972, in addition to the above schedule, estimates of plasma testosterone, 17-OHP, PRA, and ACTH were made at mean intervals of 3 months for better assessment of treatment. Urinary corticosteroids, 17-KS, and KGS were determined by the method of Appleby et al. (1955) and Few (1961). Plasma testosterone was determined by the radioimmunological method of Forest, Cathiard, and Bertrand (1973), as was plasma DHA. Plasma 17-OHP was first determined by a competitive protein-binding technique and for the last year by the radioimmunological method of

Loras et al. (1974). Plasma ACTH was also determined by radioimmunology. PRA was determined by the radioimmunological method of Vincent, Sassard, and Cier (1972) on samples obtained in recumbent position at 8 a.m., after an overnight bedrest.

Hormonal Treatment

Before 1972, a variety of glucocorticoid preparations were used in various regimens, including hydrocortisone, cortisone acetate, prednisone, and, in few patients, dexamethasone. In patients presenting clinically with sodium-losing syndrome, 11-deoxycorticosterone acetate (DOCA), administered intramuscularly or in implants, was used until 1969. Thereafter, oral 9α-fluorocortisol was used to control salt loss.

Since 1972, hydrocortisone has been used as the main glucocorticoid therapy, with a few exceptions for those patients who were previously well equilibrated with other forms of glucocorticoids. The daily dosage was given in two divided doses, with a larger portion usually given in the morning. Most patients were receiving a morning dose of 12.5 to 100 μg of 9α-fluorocortisol as the mineralocorticoid.

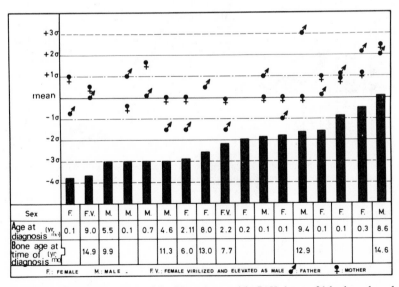

Figure 2. The final height attained in 17 patients with CAH due to 21-hydroxylase deficiency. The majority of the parents' heights are at or above the level of the mean height of the population. Only 1 of the 17 cases reached the mean height value, and all reached a height 1.5–3.5 S.D. below the mean parents' height.

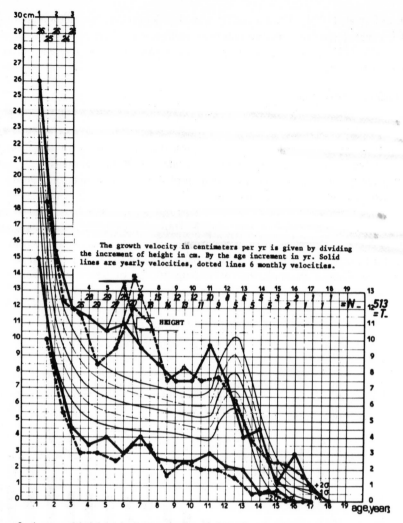

Figure 3, *A,* annual height velocity curves for 50 female patients with CAH due to 21-hydroxylase deficiency, measured by the increase in height in cm/year. Figure 3, *B,* height

RESULTS

Evaluation of Classic Method
of Control Based on Urinary Steroid Determinations

Because this method of control continued for 21 years (1951–1972), osseous maturation, statural growth, and final adult heights reached in the older patients are certainly the best way to evaluate the results.

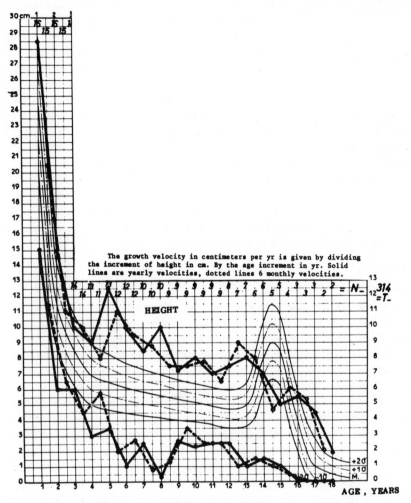

velocity curves for 25 male patients with CAH due to 21-hydroxylase deficiency. Upper and lower limits only are plotted.

The mean birth length was 49.3 cm for girls in 26 cases and 49.3 cm for boys in 19 cases, indicating normal intrauterine growth.

Figure 1, *A* and *B,* demonstrates the growth pattern for female and male patients, respectively. It is evident that the growth pattern during the first 5 years was not very different from that of the normal population, but it subsequently slowed down in both sexes. Because of the large individual variations in the growth pattern, it is inappropriate to estimate a mean curve for the entire group.

All patients in this study achieved a final adult height well below the normal mean (Figure 2), except one male child who was diagnosed late, at age 8½; his growth curve lay well above the upper limit of the group, and he was the only one to reach a normal mean height. In nine patients (six males and three females), the final adult height was below −2 S.D. Among the eight patients diagnosed and treated after the age of 2 years, the final height was below −2 S.D. in six; when treatment was given in the first few months of life, the height attained was between the mean and −2 S.D. in six out of nine patients. There was a tendency for taller patients to have taller parents. However, none of these patients reached their parents' heights, and, furthermore, most of them remained at least 2 S.D. below their parents' heights. This was particularly striking for the boys, for whom their adult heights were well below their mothers' heights.

Figure 3, *A* and *B,* shows the height velocity for female and male patients, respectively. The variations in velocities were marked, and the pubertal growth spurt normally occurring between 11 and 13 years was not present and was replaced by a rapid decrease of the growth rate.

Evaluation of New Method of Control
Based on Testosterone, PRA, 17-OHP, and ACTH Determinations

Plasma Testosterone   The concentration of plasma testosterone was always elevated at diagnosis and before institution of substitutive therapy. This was of great diagnostic value in female patients at the neonatal period. On the contrary, it was of limited value in normal neonatal males, as it is well known that plasma testosterone concentration is always elevated in normal boys and remains so until the age of 6−7 months.

During treatment, an estimation of plasma testosterone appeared to be the most accurate parameter for controlling hydrocortisone dosage, except during the period of puberty in male patients. It reflected the degree of adrenal androgen overproduction. Whereas normal levels of plasma seemed to indicate adequate control, elevated values indicated poor hormonal control and usually an inadequate dose of glucocorticoids. In several instances, elevated levels of plasma testosterone were found under apparently appropriate glucocorticoid therapy and were normalized only by an increase in mineralocorticoid dosage. However, it should be stressed that there was usually a good correlation between plasma testosterone level and urinary 17-KS and KGS values.

Plasma Renin Activity   Estimation of PRA under basal conditions and with normal dietary sodium intake is, in our experience, the best sign of salt loss. Surprisingly, high levels of PRA were found not only in cases which presented clinically with salt-losing syndrome, but also in all cases with no clinical evidence of sodium loss. Three children (2−3 years of age) had PRA values ranging between 273 and 981 ng/liter/min, compared with normal values of 103 ± 44. In later control, serial estimations of PRA were of great value in achieving adequate hormonal equilibrium. It has been found that in several patients elevated levels

Table 1. Plasma 17-OHP values before and after treatment

Chronological age	Urine		Plasma				Treatment		
	17-KS (mg/24 hr)	KGS (mg/24 hr)	Testosterone (ng/100 ml)	17-OHP (ng/100 ml)	PRA (ng/liter/min)	ACTH (pg/ml)	Hydrocortisone (mg/day)	9α-Fluorocortisol (µg/day)	Salt (g/day)
2 days	2.54	3.34	92	8,977		71			
2 months	0.76	2.59	6.6	1,488	372		10	25	2
3 months	0.70	4.05	13.2		675		10	25	2
5.5 months	0.73	5.54			240		10	50	2
6 months	0.29	3.33	7	463	435	60	10	50	2.5
10 months	0.24	2.07	6		88	76	10	50	3
11 months	0.25	2.36	5		75	92		50	2

of PRA were associated with an increase in urinary excretion of 17-KS and KGS and with elevation of plasma testosterone values, in spite of an apparently adequate dosage of glucocorticoids. An increase in mineralocorticoid dosage was then followed by a decrease in plasma testosterone concentration and in urinary 17-KS and KGS. Thus, a smaller dosage of hydrocortisone was used with a better achievement of hormonal equilibrium.

Plasma 17-Hydroxyprogesterone Plasma 17-OHP values were always very high before administration of substitutive therapy. But after treatment, normal values could not be obtained even with an apparently adequate dosage of both 9α-fluorocortisol and hydrocortisone (Table 1). A diurnal rhythm with great individual variations—even variations in the same patient from day to day—was observed before and during treatment. Furthermore, frequent estimations of 17-OHP in later treatment of the disease have demonstrated that a normal or low level is a definite sign of treatment overdosage.

Plasma ACTH Plasma ACTH values were elevated at diagnosis and before institution of treatment. They appeared to follow a pattern of variations similar to that observed for 17-OHP and were not of much help for adjusting the glucocorticoid treatment.

Analysis of the growth pattern in six new cases treated from 1972–1974 and controlled by the new method showed that linear growth was satisfactory, and the bone age to statural age ratio was 0.9. Comparatively, six children of the same chronological age treated before 1972 demonstrated a marked growth retardation, with a bone age to statural age ratio of 2.

DISCUSSION

From our data on patients treated before 1972 by the classic method, it is evident that reduction in adult height remains a major problem in CAH and that the time when treatment is started does not seem to play a major role in the final height attained. Indeed, several patients treated early reached a markedly reduced height, in agreement with several observations by other authors (Bailey and Komrower, 1974; Bergstrand, 1966; Borniche, Canlorbe, and Job, 1974; Brook et al., 1974; Rappaport et al., 1973). When analyzing individual data, it was found that, in addition to the problems of compliance and inappropriate therapy, two major factors seemed to be responsible for this short adult stature. First, as already explained by Rappaport, Cornu, and Royer (1968), the first 2 years of life are critical because of the frequent occurrence of infections and difficulties in controlling the salt loss. Second, in several older children, elevated 24-hr urinary steroid levels persisted in spite of a marked increase in glucocorticoid dosage and appeared to be mainly related to difficulties in the control of salt loss. This led to a decrease in linear growth with a paradoxical increase in osseous maturation. In these patients, it is postulated that for some unexplained reasons the badly controlled salt loss was responsible for a sustained adrenal hyperactivity. Because of dissatisfaction with these results, it was decided in early 1972 to look for a new method of control which could give more accurate information on the needs for both glucocorticoid and mineralocorticoid therapy. Plasma ACTH, 17-OHP, and testosterone levels were chosen as control parameters of the salt loss (Gillet and Francois, 1973). Of all the parameters, PRA is probably the most helpful in detecting salt loss and in adapting the 9α-fluorocortisol treatment. It certainly allowed a reduction of the mean daily amount of hydrocortisone in our patients since 1972 from 28 mg/m^2/day to 21 mg/m^2/day, with extreme values of 12 and 30 mg/m^2/day. Although frequently closely related to the amount of 24-hr urinary steroids, plasma testosterone levels appear to be a more accurate parameter for the adjustment of glucocorticoid treatment than the 17-KS and KGS urinary excretion, particularly in infancy, when 24-hr urinary collection remains a problem. However, it should be remembered that elevated levels of plasma testosterone may be related to insufficient mineralocorticoid therapy. Plasma 17-OHP does not seem to be a reliable parameter, as elevated levels are always present under appropriate therapy. Thus, in these studies, normal or low levels of plasma 17-OHP are an indication of overtreatment. Because of persistent elevated plasma 17-OHP levels and because 17-OHP is known to be a potent saliduretic steroid, it has been decided to treat the non-salt-losing form of CAH with small amounts of 9α-fluorocortisol in order to suppress the resulting increase in PRA.

Finally, plasma ACTH levels appear to be too variable to be used as a parameter in the adjustment of treatment.

CONCLUSION

It is still too early to give a definite statement on the efficacy of this new method, particularly on its long-term effect on statural growth; however, the experience gained during the last 4 years has resulted in 1) a reduction of the daily dosage of hydrocortisone; 2) a more accurate evaluation of the needs of 9α-fluorocortisol; and 3) apparently better results in growth velocity and skeletal maturation.

REFERENCES

Appleby, J. C., G. Gibson, J. N. Norymberski, and R. D. Stubbs. 1955. Indirect analysis of corticosteroids. I. The determination of 17-hydroxycorticosteroids. Biochem. J. 60:453.
Bailey, C. C., and G. M. Komrower. 1974. Growth and skeletal maturation in congenital adrenal hyperplasia: review of 20 cases. Arch. Dis. Child. 49:4.
Bergstrand, C. G. 1966. Growth in congenital adrenal hyperplasia. Acta Paediatr. Scand. 55:463–472.
Borniche, P., P. Canlorbe, and C. Job. 1974. Remarques sur la croissance staturale des hyperplasies surrénales congénitales virilisantes traitées. Ann. Pédiatr. (Paris) 21:27.

Brook, C. G. D., M. Zachmann, A. Prader, and G. Nurset. 1974. Experience with long-term therapy in congenital adrenal hyperplasia. J. Pediat. 85:12—19.

Few, J. D. 1961. A method for the analysis of urinary 17 hydroxycorticoids. J. Endocrinol. 22:31.

Forest, M. G., A. M. Cathiard, and J. A. Bertrand. 1973. Total and unbound testosterone levels in the newborn in normal and hypogonadal children: use of a sensitive radioimmunoassay for testosterone. J. Clin. Endocrinol. Metab. 36:1132.

Gillet, P., and R. Francois. 1974. L'hyperplasie surrénale congénitale, intérêt des dosages plasmatiques de testostérone, 17 hydroxyprogestérone, ACTH et activité rénine pour la surveillance du traitement de l'HSC par déficit en 21 hydroxylase. J. Parisien. Pédiatr. Paris.

Loras, B., H. Roux, L. A. Parere, M. David, and J. Bertrand. 1973. Dosage de la 17-hydroxyprogestérone plasmatique par liaison compétitive aux protéines. Biomed. 121—317.

Rappaport, R., G. Cornu, and P. Royer. 1968. Statural growth in congenital adrenal hyperplasia treated with hydrocortisone. J. Pediat. 73:760—766.

Rappaport, R., E. Bouthreuil, C. Marti-Henneberg, and A. Basmaciogullari. 1973. Linear growth, bone maturation and growth hormone secretion in prepubertal children with congenital adrenal hyperplasia. Acta Paediatr. Scand. 62:513—519.

Sempe, M., and N. P. Masse. 1965. La croissance normale: méthodes et résultats. In 20ème Congrès des pédiatres de Langue Française, Masson, Paris 21.

Sempe, M. 1972. Analyse numérique de la maturation osseuse du poignet et de la main. Commentaires et critiques de la méthode des standards pour âge osseux de. In J. M. Tanner, R. H. Witehouse, and M. Healy (eds.). Meeting of Coordinated Growth Teams, International Children's Centre, London.

Vincent, M., J. Sassard, and J. F. Cier. 1972. Méthode rapide de détermination radio-immunochimique de l'activité rénine. Rev. Eur. Etud. Clin. Biol. 17: 1001.

Wilkins, L., R. W. Lewis, R. Klein, and E. Rosemberg. 1950. The suppression of androgen secretion in a case of congenital adrenal hyperplasia. Bull. Johns Hopkins Hosp. 86:249—252.

Plasma 17-Hydroxyprogesterone in the Newborn with Congenital Adrenal Hyperplasia

Raphael David and E. Youssefnejadian

In the follow-up of our patients with congenital adrenal hyperplasia (CAH) due to 21-hydroxylase defect, it has not been found, thus far, that the measurement of plasma 17-hydroxyprogesterone (17-OHP) is particularly useful in assessing optimal therapy. Discrepancies between morning plasma 17-OHP levels, on the one hand, and urinary pregnanetriol and 17-ketosteroid excretion, on the other, have been observed. Nevertheless, the diagnostic value of plasma 17-OHP in CAH is well recognized (Barnes and Atherden, 1972; Strott, Yoshimi, and Lipsett, 1969). In our studies, plasma 17-OHP measurements have been especially useful in the newborn, in whom difficulties in diagnosis may be encountered owing to a delay in the appearance of abnormal urinary steroids characteristic of the syndrome (Shackleton, Mitchell, and Farquhar, 1972; Wilkins, 1965).

Plasma 17-OHP has been measured in this laboratory by a simple radioimmunoassay (Youssefnejadian et al., 1972) in six infants with CAH (ages 3 days to 3 months), 20 normal newborns, and in 10 samples of cord blood from normal vaginal deliveries. All but two CAH babies were salt losers. In five of the affected infants, urinary pregnanetriol was also measured. In one baby, B. B., 17-OHP was also measured in cord and in maternal blood. The data are shown in Table 1. In all CAH infants, as well as in the cord blood of B. B., plasma 17-OHP was greatly elevated at a time when urinary pregnanetriol was either undetectable or normal in at least four patients.

It should be noted that the 17-OHP level in the cord blood of B. B. was very high (36 μg/dl), whereas maternal 17-OHP was normal (1.2 μg/dl) (Youssefnejadian et al., 1972). The response to intravenous ACTH (20 U. over 4–6 hr) was brisk in the three infants studied (Table 1). Thus, the effect of ACTH may be useful when resting values of 17-OHP are not clearly abnormal.

In conclusion, it is felt that the estimation of plasma 17-OHP affords a sensitive means for early detection of CAH due to 21-hydroxylase deficiency in the newborn infant.

Table 1. Measurement of 17-hydroxyprogesterone by radioimmunoassay

Subjects	17-Hydroxyprogesterone (μg/dl) (mean ± S.D.)		Pregnanetriol (mg/24 hr)
	Before ACTH	After ACTH	
20 Normal newborns	Mean 0.22 ± 0.12 Range 0.09—0.63		
10 Samples of cord blood	Mean 1.42 ± 0.35 Range 0.74—1.87		
6 CAH babies			
B. J., 3 days old	18		Not measured
M. P., 3 days old	40	102.4	Undetectable
B. B., cord blood	36		
4 days old	26.6	80.0	0.15
B. W., 8 days old	47		Undetectable
10 days old	60.7		
F. B., 23 days old	24		Undetectable
25 days old	21		
J. W., 3 months old	33.3	175.0	0.8

REFERENCES

Barnes, N. D., and S. M. Atherden. 1972. Diagnosis of congenital adrenal hyperplasia by measurement of plasma 17-hydroxyprogesterone. Arch. Dis. Child. 47:62—65.

Shackleton, C. H., F. L. Mitchell, and J. W. Farquhar. 1972. Difficulties in the diagnosis of the adreno-genital syndrome in infancy. Pediatrics 49:198—205.

Strott, C. A., T. Yoshimi, and M. B. Lipsett. 1969. Plasma progesterone and 17-hydroxyprogesterone in normal men and children with congenital adrenal hyperplasia. J. Clin. Invest. 48:930—935.

Wilkins, L. 1965. The Diagnosis and Treatment of Endocrine Disorders in Childhood and Adolescence, Ed. 3, p. 412. Charles C Thomas, Springfield, Illinois.

Youssefnejadian, E., E. Florensa, W. P. Collins, and I. F. Sommerville. 1972. Radioimmunoassay of 17-hydroxyprogesterone. Steroids 20:773—788.

Evaluation of Congenital Virilizing Adrenal Hyperplasia Patients on Single versus Multiple Prednisone Schedules

Carol Huseman, Madan Varma, Robert M. Blizzard, and Ann Johanson

Various glucocorticoids have been used in the therapy of patients with congenital virilizing adrenal hyperplasia (CVAH) since Wilkins et al. (1950) and Bartter, Forbes, and Leaf (1950) reported successful therapy with cortisone. Although cortisone continues to be the drug of choice, it must be administered in at least two oral doses/day.

The parameters which have been used to evaluate control were growth rate, bone age, clinical signs of virilization, and measurement of urinary 17-ketosteroids (17-KS) and pregnanetriol. Evaluation of urinary 17-KS and pregnanetriol in children is inherently difficult and often inaccurate, and evaluation of the growth rate, bone age, and clinical signs of virilization does not allow for evaluation over short periods of time. Consequently, this study was established for several purposes: 1) to determine whether prednisone administered t.i.d., b.i.d., or q.d. is equally effective in the therapy of CVAH patients; and 2) to determine whether plasma 17-hydroxyprogesterone (17-OHP), progesterone, and/or testosterone, could be used more successfully than urinary 17-KS or pregnanetriol levels in the management of CVAH patients.

MATERIALS AND METHODS

Six patients, ages 5–17 years, were evaluated. All had C-21-hydroxylase deficiency. Four of the six patients were salt-losers.

During each of the three study periods, blood was drawn every 4 hr for 24 hr for measurement of plasma steroids, and 24-hr urine specimens were collected for measurement of 17-KS and pregnanetriol the day of and the day after the plasma collection.

The prednisone dosage was one-fourth of the cortisone dose the patient was receiving previous to the study. Each patient received each of the three prednisone schedules (t.i.d., b.i.d., and q.d.) for at least 1 month prior to each 2-day study period. The total dosage was unchanged in five of six patients and ranged from 4.2–8.8 mg/m^2/day. On the t.i.d. schedule, prednisone was administered at 0800, 1400, and 1800 or 2000 hr each day. The dosage was equally divided in four patients on the t.i.d. schedule. In the remaining two patients, half of the prednisone dosage was given at 1800 or 2000 hr. On the b.i.d. schedule, prednisone was administered every 12 hr at 0800 and 1800 or 2000 hr. The dosage was equally divided in three patients, and in the remaining three patients two-thirds of the total dose was given in the evening. On the q.d. prednisone schedule, each of the six patients received his total dose at 1800 or 2000 hr.

Six normal children, ages 4–12 years, were evaluated as controls. Blood was drawn every 4 hr for 24 hr for plasma steroids. Testosterone was measured by radioimmunoassay according to a method previously described (Varma et al., 1975). 17-OHP and progesterone were measured by radioimmunoassay. Briefly, 1 ml of plasma was spiced with approximately 1,000 cpm of ^{3}H-labeled 17-OHP and progesterone, extracted once with carbon tetrachloride, and washed with 0.1 N NaOH and 0.1 N HCl. The extracted sample was chromatographed on Sephadex LH-20 columns in 5-ml disposable pipettes (Corning) and eluted with benzene-methanol (95:5) solvent. In this system, the progesterone fraction came off the column in the 3–5.5-ml fraction and 17-OHP in the 5.5–8.5-ml fraction. The chromatographed samples were dried in a stream of air and resuspended in 1.5 ml of methanol. A sample (250 μl) was taken to count for recovery, and three aliquots ranging from 10 μl (high value) to 600 μl (low value) were used in binding runs for radioimmunoassay.

RESULTS AND DISCUSSION

The mean 24-hr plasma 17-OHP value was 33 ng/dl, the mean 24-hr progesterone value was 50 ng/dl, and the mean testosterone value was 31 ng/dl in the six normal children.

The peak plasma 17-OHP value occurred at 0900 hr in the normal subjects. The mean 0900-hr value for plasma 17-OHP was 54 ng/dl, and the 1700-hr mean value was 34.0 ng/dl. This diurnal variation has also been noted by other investigators (Atherden, Barnes, and Grant, 1972; Strott, Yoshimi, and Lipsett, 1969).

Plasma progesterone in the normal children did not show the diurnal variation of plasma 17-OHP, with a mean 0900-hr progesterone value of 61.0 ng/dl and a 1700-hr value of 52.0 ng/dl.

Testosterone also showed no diurnal variation in the normal subjects. The mean 0900-hr value in these subjects was 36 ng/dl, and the 1700-hr testosterone concentration was 33 ng/dl.

As in the normal children, the CVAH patients also showed the diurnal variation of plasma 17-OHP. The peak 17-OHP concentration occurred primarily at 0900 hr in the majority of patients on all prednisone schedules. The nadir of 17-OHP concentration occurred at 0100–0500 hr in the majority of patients.

Therefore, the time of day becomes a critical factor in the usefulness of a single plasma sample for 17-OHP. Samples obtained at late afternoon or evening could be misleadingly low.

Plasma progesterone showed less diurnal variation than plasma 17-OHP concentrations in these patients. In only one-third of the patients on all prednisone schedules did the peak progesterone value occur at 0900 hr. Testosterone also showed little diurnal variation.

An attempt was made to correlate plasma 17-OHP concentration with urinary pregnanetriol on each prednisone schedule. In our six CVAH patients, there were four instances in which urinary pregnanetriol was abnormal for chronological age on all prednisone schedules. In these four instances, the 0900-hr plasma 17-OHP concentration was greater than 800 ng/dl. When urinary pregnanetriol was normal, the 0900-hr plasma 17-OHP concentration was less than 800 ng/dl in all but two instances. In these two instances, both when the patients were on q.d. prednisone schedules, the urinary pregnanetriol values were at the upper limits of normal for chronological age at a time when the 0900-hr plasma 17-OHP concentration was greater than 800 ng/dl. These results could be interpreted to mean that plasma 17-OHP concentration is a more sensitive method for detecting early escape at adrenal suppression than is urinary pregnanetriol.

Therefore, a positive correlation was found between elevated urinary pregnanetriol values and a 0900-hr plasma 17-OHP concentration greater than 800 ng/dl. The 0100-hr plasma 17-OHP concentration was 108−183 ng/dl from this same group of patients with elevated urinary pregnanetriol, and 0900-hr plasma 17-OHP values were greater than 800 ng/dl. Therefore, the timing of single plasma sampling is critical.

Control of CVAH was better on the t.i.d. and b.i.d. schedules of prednisone than on the q.d. prednisone schedule, because the 0900-hr plasma 17-OHP concentration was less than 800 ng/dl and there was normal urinary 17-KS and pregnanetriol excretion for chronologic age. By these criteria, all six patients were well controlled on the b.i.d. schedule. Only two out of six patients were well controlled on the q.d. schedule.

When the mean 24-hr plasma 17-OHP concentration, rather than the 0900-hr plasma 17-OHP concentration, was compared with urinary pregnanetriol values, there were four instances in which the urinary steroids were elevated on all prednisone schedules. In these four instances, the mean 24-hr plasma 17-OHP concentration was greater than 320 ng/dl. There were two instances on the q.d. schedule, however, in which the mean plasma 17-OHP concentration was greater than 320 ng/dl with a normal urinary pregnanetriol value. Again, these were the two patients who had urinary pregnanetriol values at the upper limits of normal for their chronological age.

Therefore, there was a positive correlation between a mean 24-hr plasma 17-OHP concentration greater than 320 ng/dl and an elevated urinary pregnanetriol concentration. Using the mean 24-hr 17-OHP concentration of less than 320 ng/dl and normal urinary pregnanetriol and 17-KS excretion, control was better while the patient received prednisone twice a day. On the b.i.d. schedule, all six patients were well controlled by the above criteria, and on the q.d. schedule only two out of six were well controlled.

A 24-hr mean plasma steroid determination obviously cannot be of practical value in patient care. However, this measurement was considered essential to determine correlations between plasma and urinary steroids. Also, on the basis of this correlation, it was possible to determine that single plasma samples, rather than 24-hr plasma or urinary steroids samples or both, could be used in judging good control of CVAH.

Plasma progesterone and its correlation with urinary 17-KS and pregnanetriol on each prednisone schedule were also studied. When the mean 24-hr plasma progesterone values were correlated with urinary steroids, the mean 24-hr plasma progesterone range was elevated to 193−468 ng/dl, whereas the urinary pregnanetriol and 17-KS values were elevated. There were six prednisone schedules, however, in which the mean 24-hr progesterone value was greater than 193 ng/dl, while there were normal urinary 17-KS and pregnanetriol. In these studies, plasma progesterone could not be correlated with urinary 17-KS and pregnanetriol. These findings are in contrast with those of Lippe et al. (1974), who found a positive correlation between plasma progesterone values greater than 100 ng/dl and abnormal urinary 17-KS and pregnanetriol values. An attempt was made to correlate the plasma progesterone and 17-OHP concentrations, but no correlation was found. The correlation coefficient was 0.19 in the correlation of mean 24-hr or 0900-hr samples of plasma progesterone with the corresponding 17-OHP concentrations.

Our last study correlated the mean 24-hr plasma testosterone with urinary 17-KS and pregnanetriol on each of the prednisone schedules. Urinary 17-KS values were elevated in four instances, and in three of these four instances the plasma testosterone concentration was less than or equal to 40 ng/dl. Therefore, no correlation could be made. In four of the six patients, testosterone values were in the prepubertal range under all prednisone schedules (i.e., ≤35 ng/dl), whereas the 17-KS and pregnanetriol excretions were normal.

These studies were unable to correlate the amount of prednisone required with the degree of control. The patient with the lowest total dosage per day (4.2 mg/m^2/day) was in good control on all schedules, and a patient on one of the highest dosages per day (7.5 mg/m^2/day) was in poor control during two of the three prednisone schedules. No correlation could be made of the dosages required to control salt losers as compared to non-salt-losers.

CONCLUSIONS

Although this report concerns only six CVAH patients, the following conclusions can be made:

1. Prednisone at 1800 or 2000 hr q.d. produced adequate control in only two out of six patients.

2. Prednisone administered b.i.d. at 12-hr intervals, either as equally divided dosages or with the larger dose in the evening, produced adequate control in six out of six patients.

3. A mean 24-hr plasma 17-OHP concentration greater than 320 ng/dl or 0900-hr plasma 17-OHP concentration greater than 800 ng/dl correlated with elevated urinary pregnanetriol determinations.

4. Plasma 17-OHP concentrations were elevated more frequently than was urinary pregnanetriol excretion.

5. Plasma progesterone concentrations did not correlate with plasma 17-OHP or urinary 17-KS and pregnanetriol excretion.

6. Plasma testosterone concentrations did not correlate with plasma 17-OHP or progesterone concentrations.

REFERENCES

Atherden, A., M. Barnes, and D. Grant. 1972. Circadian variation in plasma 17-hydroxyprogesterone in patients with congenital adrenal hyperplasia. Arch. Dis. Child. 47:602–604.

Bartter, F. C., A. P. Forbes, and A. Leaf. 1950. Congenital adrenal hyperplasia associated with the adrenogenital syndrome: an attempt to correct its disordered hormonal pattern. J. Clin. Invest. 29:797–802.

Lippe, B. M., S. H. LaFranchi, N. Lavin, A. Parlow, S. Coyupta, and S. Kaplan. 1974. Serum 17-hydroxyprogesterone, progesterone, estradiol, and testosterone in the diagnosis and management of congenital adrenal hyperplasia. J. Pediatr. 85:782–787.

Strott, C. A., T. Yoshimi, and M. B. Lipsett. 1969. Plasma progesterone and 17-hydroxyprogesterone in normal men and children with congenital adrenal hyperplasia. J. Clin. Invest. 48:930–935.

Varma, M. M., R. R. Varma, A. J. Johanson, A. Kowarski, and C. J. Migeon. 1975. Long-term effects of vasectomy on pituitary-gonadal function in man. J. Clin. Endocrinol. Metab. 40:868–871.

Wilkins, L., R. A. Lewis, R. Klein, and E. Rosemberg. 1950. The suppression of androgen secretion in a case of congenital adrenal hyperplasia. Bull. Johns Hopkins Hosp. 86:249–252.

A Chronobiological Approach to the Treatment of Congenital Adrenal Hyperplasia

Walter J. Meyer, III, James P. Gutai, Bruce S. Keenan,

Gerry R. Davis, A. Avinoam Kowarski, and Claude J. Migeon[1]

The clinical management of patients with congenital adrenal hyperplasia (CAH) requires periodic 24-hr urine collections, which are inconvenient, inaccurate, and often necessitate hospitalization. The purpose of this study was to determine which adrenal hormone could be easily and accurately measured in plasma and which would also be representative of the adequacy of therapy. Meyer, Diller, and Bartter (1972) reported that, even during treatment, urinary 17-ketosteroids (17-KS) of CAH patients had a diurnal variation. Therefore, careful attention was given to circadian rhythm with the goal of finding a plasma steroid which would not fluctuate markedly throughout a 24-hr period and hence would allow evaluation at any time during the day. In this study, 17α-hydroxyprogesterone (17-OHP), the precursor of urinary pregnanetriol, and androstenedione, one of the precursors of urinary 17-KS, were the plasma adrenal steroids measured. It was observed that plasma concentration of androstenedione correlated better with urinary 17-KS than did plasma levels of 17-OHP. Furthermore, plasma androstenedione showed less fluctuation throughout the day and may, therefore, be a useful tool in assessing the therapy of CAH.

PATIENTS

Patients were admitted to the Pediatric Clinical Research Unit at the Johns Hopkins Hospital. All patients except the infants ate three meals a day and had

This work was supported by Research Grants R01-HD-06-284 and AM-00180 and Traineeship Grant T1-AM-5219 from the National Institutes of Health, United States Public Health Service. Patients were studied at the Clinical Research Center of the Department of Pediatrics, the Johns Hopkins Hospital, supported by Grant 5-M01-RR-0052 from the General Clinical Research Centers Program of the Division of Research Resources, the National Institutes of Health, United States Public Health Service.

The following trivial names are used: 17α-hydroxyprogesterone, 17-hydroxypregn-4-ene-3,20-dione; androstenedione, androst-4-ene-3,17-dione; progesterone, pregn-4-ene-3,20-dione; and pregnanetriol, 5β-pregnane-3α,17,20α-triol.

[1] Recipient of Research Career Award 5K06-AM-21855 from the National Institutes of Health, United States Public Health Service.

normal wake-sleep periods, with sleep commencing between 9 p.m. and midnight and arousal between 7 and 9 a.m. Table 1 contains a profile of each patient—his sex, age, treatment (per m^2 body surface area, in equivalent dose of oral cortisone acetate for 24 hr), urinary 17-KS and duration of study. Patients 1–10 ranged in age from 9–17 years 4 months, and in surface area from 0.96–1.74 m^2. They had been treated for time periods of at least 9 years, and their therapy was equal to the replacement dose in most cases. The duration of study was 10–24 hr in all but one subject who was studied only for 4 hr. Two patients (1 and 2) were studied first on oral therapy, then while on intramuscular therapy every 3rd day. Patient 11, a 29 years 6 months-old female, had urinary 17-KS levels ranging from 30.1–45.9 mg/24 hr and pregnanetriol levels ranging from 7.4–49.9 mg/24 hr and had never been treated.

Two young children (A and B), ages 4 months and 1 year 3 months, were studied on a different protocol. Because of their small body size, blood samples were drawn every 4–8 hr, and the concentrations of progesterone, 17-OHP, and androstenedione were determined. Both patients received adequate replacement therapy (I.M. cortisone acetate every 3rd day, calculated in accordance with their surface area).

Table 1. Profiles of patients studied

Patient	Sex	Age (years^{months})	Cortisone acetate[a] (mg/m^2/day)	Urinary 17-KS (mg/day)	Duration of study (hr)
1	M	10^1	27.3	21.1	24
		11^3	28.6[b]	7.3	24
2	F	15^8	35.0[c]	16.3	15
		16^1	26.0[b]	5.7	24
3	M	13^8	31.3	12.3	25
4	F	15^5	25.2	9.0	24
5	M	11^5	26.4[d]	3.4	25
6	F	17^4	18.7	3.8	22
7	F	9^0	26.0	6.3	16
8	F	14^3	20.8	39.2	10
9	M	11^8	27.0[c]	4.0	12
10	M	11^8	22.7	12.2	4
11	F	29^6	Untreated	35.7	24
A	M	0^4	36.9[b]	2.4	72
B	F	1^3	23.8[b]	0.6	72

[a]Equivalent oral dose.
[b]Given as intramuscular cortisone acetate.
[c]Given as hydrocortisone.
[d]Given as prednisone.

METHODS AND MATERIALS

As previously described, a nonthrombogenic catheter was inserted into an antecubital vein and connected to a portable pump that withdrew blood at a constant rate of 6 ml/hr (Kowarski et al., 1971). The blood was collected in 60-min aliquots, on ice, and the plasma was separated within 1 hr of collection. The carbon tetrachloride extract of the plasma was chromatographed on a Sephadex LH-20 column eluted with 5% methanol in benzene. Fractions containing androstenedione, progesterone, and 17-OHP were analyzed by radioimmunoassay with the use of specific antibodies for each (Gutai et al., 1975). Antibodies were obtained by conjugating the 3-ketone of the steroids to bovine serum albumin.

Urinary 17-KS were determined on 4-hr fractions collected on the day of constant blood withdrawal. They were analyzed by the Zimmermann reaction (Callow, Callow, and Emmins, 1938). Pregnanetriol levels were determined by the method of Bongiovanni and Eberlein (1958).

RESULTS

The integrated concentrations of plasma 17-OHP and androstenedione for the total period of study were compared with the corresponding 24-hr urinary

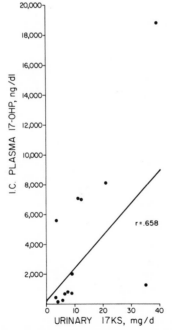

Figure 1. Integrated concentration of plasma 17-OHP versus 24-hr urinary 17-KS in 11 CAH subjects.

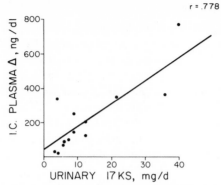

Figure 2. Integrated concentration of plasma androstenedione (Δ) versus 24-hr urinary 17-KS in 11 CAH subjects.

17-KS (Figures 1 and 2). The 24-hr integrated concentrations of plasma 17-OHP and androstenedione were both significantly correlated with the 24-hr urinary excretion of 17-KS, but the correlation of plasma androstenedione and 17-KS excretion was greater ($r = 0.778$, $p < 0.01$) than that of plasma 17-OHP ($r = 0.658$, $p < 0.05$). In spite of these correlations, patient 6 had high plasma

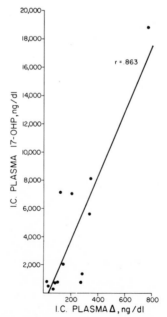

Figure 3. Integrated concentrations of plasma 17-OHP versus integrated concentration of plasma androstenedione (Δ) in 11 CAH subjects.

Table 2. Variations of plasma concentrations of hormones throughout 24 hr

Patient	Plasma 17-OHP (ng/dl)		Plasma androstenedione (ng/dl)	
	1-hr I.C.[a]	24-hr I.C.	1-hr I.C.	24-hr I.C.
1	867–16,285	8,274	200–473	344
	113–5,398	791	40–243	103
2	318–3,416	746 (15-hr)	168–508	276 (15-hr)
	37–1,735	254	56–137	72
3	2,258–11,550	7,009	122–318	203
4	303–4,703	2,120	72–254	143
5	25–4,700	477	25–66	33
6	321–13,512	5,613	159–533	337
7	117–1,679	709 (16-hr)	52–141	88 (16-hr)
8	10,339–28,554	18,840 (10-hr)	572–962	767 (10-hr)
9	40–206	82 (12-hr)	19–33	25 (12-hr)
10	5,371–9,141	7,163 (4-hr)	100–143	123 (4-hr)
11	201–8,276	1,341	121–605	286
A infant	840–14,015	(6,017)	82–752	(362)
B infant	1,612–21,878	(12,381)	60–175	(123)
Normal male	39–220	109	50–136 (95)[b]	
Normal female	11–285 (98)[c]		111–288 (180)[b]	
Prepubertal	10–77 (37)[d]		(21)[b]	

[a]I.C., integrated concentration.
[b]Range and mean (Migeon, 1972).
[c]Range and mean (Abraham et al., 1971).
[d]Range and mean (Gutai et al., 1975).

androstenedione and 17-OHP with normal 17-KS. The integrated concentrations of plasma 17-OHP and androstenedione were closely correlated ($r = 0.861, p < 0.001$), as shown in Figure 3. This would be expected, because 17-OHP is the immediate biosynthetic precursor of androstenedione.

The variation of the plasma concentrations of these hormones throughout the day is shown in Table 2. All but one patient with CAH had 24-hr integrated concentrations of plasma 17-OHP which were above the normal range. Two young children, ages 4 months and 1 year 3 months, had 17-OHP fluctuations as wide as those of the older patients. Their determinations were made on single samples over a 3-day period, and their mean value was not an integrated concentration. These mean concentrations were much greater than the mean level for normal prepubertal children.

As shown in Table 2, the 1-hr integrated concentration of plasma androstenedione in both female and male patients had fewer fluctuations than did 17-OHP and was in the normal range in six patients. Both young children had markedly elevated androstenedione for their age. The degree of diurnal variation of the 1-hr integrated concentration of plasma in all patients ranged from 1.5- to 5-fold and was smaller than the 10- to 50-fold variation for 17-OHP. Insertion of

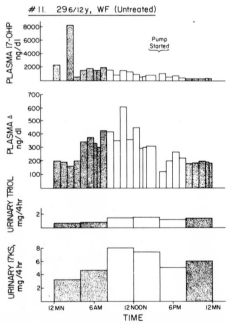

Figure 4. Circadian pattern of plasma 17-OHP, plasma androstenedione (Δ), urinary pregnanetriol (*triol*), and urinary 17-KS in a 26½-year-old untreated CAH female (patient 11). *Shaded areas* denote night.

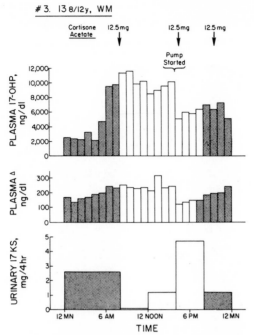

Figure 5. Circadian pattern of plasma 17-OHP, plasma androstenedione (Δ), and urinary 17-KS in a treated 13 years 8 months-old CAH male (patient 3). *Shaded areas* denote night.

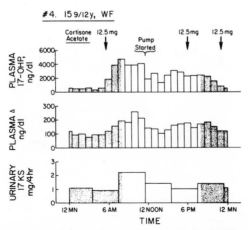

Figure 6. Circadian pattern of plasma 17-OHP, plasma androstenedione (Δ), and urinary 17-KS in a treated 15 years 9 months-old CAH female (patient 4). *Shaded areas* denote night.

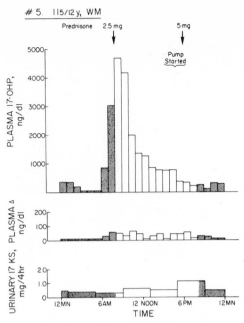

Figure 7. Circadian pattern of plasma 17-OHP, plasma androstenedione (Δ), and urinary 17-KS in a treated 11 years 5 months-old CAH male (patient 5). *Shaded areas* denote night.

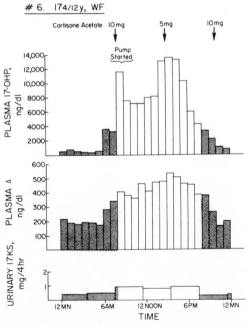

Figure 8. Circadian pattern of plasma 17-OHP, plasma androstenedione (Δ), and urinary 17-KS in a treated 17 years 4 months-old CAH female (patient 6). *Shaded areas* denote night.

the constant withdrawal catheter did not influence the concentrations of any of the hormones measured.

The pattern of variation of the plasma androstenedione and 17-OHP of untreated patient 11 is shown in Figure 4. She had a much higher 1-hr integrated concentration of 17-OHP in the early morning hours than in the afternoon and early evening, but her plasma androstenedione was highest around noon. The urinary pregnanetriol and 17-KS excretion peaked in the middle of the day.

A similar diurnal pattern with bursts of steroid secretion was also observed in treated patients (Figures 5–8). In all, the 17-OHP had a much greater variation than did androstenedione. In one study (Figure 7), plasma 17-OHP ranged from normal to 200 times normal levels; by contrast, plasma androstenedione varied only 2-fold and was in the normal range for the entire period. This particular patient was in good control by all parameters measured, with the exception of plasma 17-OHP between 7 and 10 a.m.

The diurnal patterns of plasma 17-OHP and androstenedione were synchronous ($p < 0.01$). All studies showed a rise in plasma 17-OHP between 5 and 7 a.m., which was a few hours later than the time of 17-OHP rise in normal subjects (Gutai et al., 1975) and also later than the highest concentration observed in the untreated subject. The relatively late normal surge of plasma

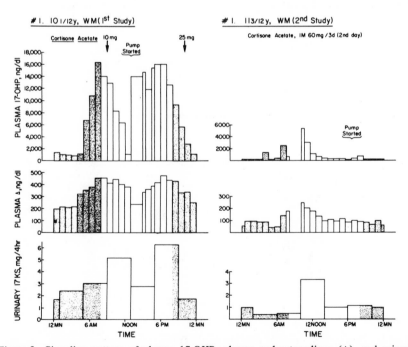

Figure 9. Circadian pattern of plasma 17-OHP, plasma androstenedione (Δ), and urinary 17-KS for a CAH male (patient 1) treated with oral cortisone acetate (*left*) and intramuscular cortisone acetate every 3rd day (*right*). *Shaded areas* denote night.

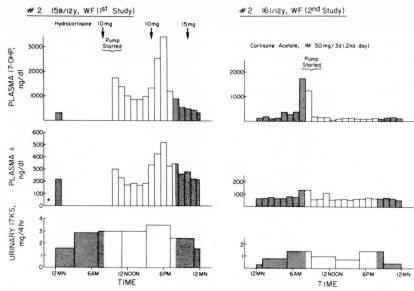

Figure 10. Circadian pattern of plasma 17-OHP, plasma androstenedione (Δ), and urinary 17-KS for a CAH female (patient 2) treated with oral hydrocortisone (*left*) and with intramuscular cortisone acetate every 3rd day (*right*). *Shaded areas* denote night.

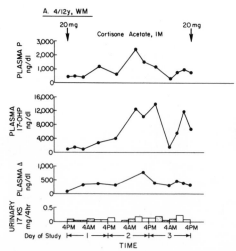

Figure 11. Plasma progesterone, (*P*), plasma 17-OHP, plasma androstenedione (Δ), and urinary 17-KS measured every 4–8 hr for 3 days between successive doses of intramuscular cortisone acetate in a 4-month-old CAH male (patient A).

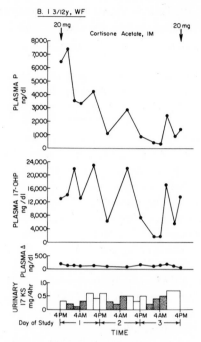

Figure 12. Plasma progesterone (*P*), plasma 17-OHP, plasma androstenedione (Δ), and urinary 17-KS measured every 4–8 hr for 3 days between successive doses of intramuscular cortisone acetate in a 1 year 3 months-old CAH female (patient B).

17-OHP and androstenedione is similar to the relatively late peak in urinary 17-KS excretion observed in treated patients by Meyer et al. (in press). Perhaps treatment altered the diurnal rhythm of adrenal function in these patients.

Two patients were studied on two treatment regimens—oral medication and intramuscular medication every 3rd day. Both patients were in much better control while taking the intramuscular medication. In spite of that, a diurnal pattern in plasma concentrations of 17-OHP and androstenedione was evident during both types of treatment (Figures 9 and 10).

The two youngest children were studied with single plasma samples drawn every 4–8 hr and, therefore, diurnal patterns could not be analyzed (Figures 11 and 12). In these studies, the androstenedione had fewer fluctuations than progesterone and 17-OHP. These variations during the 3-day study period are similar to the variation seen in the other patients during 1 day.

DISCUSSION

Elevated values of plasma 17-OHP concentration have been reported in patients with CAH (Barnes and Atherden, 1972; Simopoulos et al., 1971; Strott,

Yoshimi, and Lipsett, 1969). Subsequent reports (Atherden, Barnes, and Grant, 1972; Lippe et al., 1974), as well as the present study, have demonstrated a marked circadian variation (10- to 50-fold changes) of plasma 17-OHP in subjects with CAH. This contrasts with a 2- to 3-fold variation in normal men (Gutai et al., 1975). The variation was present in all patients studied, regardless of the degree of clinical control, as judged by the excretion of urinary 17-KS, suggesting that plasma 17-OHP levels are probably a poor index of clinical control.

Plasma concentrations of androstenedione are elevated in patients with CAH (Horton and Frasier, 1967; Rivarola, Saez, and Migeon, 1967). Androstenedione is probably the result of the conversion of 17-OHP (Loriaux, Ruder, and Lipsett, 1974) and, hence, the high correlation between plasma levels of 17-OHP and levels of androstenedione. The proportionally higher levels of plasma 17-OHP when compared to androstenedione may be related to the faster clearance of 17-OHP from the plasma (Horton and Frasier, 1967; Strott, Yoshimi, and Lipsett, 1969) or to a rate-limiting conversion of 17-OHP to androstenedione. There are no reports of circadian studies of plasma androstenedione in normal subjects or patients with CAH. Our study demonstrates that plasma androstenedione has much less diurnal variation than 17-OHP and has a better correlation than 17-OHP with urinary 17-KS. Plasma androstenedione is also not immediately affected by a dose of medication.

The concentration of plasma 17-OHP is an excellent indicator of 21-hydroxylase deficiency and is usually elevated at some time during the day even in well controlled patients. Androstenedione is secreted in large amounts in CAH patients and contributes 50% or more of the blood production of testosterone (Rivarola, Saez, and Migeon, 1967). Because androstenedione plays an important role in the excessive virilization in CAH and because its levels fluctuate less than those of 17-OHP, it may be a useful parameter in evaluating treatment of CAH patients.

REFERENCES

Abraham, G. E., R. S. Swerdloff, D. Tulchinsky, K. Hooper, and W. D. Odell. 1971. Radioimmunoassay of plasma 17-hydroxyprogesterone. J. Clin. Endocrinol. Metab. 33:42–46.

Atherden, S. M., N. D. Barnes, and D. B. Grant. 1972. Circadian variation in plasma 17-hydroxyprogesterone in patients with congenital adrenal hyperplasia. Arch. Dis. Child. 47:602–604.

Barnes, N. D., and S. M. Atherden. 1972. Diagnosis of congenital adrenal hyperplasia by measurement of plasma 17-hydroxyprogesterone. Arch. Dis. Child. 47:62–65.

Bongiovanni, A. M., and W. R. Eberlein. 1958. Critical analysis of methods for measurement of pregnane-3-alpha,17-alpha,20-alpha-triol in human urine. Anal. Chem. 30:388–393.

Callow, N. H., R. K. Callow, and C. W. Emmins. 1938. Colorimetric determination of substances containing the grouping—CH_2—CO—in urine extracts as an indication of androgen content. Biochem. J. 32:1312—1331.

DeLacerda, L., A. Kowarski, and C. J. Migeon. 1973. Integrated concentrations and diurnal variation of plasma cortisol. J. Clin. Endocrinol. Metab. 36:227—238.

Gutai, J. P., W. J. Meyer, A. Kowarski, and C. J. Migeon. 1975. Circadian variation of 17-hydroxyprogesterone (17-OHP); progesterone (P) and cortisol (F) in the plasma of normal adult male subjects. Cronobiologia 2 (Suppl. 1):26.

Horton, R., and S. D. Frasier. 1967. Androstenedione and its conversion to plasma testosterone in congenital adrenal hyperplasia. J. Clin. Invest. 46: 1003—1009.

Kowarski, A., R. G. Thompson, C. J. Migeon, and R. M. Blizzard. 1971. Determination of integrated plasma concentrations and true secretion rates of human growth hormone. J. Clin. Endocrinol. Metab. 32:356—360.

Lippe, B. M., S. H. LaFranchi, N. Lavin, A. Parlow, J. Coyotupa, and S. A. Kaplan. 1974. Serum 17α-hydroxyprogesterone, progesterone, estradiol and testosterone in the diagnosis and management of congenital adrenal hyperplasia. J. Pediatr. 85:782—787.

Loriaux, D. L., H. J. Ruder, and M. B. Lipsett. 1974. Plasma steroids in congenital adrenal hyperplasia. J. Clin. Endocrinol. Metab. 39:627—630.

Meyer, W. J., E. C. Diller, and F. C. Bartter. 1972. The circadian periodicity of urinary 17-ketosteroids in congenital adrenal hyperplasia. Endocrinology 32 (Abstr.).

Meyer, W. J., E. C. Diller, F. C. Bartter, and F. Halberg. The circadian periodicity of urinary 17-ketosteroids in congenital adrenal hyperplasia. J. Clin. Endocrinol. Metab., in press.

Migeon, C. J. 1972. Adrenal androgens in man. Am. J. Med. 53:606—626.

Rivarola, M. D., J. M. Saez, and C. J. Migeon. 1967. Studies of androgens in patients with congenital adrenal hyperplasia. J. Clin. Endocrinol. Metab. 27: 624—630.

Simopoulos, A. P., J. R. Marshall, C. S. Delea, and F. C. Bartter. 1971. Studies on the deficiency of 21-hydroxylation in patients with congenital adrenal hyperplasia. J. Clin. Endocrinol. Metab. 32:438—443.

Strott, C. A., T. Yoshimi, and M. B. Lipsett. 1969. Plasma progesterone and 17-hydroxyprogesterone in normal man and children with congenital adrenal hyperplasia. J. Clin. Invest. 48:930—939.

Corticotropin-Releasing Hormone–Adrenocorticotropin Suppression by an Antiandrogenic Drug (Cyproteronacetate)
A Therapeutic Possibility for Congenital Adrenal Hyperplasia

Jürg Girard and Joyce B. Baumann

Therapy and control of patients with congenital adrenal hyperplasia (CAH) are mainly complicated by two problems: first, life-threatening crises of salt loss, induced by stress situations, appear in individual patients with or without a primary salt-losing form of CAH; and second, continuous androgen production is suppressed without the use of an overdose of cortisol. Although virilization in girls is usually well controlled, the achievement of an adequate growth rate is difficult. An impaired adult height prognosis can result from excessive bone maturation or excessive suppression of bone maturation.

These complications are presumed to be due to an insufficient suppression of adrenocorticotropic hormone (ACTH) secretion, which leads to ACTH stimulation of the enzyme-deficient adrenal cortex. The subsequent excessive secretion of androgenic steroids or the secretion of competitive inhibitors of aldosterone or both results in salt-losing crises.

Cyproteronacetate (CA) is a powerful antiandrogenic and progestogenic drug (Neumann and Steinbeck, 1974a). It is assumed that its inhibition of luteinizing hormone and follicle-stimulating hormone secretion is mediated through the progestogenic action (Neumann and Steinbeck, 1974b). A competitive receptor inhibition of androgens explains why its antiandrogenic action (Walsh and

Supported by Schweiz National fonds Credit No. 3. 0690. 73.

217

Korenman, 1970) is mainly peripheral. The drug is currently used in psychiatry in sexual deviation (Laschet and Laschet, 1971) and in pediatrics in precocious puberty (Rager et al., 1973). It has also been used for the treatment of hirsutism (Braendle et al., 1974).

In precocious puberty, Cyproteronacetate can certainly suppress the development of secondary sex characteristics both in boys and in girls. The dose is around 75–100 mg/m^2/day. Whether or not the acceleration in bone maturation in these cases can be inhibited is not yet settled (Bossi, Joss, and Zurbrügg, 1973; Helge, 1973).

In the experience of these authors, weakness and striking fatigability are reported in many of the children treated with CA. This observation and the known adrenal-suppressing effect of progestational agents (Sadeghi-Nejad, Kaplan, and Grumbach, 1971) lead to the suspicion of adrenal insufficiency induced by CA. Findings in an individual girl are shown in Figure 1. A decrease in free urinary cortisol excretion, low morning plasma cortisol and ACTH values, and an impaired response of plasma cortisol to exogenous ACTH are general findings in the majority of children treated with CA for precocious puberty. A diminished

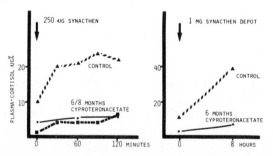

Figure 1. Free urinary cortisol excretion before and after 2, 8, and 12 months of treatment with CA in a girl with precocious puberty. Random morning plasma cortisol and ACTH values before and 3 and 12 months after starting therapy are given. The graphs (*bottom*) give the plasma cortisol response to synthetic 1–24 ACTH (Synacthen (*left*) and to a Synacthen Depot preparation (*right*). The patients' values are compared to control values in children of similar age.

response of plasma cortisol to ACTH has been reported in similarly treated patients (Bossi, Zurbrügg, and Joss, 1973). Early animal experiments demonstrated a decreased adrenal weight in CA-treated rats (Hamada, Neumann, and Junkmann, 1963).

The above observations strongly suggested, therefore, an adrenal insufficiency induced by CA. Obviously, the most important question for the patients was whether or not stress-induced corticotropin-releasing hormone (CRH) or CRH-ACTH adrenal activity would be impaired in CA-treated patients. Only a dynamic test with a stimulation of CRH-ACTH adrenal activity, such as insulin-induced hypoglycemia, would possibly help to answer the question. For ethical reasons, an animal model was taken to investigate whether Cyproteronacetate treatment leads to an impaired ACTH secretion and consequently to impaired adrenocortical steroid secretion in response to stress.

EXPERIMENTAL PROTOCOL

Male albino rats, approximately 300 g in weight, were given a daily subcutaneous injection of Cyproteronacetate. Control rats were injected with saline solution

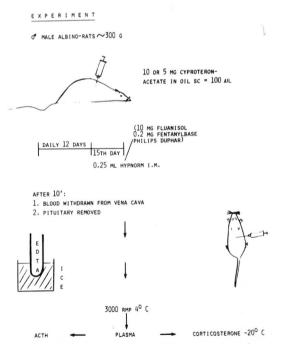

Figure 2. Flow sheet of the investigation protocol. A hypnorm injection was given 10–15 min before opening the abdominal cavity and bleeding the animal. This timing was found to give a reproducible stress reaction.

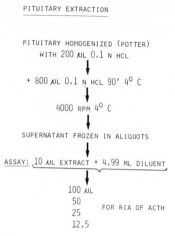

PITUITARY EXTRACTION

PITUITARY HOMOGENIZED (POTTER)
WITH 200 ᴫL 0.1 N HCL

+ 800 ᴫL 0.1 N HCL 90' 4° C

4000 RPM 4° C

SUPERNATANT FROZEN IN ALIQUOTS

ASSAY: 10 ᴫL EXTRACT + 4.99 ML DILUENT

100 ᴫL
50
25
12.5   FOR RIA OF ACTH

Figure 3. Pituitary extract procedure for ACTH content.

because the carrier oil was not available. Twenty-four hr after the last injection, the animals were anesthetized with "Hypnorm," administered intramuscularly. The abdominal cavity was opened 10–15 min after injection and trunk blood was collected in EDTA on ice, centrifuged at 4°C, and the supernatant plasma was frozen in aliquots for assays of ACTH and corticosterone. Plasmas were kept frozen at −20°C until assayed (Figure 2).

Animals were weighed daily from the beginning to the end of the experiment. Adrenal glands and pituitaries were removed at the end of the experiment and their weights related to the body weight of the animal. Pituitaries were

Table 1. Cross-reactivity of antiserum used in cortisol assay

	Percentage of cross-reaction
Corticosterone	89.0
20β-Hydroxyprogesterone	3.7
Progesterone	2.0
17-Hydroxyprogesterone	1.8
20α-Hydroxyprogesterone	1.8
Deoxycortisol	1.8
Aldosterone	1.6
Deoxycorticosterone	1.5
Cortisone	0.8
Tetrahydrocortisone	<0.1
Tetrahydrocortisol	<0.1
Tetrahydrodeoxycortisol	<0.1

submitted to a simple extraction procedure for measuring the pituitary ACTH content (Figure 3).

For studying the duration of treatment required to suppress ACTH secretion, rats were investigated daily after 1–12 injections. Animals were killed and investigated as above 24 hr after the last injection.

For the study of concomitant ACTH treatment, animals were studied in four different groups: saline control, Cyproteronacetate, ACTH "control," and Cyproteronacetate and ACTH. For the ACTH treatment, a synthetic α_1–24 preparation (Synacthen Depot, CIBA) was used in a dose of 100 μg daily, injected subcutaneously. In order to avoid a "contamination" of the circulating ACTH by exogenous Synacthen, the last ACTH injection was given 48 hr before killing the animal.

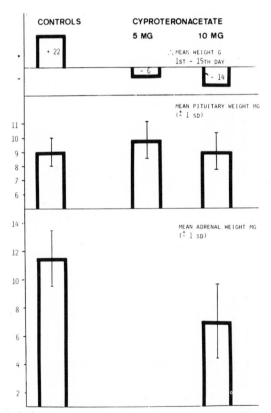

Figure 4. Body, pituitary, and adrenal weights of CA-treated rats. *Top,* mean difference in body weight from day 1 to day 15, six rats in each group; *middle,* mean ± 1 S.D. of pituitary weights in mg/rat, six rats in each group; *bottom,* mean ± 1 S.D. of adrenal weights in mg/100 g of rat, six rats in the control group and six rats after 10 mg of CA daily.

RADIOIMMUNOASSAYS

Synthetic human 1–39 ACTH (CIBA) was iodinated according to the method of Greenwood, Hunter, and Glover (1963), and labeled ACTH was purified on Quso (Berson and Yalow, 1968) with an additional purification step (adsorption to Florisil and elution with 0.1 N HCl) immediately before using the label in an assay. The antibody used was a gift from Professor Despieds, Marseilles, France, and has been characterized by Oliver (1971). Synthetic human 1–39 ACTH was used as a reference preparation. Dextran-coated charcoal was used for phase separation. Each plasma was assayed at three to four different dilutions.

For the corticosterone assay, a cortisol antiserum with the cross-reacting activities given in Table 1 was used. The assay was performed in duplicate or

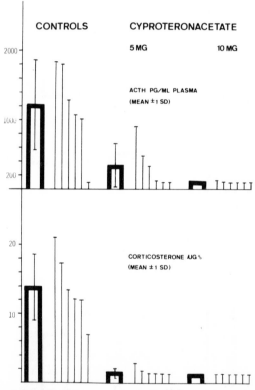

Figure 5. Mean and individual plasma concentrations for corticosterone and ACTH. *Top,* plasma ACTH concentrations in pg/ml (mean ± 1 S.D. and individual values). Controls, 1,215 ± 647.6 (range 100–1,830); CA (5 mg), 337.5 ± 315.9 (range ≤100–900); and CA (10 mg), 105.8 ± 10.2 (range ≤100–125). *Bottom,* plasma corticosterone concentration in μg% (mean ± 1 S.D. and individual values). Controls, 13.8 ± 4.8 (range 7–21). CA (5 mg), 1.6 ± 0.5 (range undetectable, ≤1.4–2.8); CA (10 mg), all undetectable, below sensitivity of the assay, 1.4 μg%.

triplicate. Charcoal dextran was used for the separation of bound and free fractions.

RESULTS AND DISCUSSION

As is evident from Figure 4, rats treated with CA gained less in body weight in comparison to the controls. No difference in pituitary weight was apparent. Adrenal weight in relation to body weight was found to be definitively diminished in CA-treated rats. Figure 5 gives the mean and individual plasma concentrations for corticosterone and ACTH. The stress response, due to hypnorm anesthesia and the blood sampling procedure described, is evident from the corticosterone and ACTH values in control rats. CA treatment with either 5 or 10 mg of CA/day over 14 days resulted in undetectable corticosterone concentrations. In

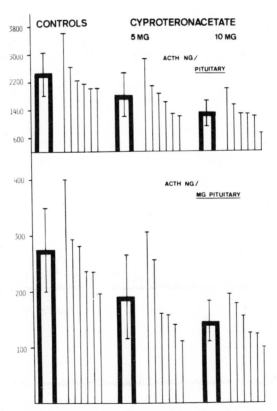

Figure 6. Pituitary ACTH content. *Top,* ng of ACTH/pituitary; *bottom,* ng of ACTH/mg of pituitary (mean ± 1 S.D. and individual values). Controls, 273 ± 71.6 ng/mg of pituitary (range 194–400); CA (5 mg), 190.7 ± 75.1 (range 111–309); CA (10 mg), 145.7 ± 36.3 (range 100–194).

some rats, an ACTH stress response is still evident, but the mean ACTH concentration and individual ACTH values are well below the controls among those treated with 10 mg.

The pituitary ACTH content in ng/mg of pituitary is shown in Figure 6. It is obvious that CA treatment not only inhibits ACTH secretion but also diminishes pituitary ACTH content after the 10-mg regimen.

From these experiments, it can be concluded that CA in a dose of 5 or 10 mg/rat applied over 14 days leads to adrenal atrophy and an impaired stress CRH-ACTH release and subsequently an impaired or absent corticosterone response.

For the investigation of the duration of treatment required to suppress CRH-ACTH adrenal activity, rats were similarly treated and investigated 24 hr after each injection. From Figure 7, it is apparent that two injections are sufficient to induce a diminished ACTH and corticosterone response to stress 24 hr after injection.

Analysis of the data from the experiments which used CA and ACTH treatment simultaneously requires a more complicated interpretation. From Figure 8 it can be seen that, compared to controls, body weight increased less in animals treated with CA or ACTH alone or in combination. ACTH treatment alone induced hypertrophy of the adrenal glands as judged by the weight in

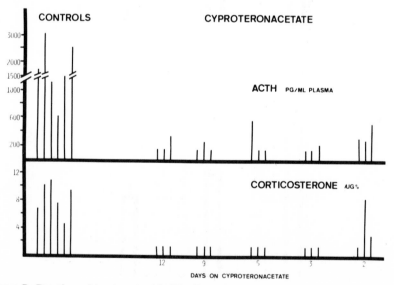

Figure 7. Duration of treatment with CA. *Top,* plasma ACTH in pg/ml; *bottom,* plasma corticosterone in μg%. Individual values in controls are given in comparison to values in response to the anesthesia and bleeding stress (see Figure 2) 24 hr after 12, 9, 5, 3, and 2 injections, respectively.

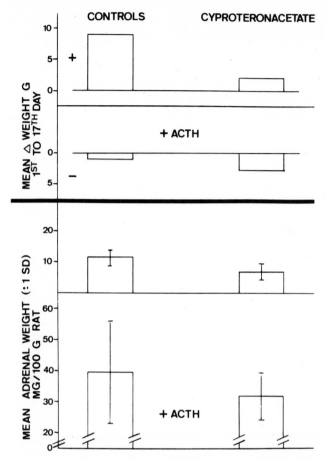

Figure 8. Effect of concomitant treatment with Cyproteronacetate (10 mg/day) and Synacthen (100 μg/day). *Top,* body weight change is the mean of the body weight increase (9.1 g) of six animals (range +3–+16). CA (10 mg). mean +2.1 g (range –4–+7); ACTH, mean –1 g (range +17– –12); CA and ACTH, mean – 2.8 g (range +9– –16). *Bottom,* mean adrenal weight in mg/100 g of rat ± 1 S.D. Controls, 11.5 ± 2 (range 8.5–14.7); CA (10 mg), mean 6.9 ± 2.7 (range 3.1–12.4); ACTH (100 μg), mean 39.5 ± 16.6 (range 24.5–74.2); CA and ACTH, mean 31.8 ± 7.6 (range 18–43.7).

relation to body weight; there was a less pronounced hypertrophy in animals treated concomitantly with ACTH and CA. Adrenal weights of these animals were above control weights, but below the adrenal weights of animals treated with ACTH only. Plasma ACTH concentrations in response to stress were impaired in animals treated with ACTH alone, as compared to controls. ACTH response to stress was practically absent in CA-treated rats and only slightly altered by a concomitant treatment with CA and ACTH. Plasma corticosterone concentrations were again inhibited in ACTH-treated animals, as compared to the controls. CA treatment completely abolished corticosterone response to stress. Simultaneous treatment with CA and ACTH could not restore the CRH-ACTH adrenocortical stress response (Figure 9). Results from these experiments suggest that under the experimental conditions ACTH can restore the adrenal weight but cannot restore the CRH-ACTH adrenal response to stress. This is probably due to a "Cushing's state" induced by the high dose ACTH

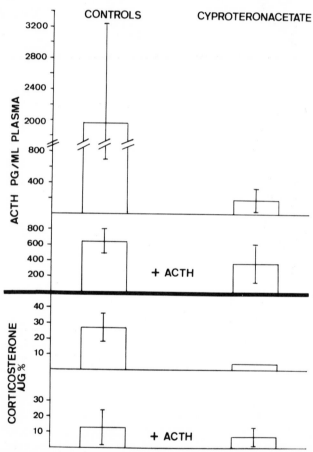

Figure 9. Effect of concomitant treatment with CA (10 mg) and ACTH (Synacthen, 100 μg). *Top*, plasma ACTH concentration in pg/ml (mean ± 1 S.D.). Controls, mean 1,960.6 ± 1,271.3 (range 320–3,380); CA (10 mg), mean 176.7 ± 153.9 (range 45–450); Synacthen, mean 644.8 ± 156.3 (range 496–940); CA and ACTH, mean 369.5 ± 247 (range 195–760). *Bottom*, plasma corticosterone measured in μg% (mean ± 1 S.D.). Controls, mean 27.3 ± 9.1 (range 13–36); CA (10 mg), mean ≤4 μg% (range of animals was at or below lower limit of assay); ACTH, mean 12.8 ± 11.1 (range 4–31); CA and ACTH, mean 7.3 ± 6.3 (range 4–20).

treatment. A short loop feedback of exogenous ACTH on endogenous ACTH production and secretion must be considered.

A few data, which were available from children with congenital adrenal hyperplasia treated with CA, were analyzed in retrospect. In all cases, the indication for such a treatment was considerably advanced bone age. The purpose of the treatment, therefore, was to suppress the plasma androgenic activity by the antiandrogenic action due to a peripheral receptor inhibition of CA. From six patients treated with CA, the best example is shown in Figure 10. At diagnosis, the girl showed advanced bone age and was initially overtreated with cortisone. The cortisone dose was reduced subsequently and secondary sexual characteristics began to develop. Urinary pregnanetriol and ketosteroid excretion were not suppressible to levels judged to indicate a well controlled state. These

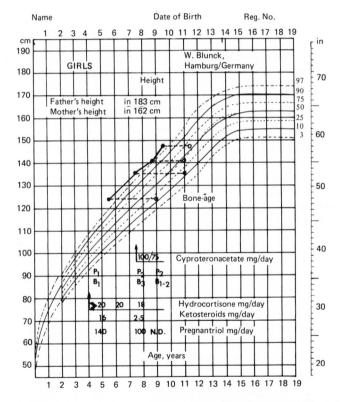

Figure 10. Growth, bone age, puberty ratings, ketosteroid and pregnanetriol excretion in a girl (patient of Professor W. Blunck, Hamburg, Germany) treated initially with hydrocortisone only and at the age of 7½ years with Cyproteronacetate. The decrease in bone age acceleration after CA treatment and in ketosteroid and pregnanetriol excretion is evident. (ND = nondetectable.)

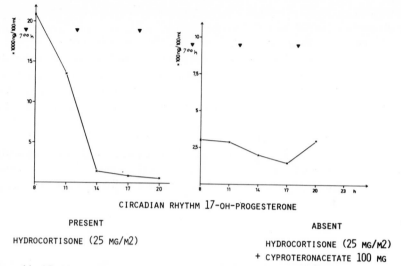

CIRCADIAN RHYTHM 17-OH-PROGESTERONE

PRESENT

HYDROCORTISONE (25 MG/M2)

ABSENT

HYDROCORTISONE (25 MG/M2)
+ CYPROTERONACETATE 100 MG

Figure 11. 17α-Hydroxyprogesterone concentration in plasma throughout the day in two patients with CAH receiving an equal amount of hydrocortisone, divided into three doses. *Left,* patient receiving hydrocortisone only; *right,* patient receiving hydrocortisone and CA. (Data from Petrykowski, 1975.)

findings together with the very rapid bone maturation were the indication for Cyproteronacetate therapy. Secondary sex characteristics diminished and bone age advanced very slowly over the next treatment period. This, together with the height velocity judged as normal for bone age, considerably improved the adult height prognosis. An indication for the ACTH-suppressive effect of CA in CAH is given by a series of patients described by Petrykowski. Under a treatment of 20 mg of hydrocortisone/m^2/day, all patients investigated showed a more or less marked circadian rhythm of plasma 17α-hydroxyprogesterone. The one patient showing no circadian rhythm and low 17α-hydroxyprogesterone values was under simultaneous treatment with hydrocortisone and CA (Figure 11).

CONCLUSIONS

ACTH-dependent steroid secretions from enzyme-deficient adrenals in CAH are the pathogenetic factors causing the difficulties in the control of CAH patients, as opposed to simple adrenal insufficiency, which is much easier to manage. It is for these reasons that a surgical adrenalectomy can be considered for treatment of CAH. As an alternative, a chemical adrenalectomy using aminoglutethimide may be considered. If ACTH must be suppressed by the glucocorticoid therapy alone, a dose somewhere between a replacement and an excess has to be carefully adjusted to each patient's "sensitivity" to glucocorticoids in respect to the ACTH-suppressive effect. Furthermore, an unforeseen stressful event will lead to an endogenous ACTH secretion with its consequences. It is unquestionable that an efficient, reversible suppression of ACTH secretion by another drug would help to solve some of the problems. Under an effective suppression of ACTH stimulation, glucocorticoid replacement could be applied in a dose equivalent to the daily requirement to substitute the lacking cortisol secretion. It would allow a circadian rhythm of cortisol application without the fear of rising ACTH concentrations during the night. Stress could be handled by increased cortisol alone, and the danger of salt-losing crises would be diminished.

Results presented in animal experiments provide evidence that CA is an effective drug for suppressing ACTH secretion. The dose used in rats is, however, well above the dose used in humans with precocious puberty or hypersexuality. Signs of ACTH suppression and subsequent secondary adrenal insufficiency are, however, evident in children treated with Cyproteronacetate in a dose of 75 mg/m^2/day. Furthermore, the antiandrogenic action of Cyproteronacetate is desirable during the most critical time of CAH treatment, that is, until early puberty, at which time, however, the gonadotropin-suppressive effect of CA would probably not allow a continuous treatment with the drug.

The mode of action of the ACTH-inhibiting effect of CA is unknown. A glucocorticoid-like effect of CA is present only in terms of adrenal involution and thymolysis in rats; other typical corticoid effects are lacking. Cyproteronacetate and Cyproterone do not have an antiphlogistic effect; they are not gluconeogenetic and do not lead to a reduction of the eosinophilic blood cell count (Neumann and Steinbeck, 1974c). There is no observation of a development of Cushingoid features, either in animals or in man. If its mode of action is to be looked for in the hypothalamic area, possible influences upon other releasing and inhibiting factors have to be investigated.

The present observations allow, however, the conclusion that CA, in addition to its powerful antiandrogenic action and its suppressive effect on gonadotropin secretion, is definitely capable of inhibiting ACTH production and secretion. The drug can, therefore, be used in CAH patients (who are difficult to control). Whether or not the drug is effective in limiting the speed of bone maturation in CAH remains to be shown. The drug itself or an analogue thereof could, however, provide a possible means of effectively and reversibly suppressing excessive or undesired ACTH secretion. Its application would not be limited to treatment of CAH.

Cyproteronacetate, by its androgenic action on one hand and more effectively by its ACTH-suppressive effect on the other hand, offers a therapeutic possibility in congenital adrenal hyperplasia.

ACKNOWLEDGMENTS

We gratefully acknowledge the technical assistance of S. Graf, G. van Hees, and M. Käslin.

REFERENCES

Berson, S. A., and R. S. Yalow. 1968. Radioimmunoassay of ACTH in plasma. J. Clin. Invest. 47:2725–2751.

Bossi, E., E. E. Joss, and R. P. Zurbrügg. 1973. Evaluation of the effectiveness of treatment on adult height prognosis in disorders with advanced and retarded bone age. Acta Paediatr. Scand. 62:401–404.

Bossi, E., R. P. Zurbrügg, and E. E. Joss. 1973. Cyproteronacetat und Pubertas praecox. Med. Mitt. Schering, Nr. 2. 19–25.

Braendle, W., H. Boess, M. Breckwoldt, C. Leven, and G. Bettendorf. 1974. Wirkung und Nebenwirkung der Cyproteronacetatbehandlung. Arch. Gynaekol. 216:335–345.

Greenwood, F. C., W. M. Hunter, and J. S. Glover. 1963. The preparation of ^{131}I-labeled human growth hormone of high specific radioactivity. Biochem. J. 89:114–123.

Hamada, H., F. Neumann, and K. Junkmann. 1963. Intrauterine antimaskuline Beeinflussung von Rattenfeten durch ein stark gestagen wirksames Steroid. Acta Endocrinol. 44:380–388.

Helge, H. 1973. Frühreife. Monatsschr. Kinderheilkd. 121:636–646.

Laschet, U., and L. Laschet. 1971. Psychopharmacotherapy of sexual offenders with cyproterone acetate. Pharmakopsychiatrie-Neuro-Psychopharmakologie 4:99–104.

Neumann, F., and H. Steinbeck. 1974a. Antiandrogen. In O. Eichler, A. Farah, H. Herken, and A. D. Welch (ed.), Androgens II and Antiandrogens: Handbook of Experimental Pharmacology, Vol. XXXV/2, Section VI, pp. 235–237. Springer, Berlin.

Neumann, F., and H. Steinbeck. 1974b. Neural-gonadal feedback system. In O. Eichler, A. Farah, H. Herken, and A. D. Welch (eds.), Androgens II and Antiandrogens: Handbook of Experimental Pharmacology, Vol. XXXV/2, Section VI, pp. 278–304. Springer, Berlin.

Neumann, F., and H. Steinbeck. 1974c. Fertility. In O. Eichler, A. Farah, H. Herken, and A. D. Welch (eds.), Androgens II and Antiandrogens: Handbook of Experimental Pharmacology, Vol. XXXV/2, Section VI, pp. 339–344. Springer, Berlin.

Neumann, F., and H. Steinbeck. 1974d. Various further effects of Antiandrogens (influence of cyproterone acetate on adrenal function). In O. Eichler, A. Farah, H. Herken, and A. D. Welch (eds.), Androgens II and Antiandrogens: Handbook of Experimental Pharmacology, Vol. XXXV/2, Section VI, 424–425. Springer, Berlin.

Oliver, C. 1971. Le Dosage Radio-Immunologique de l'A.C.T.H. Plasmatique. Ph.D. thesis, Faculté de Médecine, Marseilles, France.

Rager, K., R. Huenger, D. Gupta, and J. Bierich. 1973. The treatment of precocious puberty with Cyproterone Acetate. Acta Endocrinol. 74:399–408.

Sadeghi-Nejad, A., S. L. Kaplan, and M. M. Grumbach. 1971. J. Pediatr. 78:616–624.

Walsh, P. C., and S. G. Korenman. 1970. Action of antiandrogens: preservation of 5α-reductase activity and inhibition of chromatin-dihydrotestosterone complex formation. Clin. Res. 18:126.

LONG-RANGE FOLLOW-UP

Growth and Sexual Maturation in Treated Congenital Adrenal Hyperplasia

Songja Pang, Frederic M. Kenny, Thomas P. Foley, and Allan L. Drash

Since the institution of steroid therapy for the treatment of congenital adrenal hyperplasia (CAH) was reported in 1950 (Wilkins et al.), successful linear growth and normal sexual maturation in these patients have become the important aims of therapy. It is, therefore, worthwhile to review growth and development of children with CAH to establish the effects of long-term steroid therapy. Three important aspects of linear growth in the treatment of CAH previously have been reported: 1) the dosages of glucocorticoid hormones recommended in the earlier years were excessive, resulting in growth retardation (Raiti and Newns, 1971; Rappaport, Gornu, and Royer, 1968; Riddick and Hammond, 1975; Sperling et al., 1971); 2) the potent glucocorticoid hormones such as prednisone, prednisolone, dexamethasone, and triamcinolone caused greater growth suppression, despite normalization of androgen levels (Bailey and Komrower, 1974; Laron and Pertzelon, 1968; Stemfel et al., 1968); and 3) either excess (Rappaport et al., 1973) or inadequate treatment (Brook et al., 1974) ultimately may cause smaller stature.

Premature sexual maturation in CAH patients after the initiation of treatment was observed when the bone age was already advanced (Penny, Olambi-wonnu, and Frasier, 1973; Wilkins et al., 1951, 1952; Wilkins and Cara, 1954). In contrast, others have described decelerated maturation in similar cases (Bongiovanni, Moshang, and Parks, 1973). The problems of menarche, menses, and testicular function have been discussed (Grayzel, 1974; Jones and Verkauf, 1971; Molitor, Chestow, and Fariss, 1973), although more recently there are reports of successful pregnancies in treated patients (Mori and Miyakama, 1970; Riddick and Hammond, 1975). Nonetheless, normal growth and sexual maturation seem possible with early diagnosis and adequate therapy in CAH. Therefore, this study evaluates the following: 1) the effects of long-term steroid therapy on linear, skeletal, and sexual maturation in past and current medical control of the disease; 2) the effects of the age at which therapy began and the type of defect on subsequent growth and development; and 3) the possible factors of linear growth involved in the pubertal maturation in patients with CAH.

PATIENTS AND METHOD

Twenty-four adolescent or young adult patients, aged 12–20.6 years, with virilizing CAH due to 21-hydroxylase deficiency were retrospectively evaluated. The duration of follow-up was 7–20.5 years at Children's Hospital of Pittsburgh.

For both sexes, patients with salt-losing CAH comprise 60% of the total. Eleven females and six males were diagnosed before age 2 years, five males between ages 3 and 7 years, and two females at ages 7 and 13 1/2 years. The diagnosis was based on clinical and biochemical abnormalities, including elevated 24-hr urinary 17-ketosteroid and pregnanetriol, which were normally suppressed on glucocorticoid replacement therapy. All patients without palpable gonads had sex chromatin studies. The treatment consisted of either oral cortisone acetate (15–20 mg in two or three divided doses/day) or I.M. cortisone acetate (25 mg every 3 days below age 2 years), and, in the majority of patients, oral cortisone acetate (39 ± 11 $mg/m^2/24$ hr in two or three divided doses during prepuberty). Two patients were treated with prednisone in doses equivalent to cortisone acetate prior to the onset of puberty, and one patient received hydrocortisone. During and after the onset of puberty, half of the patients were receiving either prednisone (5–9 $mg/m^2/day$) or hydrocortisone (19–20 $mg/m^2/day$). The remainder of the patients received oral cortisone acetate in a dose of 28 ± 11 $mg/m^2/24$ hr after the onset of puberty. Clinical and biochemical assessments of the patients were evaluated every 6 months in most patients. Glucocorticoid dosage was adjusted to maintain the excretion of urinary 17-ketosteroids (17-KS) at less than 6 mg/24 hr prior to puberty and at less than 15 mg in females and 17 mg in males during puberty. However, these criteria were slightly modified later in order to allow catch-up or normal growth in some individuals. Urinary 17-ketosteroids were measured by the Zimmerman method without the Allen correction, and bone age was determined every 1–2 years by the hand and wrist standards of the Greulich and Pyle atlas (Greulich and Pyle, 1959). Height and weight age were determined by using the standard of Wilkins (1962). Stages of pubertal development were determined by the Tanner scale (Tanner, 1974).

The degrees of medical control of the patients were classified as good, fair, and poor by the following criteria: clinical growth rate, presence or absence of virilization and bone maturation, and 17-ketosteroid excretion. The patients under good control had a growth rate which was parallel to the normal percentile or an initially decreased growth rate followed by parallel growth, absence of virilization, bone age within 2 S.D. of chronological age, and a mean urinary 17-ketosteroid excretion determined from early age which was less than 6 mg/24 hr during prepuberty and less than 17 mg/24 hr after the onset of puberty. By contrast, the patients with acceleration of growth and bone maturation (bone age > 2 S.D. of chronological age) with or without presence of virilization and generally elevated urinary 17-ketosteroids were classified as poorly controlled. Those under fair control were between the good and poor group, clinically and

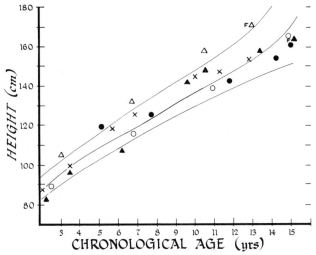

Figure 1. Representative growth curves of male patients in three degrees of control. △ and ▲, poor; ● and ○, good; X, fair; F, final height.

biochemically. Representative growth curves of actual patients are illustrated for the three different groups of patients (Figure 1). Biochemical studies and skeletal maturation in the group of patients classified according to the degree of control are shown in Table 1.

RESULTS

Linear and Skeletal Growth at Onset of Puberty in Total Group of Patients

In females, the mean age of onset of thelarche was 11.5 years (range 8.5–15) (Table 2). In males, the mean age of onset of increased testicular size was 11.6 years (range 9.4–13.5). These ages do not differ ($p > 0.1$) from the normal, as established by Marshall and Tanner (1969, 1970). The correlation between chronological, bone, weight, and height ages at onset of puberty and the degree of control (Figure 2) showed the normal chronological age range of thelarche and increased testicular size in all patients except three poorly controlled females. Height and weight ages were variable, as no correlation could be made with the degree of control. The definite abnormality was, however, the markedly advanced bone age in the poorly controlled patients. Skeletal ages in three girls were 14.5 years, >15 years, and 18 years at chronological ages of 11, 13.58, and 15 years, respectively, and in three males were 15, 16, and 16 years at chronological ages of 9.4, 10.3, and 10.5 years, respectively.

Table 1. Biochemical and skeletal maturation in the group of patients classified according to degree of control

Patients and degree of control	CA^a at time of analyses	Urinary 17-KS (mg/day)				Last growth determination		
		Prepuberty		Puberty		BA^a at CA		M-M
		Average	Range	Average	Range	BA^a	at CA	
Good								
Female								
Mc. E.	12.66	3.7	(0.8–8.2)	6.2	(4.6–8.0)	11.5	11.4	
W. K.	17.16	6.1	(2.5–12.6)	17.5	(8–28)	15	15.3	
W. L.	18.83	5.1	(2.1–6.1)	11.2	(5–13.6)			
Male								
M. R.	12.41	4.8	(4.4–5.5)	7.8				
F. J.	14.58	3.9	(1.6–5.8)	9.5	(9.1–10)			
S. D.	14.58	4.8	(2.4–7.5)	4.1		13	14.5	
Mc. J.	14.83	2.8	(2.2–3.5)	6.0	(5.1–7.9)	16	14.8	
Mean ± S.E.M.		4.4 ± 0.63		8.9 ± 1.32		13.8 ± 1	13.9 ± 0.85	−0.1
Fair								
Female								
M. J.	16	5.7	(1.6–15.4)	18.4	(10.4–22.6)	13.5	13.9	
S. M.	16	7.0	(3.0–12.2)	17.1	(12.4–20)	15	13.16	
G. L.	16.41	13.3	(3.8–26.5)	19.2	(4.2–49)	14	13	
Y. C.	17.5	3.1	(1.7–5.1)	18.7	(15–27)	12.5	11.5	
Male								
M. R.	12.0	6.1	(3.8–8.4)	28	(7–49)	12.5	10.9	
K. G.	12.58	7.5	(5.0–12)	10.3		13	12	
S. R.	17.5	7.5	(3.2–16.5)	22.5	(14.4–32)	15.5	15.5	
Mean ± S.E.M.		7.2 ± 1.14		19.1 ± 2.0		13.7 ± 0.3	12.9 ± 0.6	0.8

	CA		Poor medication		
Poor					
Female					
F.S.	12.0	6.4 (1.5–13.5)	13	15	11.6
W.E.	13.58	6.8 (4–9.6)	(11–15)[b]	15	13.6
		Medication at age 7			
H.P.	14.66	14.8 (7–26.3)	11.1 (7.8–16)[b]	18	13.16
W.M.	16		38.2 (14.6–64)	15	12.4
G.C.	17.66	No medication	17.9 (5.6–40.8)	18	13.5
Mc.G.	20.5		23.5 (7.1–52.6)	16	12.4
Male					
S.P.	16.91	34.4 (10–77)	41.6 (27.4–57.9)	17	14.9
M.J.	17.16	12.4 (3.4–25.3)	16.6 (9.0–23.6)	16	10.5
P.L.	20.58	9.1 (6.0–13)	19.5 (14–25)	15	11
S.J.	21.0	29.2	25.0 (15.2–39.8)	18	12.8
Mean ± S.E.M.	16.2 ± 1.84		23 ± 1.38	16.3 ± 0.42	12.5 ± 0.4 +3.7

[a]The abbreviations are as follows: CA, chronological age; BA, bone age.
[b]Despite normal range of 17-KS, clinically uncontrolled.

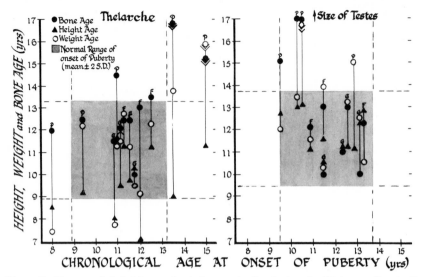

Figure 2. Linear and skeletal growth at the onset of puberty, classified according to the degree of control. ≪, same or greater; control G, good; F, fair; P, poor.

Linear and Skeletal Growth at Menarche

In four females, menarche occurred between the ages of 10 and 12.75 years, and, in five, between ages 13.6 and 16.7 years (Table 2). Two patients with ages greater than 16 years are still premenarchial. The mean menarchial age was statistically insignificant ($p > 0.05$), but was delayed when two premenarchial patients were included. The bone age and total body weight at menarche are illustrated with degree of control (Figure 3). All but one patient were within 2 S.D. of the normal critical body weight (Frisch and Revelle, 1971). However, six of eight patients had advanced bone age, particularly in poorly controlled patients at menarche. Bone ages in four patients with poor control were 15, >15, 16.8, and 18 years. The bone ages in two patients in good control and two in fair control were 12 and >15 and >13 and 15 years, respectively. Body composition, calculated as previously described (Crawford and Osler, 1975) and expressed as the percentage of fat weight of total body weight, was 33.5 ± 8.34 (2 S.D.). This is significantly greater than normal ($p < 0.05$), as reported by Crawford and Osler, 1975.

Menarchial Age and Gonadal Function with Degree of Control

Adequate comparison of menarchial ages among groups could not be made because of the limited number of patients with each degree of control (Table 3). However, only the poorly controlled patients had either menstrual abnormalities or small testicular size.

Table 2. Chronological age at onset of sexual maturation in total group of patients

| | Thelarche | | Menarche | | ↑ Testicular size | |
	Normal	Patient	Normal	Patient	Normal	Patient
Chronological age (Mean ± 2 S.D.)	11.15 ± 2.15 (n = 192)	11.5 ± 3.6 (n = 13)	12.9 ± 2.4	13.45 ± 4.26	11.64 ± 2.14 (n = 228)	11.7 ± 2.6 (n = 11)

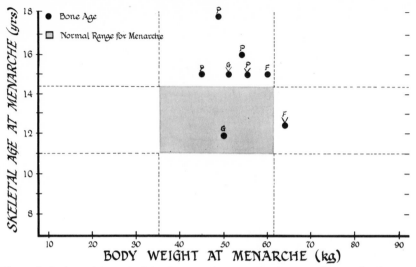

Figure 3. Body weight and skeletal maturation at menarche according to the degree of control. Control G, good; F, fair; P, poor.

Sexual Maturation According to Type of Defect (Salt Losers and Non-salt-losers)

The mean ages at onset of puberty in the patients with salt-losing CAH (11.68 ± 1.5 in females and 11.77 ± 1.2 in males) were the same as the ages in patients with non-salt-losing CAH (11.08 ± 2.3 in females and 11.73 ± 1 in males) (Table 4). The menarchial ages were the same for patients with salt-losing CAH (13.89 ± 2) and with non-salt-losing CAH (13.08 ± 2.4). Analysis according to early or late onset of therapy showed no differences in the ages of sexual maturation. However, because of the small series of late treated females, statistical comparisons were not possible.

Relationship Between Long-term Linear Growth and Degree of Control

The last height determination or the final height was compared to the corresponding chronological age and bone age (Figure 4). Final height was confirmed by x-ray by complete epiphyseal fusion or by growth arrest for more than 1 year in late adolescent patients. In all poorly controlled patients and in 7 of 14 patients in fair or good control, there was definite retardation of height age. In 12 patients (7 female, 5 male) whose growth had ceased, the mean final height was 147.7 cm (height age, 11.2 years) in females and 163.8 cm (height age, 13.8 years) in males. Eight poorly controlled patients reached final height between chronological ages 13–15.5 years in females and 12–16.8 years in males. Final heights occurred in late adolescence in four patients in good control, and their final height ages were greater than those of the patients in poor control.

Table 3. Gonadal maturation in group of patients classified by degree of control

Degree of control	Female			Male	
	Chronological age	Menarche	Menses	Chronological age	Current size
Good	12.66	Not yet		12.41	Normal
	17.16	12.33	Normal	14.58	Normal
	18.83	16.66	Normal	14.58	Normal
Mean ± S.D.		14.49 ± 3.06			
Fair	16	Not yet		12	Normal
	16	13.58		12.58	Normal
	16.44	Not yet	Moderately irregular	17.5	Small (on marihuana)
	17.5	16.58	Normal		
Mean ± S.D.		15.08 ± 2.12			
Poor	12	Not yet		16.91	Normal
	13.58	12.75	Second amenorrhea	17.16	
	14.66	10	Menorrhagia	20.58	Normal
	16	13.66	Second amenorrhea	21.08	Small
	17	13.66	Very irregular		
	20.5	11.75	Very irregular		
Mean ± S.D.		12.36 ± 1.54			

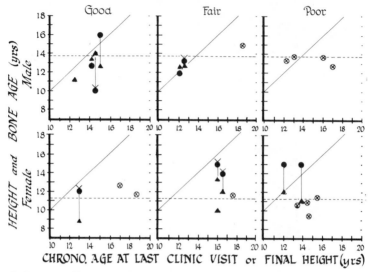

Figure 4. Long-term linear growth classified according to the degree of control. •, bone age; ▲, height age; ⊗, final height age; ——, 50th percentile; – – –, mean final height age; V, same or greater.

DISCUSSION

This study of growth and sexual maturation performed during long-range follow-up of our treated patients emphasizes the importance of adequate control in order to achieve a normal adult height and intact gonadal function. To date, glucocorticoid replacement therapy in amounts sufficient to suppress adrenal androgen secretion while allowing normal growth and sexual maturation is the only method of treatment widely employed in congenital adrenal hyperplasia. With early diagnosis and good control of the disease, normal growth and sexual maturation are possible, as seen in 50% of our patients in good control. Surprisingly, most of the poorly controlled patients who reached a short final height during early pubertal years were diagnosed at a young age. The families of these patients were in either a lower economic or intellectual group and had poor compliance. Therefore, early diagnosis and careful follow-up with good parent and patient education and cooperation are essential.

Recently Rappaport et al. (1973) have reported failure of catch-up growth with or without bone age retardation in the patients treated with excessive dosages of cortisol before age 18 months. The amount of glucocorticoid prescribed for patients in this study was gradually lowered throughout the years of follow-up, suggesting possible excess therapy in early years. In none of our patients was the bone age during adolescence more than 1.58 years below chronological age, suggesting that long-term therapy with excessive glucocorti-

Table 4. Sexual maturation in the group of patients

A. Salt loser versus non-salt-loser

| | Age of onset and follow-up | | | | |
| | Female | | | Male | |
Type	Thelarche (Mean ± S.D.)	Menarche (Mean ± S.D.)	Menses	Testes (Mean ± S.D.)	Current size
Salt loser	11.68 ± 1.5 (8)	13.89 ± 2 (4)	2 Abnormal	11.77 ± 1.2 (7)	1 small testes on drug
Non-salt-loser	11.08 ± 2.3 (4)	13.08 ± 2.4 (5)	2 Abnormal	11.72 ± 1 (4)	1 small testes

B. Early versus late initiation of therapy

| | Age of onset and follow-up | | | | |
| | Female | | | Male | |
Onset of therapy	Thelarche (Mean ± S.D.)	Menarche (Mean ± S.D.)	Menses	Testes (Mean ± S.D.)	Current size
<1 year	11.68 ± 1.5 (9)	13.7 ± 2.62 (6)	2 Abnormal	11.76 ± 1.06 (6)	1 small on drug
1.5 year	11 (1)	12.33 (1)	Very irregular		
3–4 years				11.24 ± 2.59 (2)	Normal
5–6 years				11.77 ± 1.25 (3)	1 small
7 years	8 (1)	12.75 (1)	Abnormal		
13.5 years	13.58 (1)	13.66 (1)	Very irregular		

coid dosage was less of a problem than inadequate suppression of androgens. Height age was significantly retarded ($p < 0.05$) below corresponding bone age and chronological age in 50% of patients in good or fair control. This effect may result from excessive steroid therapy during the first few years of life. However, genetic and constitutional factors and sensitivity of individuals to administered amounts of glucocorticoid therapy may be more important contributing factors in the attainment of final height, because seven other patients in good control showed parallel growth. The higher incidence of adrenal crises in salt losers did not have an effect on the age at which the various maturational events occurred. Thelarche and onset of testicular enlargement occurred at the expected chronological age in all but three poorly controlled patients in the study population. Therefore, prenatal or a mild degree of postnatal exposure to circulating androgen is not associated with early pubertal maturation. Previously, Wilkins et al. (1952) and Wilkins and Cara (1954) have reported the effect of cortisone therapy on the sexual maturation of the patient with late initiation of therapy; the onset of puberty in both sexes and menarche were established promptly when the bone age was advanced between ages of 11–14 years. Later, Penny, Olambiwonnu, and Frasier (1973) also reported a case of precocious puberty. However, Bongiovanni, Moshang, and Parks (1973) described an inconsistency of previous reports in which decelerated sexual maturation occurred in similar patients. Advanced bone ages at the onset of puberty were observed in our patients. It is of interest that the poorly controlled patients with similar heights or body weights when compared to the well controlled patients showed greatly advanced skeletal age at normal or delayed onset of puberty. The critical body weight and bone age have been reported as closely correlating factors at menarche. The body weights of our patients with CAH were within the range observed in normal controls in all except one patient. Bone age at normal menarche is not well established in American girls. However, in an English study, menarche occurred between bone ages 12–14.5 years, with highest correlation at 13–13.5 years, at mean menarchial age 13.4 years. This suggests that bone age is advanced and was not correlated with menarche in CAH patients in this study. Recently, Crawford and Osler (1975) revised the hypothesis of critical body weight at menarche and expressed body composition of fat as percentage of body weight. In patients in these studies, significantly greater fat weights were noted. However, total body weight was in the range of critical body weight observed by Frisch and Revelle (1971). This suggests either that critical body size may be an important factor or that the bone age is a much less reliable indicator of the onset of puberty and menarche when under the influence of excess adrenal androgens. Delayed menarche in girls with CAH in our limited number of patients is in accordance with the report of Jones and Verkauf (1971). However, their explanation for late onset of menarche was delayed maturation of bone age, an observation which differs from the data from these studies. Similarly, menarche might not be related to either bone age, body weight, or body composition. These factors may be secondary phenomena resulting from the hormonal and nutritional effects. Whether the delayed menarche in patients with CAH is a consequence of the prenatal exposure to excessive androgens which may have affected the programing of the CNS-hypothalamic-pituitary axis during fetal life or whether it is influenced by the elevated circulating androgens during postnatal life is not understood. Poor control resulted in abnormal menses or small testicular size in adolescent patients with CAH, and this observation suggests that an alteration of the hypothalamic-pituitary axis may be related to the persistent elevation of circulating adrenal sex hormones.

SUMMARY

The effect of long-term glucocorticoid therapy on linear growth of patients with CAH depends upon the degree of control. Thelarche and increase in testicular size occurred at the expected chronological age in the treated patient. Menarche, although delayed, seemed to correlate with body weight. Therefore, the prenatal and mild-to-moderate degree of postnatal exposure to elevated circulating androgens is not associated with early pubertal maturation. Poor control may primarily alter the secretory pattern of gonadotropins because of high adrenal androgens and may result in abnormal gonadal function in patients with CAH.

ACKNOWLEDGMENT

The authors wish to thank Lois R. Pischke for secretarial assistance.

REFERENCES

Bailey, C. G., and G. M. Komrower. 1974. Growth and skeletal maturation in congenital adrenal hyperplasia: review of 20 cases. Arch. Dis. Child. 49:4—7.

Bongiovanni, A. M., T. Moshang, Jr., and J. S. Parks. 1973. Maturational deceleration after treatment of congenital adrenal hyperplasia. Helv. Paediatr. Acta 28:127—134.

Brook, C. G., M. Zachmann, A. Prader, and G. Mürset. 1974. Experience with long term therapy in congenital adrenal hyperplasia. J. Pediatr. 85:12—19.

Crawford, J. D., and D. C. Osler. 1975. Body composition at menarche: the Frisch-Revelle hypothesis revisited. Pediatrics 56:449—458.

Frisch, R. E., and R. Revelle. 1971. Height and weight at menarche and a hypothesis of menarche. Arch. Dis. Child. 46:695—701.

Grayzel, E. F. 1974. Postpubertal adrenogenital syndrome: treatable cause of infertility. N. Y. State J. Med. June (4):1038—1039.

Greulich, W. W., and S. I. Pyle. 1959. Radiographic Atlas of Skeletal Development of the Hand and Wrist, Ed. 2. Stanford University Press, Stanford, California.

Jones, H., and B. Verkauf. 1971. Congenital adrenal hyperplasia: age at menarche and related events at puberty. Am. J. Obstet. Gynecol. 109:292—298.

Laron, Z., and A. Pertzelon. 1968. The comparative effect of 6 α-fluoroprednisolone, 6α-methylprednisolone, and hydrocortisone on linear growth of children with congenital adrenal virilism and Addison's disease. J. Pediatr. 73:774–782.

Marshall, W. A., and J. M. Tanner. 1969. Variation in pattern of pubertal changes in girls. Arch. Dis. Child. 44:291–303.

Marshall, W. A., and J. M. Tanner. 1970. Variations in the pattern of pubertal changes in boys. Arch. Dis. Child. 45:13–23.

Molitor, J. T., B. S. Chestow, and B. L. Fariss. 1973. Long term follow up of a patient with congenital adrenal hyperplasia and failure of testicular development. Fertil. Steril. 24(4):319–323.

Mori, M., and I. Miyakama. 1970. Congenital adrenogenital syndrome and successful pregnancy: report of a case. Obstet. Gynecol. 35:394–400.

Penny, R., O. Olambiwonnu, and S. D. Frasier. 1973. Precocious puberty following treatment in a six-year-old male with congenital adrenal hyperplasia: studies of follicle-stimulating hormone and plasma testosterone. J. Clin. Endocrinol. Metab. 36:920–924.

Raiti, S., and G. H. Newns. 1971. Linear growth in treated congenital adrenal hyperplasia. Arch. Dis. Child. 46:376.

Rappaport, R., G. Gornu, and P. Royer. 1968. Statural growth in congenital adrenal hyperplasia treated with hydrocortisone. J. Pediatr. 73:5, 760–766.

Rappaport, R., E. Bouthreuil, C. Marti-Hennelberg, and A. Basmaciogullari. 1973. Linear growth rate, bone maturation and growth hormone secretion in prepubertal children with congenital adrenal hyperplasia. Acta Paediatr. Scand. 62:513–519.

Riddick, D. H., and C. B. Hammond. 1975. Long term steroid therapy in patients with adrenogenital syndrome. Obstet. Gynecol. 45(1):15–20.

Sperling, M. A., F. M. Kenny, J. C. Schutt-Aine, and A. L. Drash. 1971. Linear growth and growth hormonal responsiveness in treated congenital adrenal hyperplasia. Am. J. Dis. Child. 122:408–413.

Stemfel, R. S., B. M. Shefkholislam, H. E. Leibowitz, E. Allen, and R. C. Franks. 1968. Pituitary growth hormone suppression with low-dosage long-acting corticoid administration. J. Pediatr. 73:767–773.

Tanner, J. M. 1974. Sequence and tempo in the somatic changes in puberty. In M. M. Grumbach (ed.), Control of the Onset of Puberty, pp. 448–470. A Wiley biomedical health publication.

Wilkins, L. 1962. The evaluation of the level of growth and development, standards for comparison. In The Diagnosis and Treatment of Endocrine Diseases in Childhood and Adolescence, Ed. 3, pp. 30–41.

Wilkins, L., and J. Cara. 1954. Further studies on the treatment of congenital adrenal hyperplasia with cortisone. V. Effects of cortisone therapy on testicular development. J. Clin. Endocrinol. Metab. 14:287–296.

Wilkins, L., R. A. Lewis, R. Klein, L. I. Gardner, J. F. Crigler, Jr., E. Rosenberg, and C. J. Migeon. 1951. Treatment of congenital adrenal hyperplasia with cortisone. J. Clin. Endocrinol. Metab. 11:1–25.

Wilkins, L., R. A. Lewis, R. Klein, and E. Rosenberg. 1950. The suppression of androgen secretion by cortisone in a case of congenital adrenal hyperplasia. Bull. Johns Hopkins Hosp. 86:249–252.

Wilkins, L., J. F. Crigler, Jr., S. H. Silverman. L. I. Gardner, and C. J. Migeon. 1952. Further studies on the treatment of congenital adrenal hyperplasia with cortisone. II. The effects of cortisone on sexual and somatic development with an hypothesis concerning the mechanism of feminization. J. Clin. Endocrinol. Metab. 12:277–295.

Growth Patterns in Congenital Adrenal Hyperplasia
Correlation of Glucocorticoid Therapy with Stature

Dennis M. Styne,[1] Gail E. Richards,[1] Jennifer J. Bell, Felix A. Conte,
Akira Morishima, Selna L. Kaplan, and Melvin M. Grumbach

Therapeutic use of cortisone acetate in congenital adrenal hyperplasia has favorably changed the natural history of the disease, but cortisone acetate can cause growth suppression, even if used in recommended doses. The optimal dosage of oral or intramuscular cortisone acetate was mainly established by the work of Wilkins and associates between 1951 and 1955 (Wilkins et al., 1954, 1955; Wilkins et al., 1952a, 1952b; Wilkins et al., 1951). Their recommendations were based upon the effects of cortisone treatment on the excretion of urinary 17-ketosteroids, rate of growth, bone maturation, and signs of virilization. Later, the use of potent cortisol analogues was described (Blizzard and Wilkins, 1957; Hubble, 1965; Laron and Pertzelan, 1968). However, information on the final heights achieved in treated patients is limited. Recently Brook et al. (1974) reported decreased final heights in children with congenital adrenal hyperplasia first treated after 1.3 years of age at the Children's Hospital of Zurich.

This study presents longitudinal growth data on patients with congenital adrenal hyperplasia who were treated during and after infancy, the effect of treatment upon final height, and an analysis of the dose of glucocorticoids necessary for optimal growth.

MATERIALS AND METHODS

Retrospectively, 39 patients (10 male and 29 female) with 21-hydroxylase deficiency, with or without the salt-losing variant, were studied for a minimum

[1] Recipient of a Research Fellowship in Pediatric Endocrinology from the National Institute of Arthritis, Metabolism, and Digestive Diseases and the National Institute of Child Health and Human Development, National Institutes of Health, United States Public Health Service.

This work was supported in part by grants from the National Institute of Child Health and Human Development and the National Institute of Arthritis, Metabolism, and Digestive Diseases, National Institutes of Health, United States Public Health Service.

Table 1. Patients with 21-hydrox-
ylase deficiency

	Male	Female
Patients Treated	10	29
Salt-losing	3	17
Non-salt-losers	7	12
Early treatment	4	21
Late treatment	6	8
Untreated	3	8

of 8 years prior to epiphyseal fusion (Table 1). Their ages at time of diagnosis ranged from 1 week to 9 years. The patients were seen every 3–6 months at Babies Hospital, Columbia Presbyterian Medical Center, or at the University of California, San Francisco, from 1955 to 1975. The patients received cortisone acetate, either orally or intramuscularly, hydrocortisone, prednisone, 6α-methyl-prednisolone, or dexamethasone. Twenty-four of the patients were changed from cortisone to at least one of the synthetic glucocorticoids during their treatment. Glucocorticoid dosage was adjusted to achieve normal linear growth, skeletal age (Greulich and Pyle, 1959) equal to chronological age, and urinary 17-ketosteroid excretion of 1 mg or less/24 hr/year of age up to 5 years, and normal excretion thereafter. Although some patients spent years under treatment at other centers, only the data obtained while they were attending our clinics were used.

Patients were divided into 25 early-treated children (started before 2 years of age) and 14 late-treated children (started after 2 years of age). The mean period of follow-up for the entire group was 11.8 years (12.5 years for the early-treated; 10.6 years for the late-treated group). Children with the salt-losing form, in addition to glucocorticoid treatment, were given deoxycorticosterone acetate by pellet or 9α-fluorohydrocortisone acetate and added salt in amounts sufficient to maintain the concentration of sodium and potassium within normal limits and to maintain a normal blood pressure.

Growth curves using the mean ± 1 S.D. of the pooled longitudinal patient data were plotted on growth charts drawn from the data of Simmons (1944) on normal boys and girls. Height velocity curves using the pooled patient data were drawn on the whole year height velocity standards of Tanner, Whitehouse, and Takaishi (1966). The annual height velocity was correlated with type and dose of glucocorticoid administered during that year.

Table 2. Mean final heights of early-treated, late-treated, and untreated patients

	Male		Female	
	cm ± 1 S.D.	No. of patients	cm ± 1 S.D.	No. of patients
Normal adults[a]	176.0 ± 6.5		163.0 ± 6.8	
Early-treated	164.7 ± 5.5	3	149.4 ± 9.0	9
Late-treated	158.3 ± 4.8	5	149.0 ± 6.3	7
Salt losers	164.6 ± 6.7	4	149.5 ± 8.3	9
Non-salt-losers	158.7 ± 4.6	4	151.2 ± 7.0	7
Untreated	153.5 ± 2.0	3	146.2 ± 7.2	8

[a]Hamill, Johnston, and Lemeshow (1973).

Final heights, available in 24 patients, were compared with those of 8 untreated females and 1 untreated male; 2 untreated males reported elsewhere (Brook et al., 1974) were also included (Table 2). The patients' final heights were compared with the mean and standard deviation of normal adult heights compiled by Hamill, Johnston, and Lemeshow (1973).

RESULTS

Figure 1 shows that early-treated girls grew in a normal manner at 1 S.D. below the mean until 10 years of age; subsequent growth slowed and ceased at 15

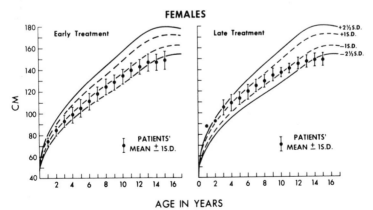

Figure 1. Growth data of girls with congenital CAH treated before and after 2 years of age, superimposed upon normal growth curves (Simmons, 1944).

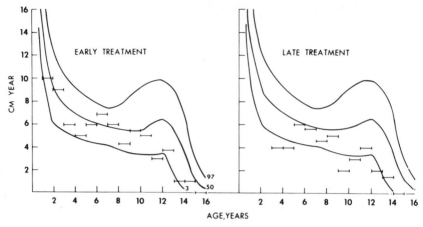

Figure 2. Height velocity charts derived from data in Figure 1, showing mean growth rate in cm/year. Each *bar* indicates the ages which start and end each annual period; the bars are superimposed upon Tanner's curves (Tanner, Whitehouse, and Takaishi, 1966) showing the mean, third, and ninety-seventh percentiles (or mean ± 1.9 S.D.) for normal height velocity for age. Note that growth ceased at 14–15 years.

years. The late-treated girls showed early excessive growth, with cessation of growth at 14 years. Both groups reached mean final heights of 149 cm (Table 2), which is 2 S.D. below the mean of normal adult female height (163 cm) and not significantly different from the untreated girls who reached 146 cm (2.5 S.D. below the mean).

One important difference between growth curves of our study group and the normal was the lack of or decreased pubertal growth spurt, best seen on the growth velocity curves in Figure 2. Normally, the peak height velocity occurs at about 12 years of age in girls, but a spread of individual patients' growth spurts over several years would spuriously decrease the peak height velocity on the

Table 3. Age at menarche of female patients with CAH[a]

Age	Menstruating	Not menstruating
13	5/17	12/17
14	6/17	11/17
15	9/13	4/13
16	9/13	4/13
17	9/12	3/12

[a]Mean age of menarche was 12.99 years ± 1.1 S.D.

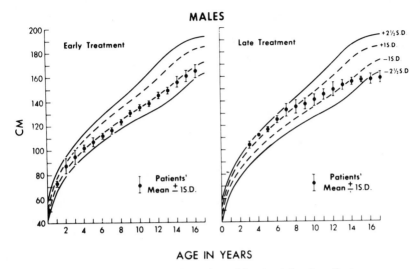

Figure 3. Growth curves for early- and late-treated male patients.

composite growth curve. Three factors are against this possibility as a major explanation: 1) skeletal age was comparable to chronological age in most cases, especially in early-treated girls; 2) the mean age of menarche (13 years) (Table 3) was close to the normal of menarche of 12.8 years (Zacharias, Rand, and Wurtman, 1976); and 3) blunted or absent growth spurts were noted on individual patients' growth velocity charts when plotted from longitudinal data (normally menarche follows peak height velocity by 1 year).

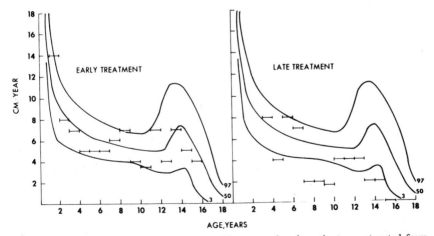

Figure 4. Height velocity charts for early- and late-treated male patients constructed from data in Figure 3.

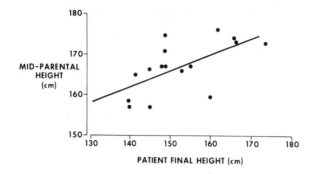

Figure 5. Relationship between each patient's final height and the average of their parental heights (mid-parental height). The linear regression line is determined by the method of lease squares. $r = 0.63$, $p < 0.01$.

The early-treated boys followed the growth curve of 1 S.D. below the mean, whereas late-treated boys showed early excessive growth and premature cessation of growth by age 15 years (Figure 3). Early-treated boys reached a final height of 164.7 cm (1.8 S.D. below the mean height for adult males), whereas late-treated boys reached a height of 158.3 cm (3.5 S.D. below the mean for normal boys).

Height velocity curves (Figure 4) show that late-treated boys had no significant growth spurt, whereas early-treated boys demonstrated a small growth spurt. However, statistical comparison is not possible, because there were only three early-treated boys studied through puberty.

There was a positive linear relationship (Figure 5) between final heights of 14 patients (12 girls and 2 boys) and the mean of the heights of their parents, where available (midparental height). The final height in all children was below the paternal height, and in 11 of 12 girls it was below the maternal height. Both boys' final heights were greater than maternal height, and in 1 boy and 11 girls it was below midparental height. The mean height of mothers was 163 cm (0.5 S.D. below normal mean female adult height) with a range of 150–173 cm; the mean height of fathers was 172.7 cm (0.5 S.D. below the normal mean of male adult height) with a range of 157–183 cm.

The estimated "optimal dose" of glucocorticoid necessary to produce height velocity closest to the normal for age was determined by comparison of height velocity with dose. There was considerable individual variation in response to glucocorticoids, as shown for oral cortisone (Figure 6, *A–D*), hydrocortisone (Figure 7), prednisone (Figure 8, *A* and *B*), 6α-methylprednisolone (Figure 9), and dexamethasone (Figure 10). The average estimated optimal dose for each glucocorticoid in terms of growth is listed in Table 4. For comparison, potencies in relation to anti-inflammatory effects are included.

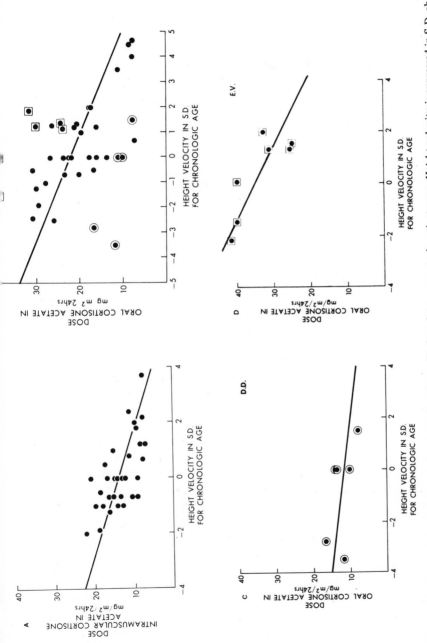

Figure 6. Height velocities of cortisone acetate–treated patients. Each *point* represents 1 patient year. Height velocity is expressed in S.D. above or below the mean for age (Figures 2 and 4). A *perpendicular line* from 0 S.D. or normal height velocity for age intercepts the *linear regression line* at a dose most closely associated with normal growth (estimated optimal dose). *A,* Estimated optimal dose of intramuscular cortisone acetate is 14 mg/m² /day. *r* = 0.66, *p* < 0.01. *B,* Estimated optimal dose of oral cortisone acetate is 22 mg/m² /day. *r* = 0.49, *p* < 0.01. *C,* Estimated optimal dose of a salt-losing female patient, noted with ○, is 11.6 mg/m² /day. *r* = 0.71, *p* < 0.05. *D,* Estimated optimal dose of a salt-losing female patient, noted with □, is 33.5 mg/m³ /day. *r* = 0.82, *p* < 0.01.

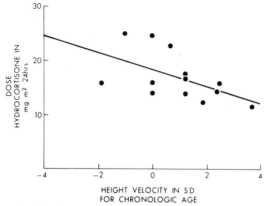

Figure 7. Estimated optimal dose of hydrocortisone is 18.4 mg/m^2/day. $r = 0.53, p < 0.05$.

DISCUSSION

Longitudinal Growth Data

Analysis of longitudinal growth data reveals several interesting and disquieting characteristics in these patients. The early-treated girls demonstrated a decreased pubertal growth spurt in spite of normal prepubertal growth, although no influence of treatment upon final height could be detected. The early-treated boys demonstrated better growth through the pubertal period than the girls, and their final heights were 10 cm greater than for untreated males. However, more male patients must be studied before the influence of treatment upon growth can be determined.

The cause of the blunted pubertal growth spurts is not clear. Because skeletal age was not significantly advanced over chronological age and neither excessive virilization nor elevation of urinary 17-ketosteroids was observed, it is unlikely that glucocorticoid treatment was inadequate. Also, the proportionate doses of glucocorticoids during the pubertal period were not larger than those given during the prepubertal period. Although none of the patients became Cushingoid, the doses could have been in excess of physiological requirements so that subtle overtreatment may have led to a diminished growth spurt.

Glucocorticoid Dosage

The growth velocity versus dose showed significant individual variation and the estimated optimal doses for growth (shown in Table 4) are general guidelines for each patient. However, the negative linear relationship between growth and dose in mg/m^2/day supports the use of dosage calculated in terms of body surface area rather than the usual recommendation of dose based on age (Wilkins et al., 1952 a and b; Hubble, 1965).

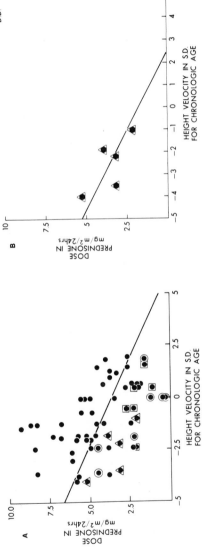

D.D.

Figure 8. *A,* Estimated optimal dose of prednisone is 3.7 mg/m³/day. $r = 0.55$, $p < 0.01$. Each of the three geometric shapes (□, ○, △) represents one of three patients who acquired doses of prednisone below the average for the group. *B,* Estimated optimal dose for a salt loser is 1.7 mg/m²/day. $r = 0.75$, $p < 0.01$. (This is the same patient shown in Figure 6c.)

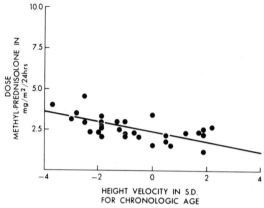

Figure 9. Estimated optimal dose of 6α-methylprednisolone is 2.4 mg/m²/day. $r = 0.65, p < 0.01$.

Synthetic glucocorticoids were used in many patients with the expectation that their slower metabolic clearance rates would allow the administration of fewer doses per day than is necessary for oral cortisone acetate and would thereby increase compliance. Furthermore, synthetic glucocorticoids contribute less to excretion of urinary 17-ketosteroids than equivalent doses of cortisone acetate. Parenthetically, these potent cortisol analogues are useful in the treatment of postmenarchial patients experiencing menstrual irregularity secondary to lack of adequate suppression of adrenal androgens on conventional cortisone therapy (Richards et al., 1976).

The present study shows that estimation of dosage of dexamethasone, prednisone, and 6α-methylprednisolone by the usual method (multiplying the

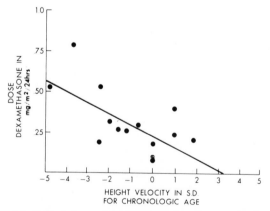

Figure 10. Estimated optimal dose of dexamethasone is 0.23 mg/m²/day. $r = 0.65, p < 0.01$.

Table 4. Mean estimated optimal doses for growth and relative potencies of growth effects and anti-inflammatory effects when compared to cortisone acetate

Glucocorticoid	No. of patients	Patient years	Mean estimated optimal dose (mg/m²/24 hr)	Relative potency of growth effects	Relative potency of anti-inflammatory effects[a]
Cortisone acetate (oral)	6	50	22.0	1	1
Cortisone acetate (intramuscular)	11	35	13.9	1.6	
Hydrocortisone	2	13	18.4	1.2	1.25
Prednisone	11	90	3.7	6	5
6α-Methylprednisolone	6	32	2.4	9	6.25
Dexamethasone	2	19	0.23	96	31.0

[a]Haynes and Larner (1975).

appropriate dose of cortisone by the ratio of anti-inflammatory or glucocorticoid effects between cortisone and the synthetic preparation) may lead to severe overtreatment. A dose of any of these three synthetic glucocorticoids, when compared with a dose of cortisone, shows a growth-suppressive effect out of proportion to the anti-inflammatory effect.

Data from these studies suggest that dexamethasone is 96 times more potent than cortisone acetate in its growth-suppressive effects, a ratio similar to that proposed by Wilkins (1965). This correlates with Van der Veer and Moolenaar's preliminary findings (1970) that dexamethasone is 100 times more potent than cortisone in reduction of androgenic substances in the urine of patients with congenital adrenal hyperplasia. However, it contrasts with data that indicate that dexamethasone is only 31 times more potent than cortisone in its anti-inflammatory effects (Haynes and Larner, 1975).

The mean estimated optimal dose of oral cortisone acetate in relation to growth is approximately double the cortisol secretion rate (Kenny et al., 1966), and the ratio of intramuscular to oral cortisone dosage is slightly higher than the 2–3:1 ratio suggested by Wilkins et al. (1952a and b). Our average optimal dose of 22 mg/m^2/day is in the range recommended by Migeon (1968), Sperling et al. (1971), and Raiti and Newns (1970), but it is lower than that suggested by Brook et al. (1974), as well as by Wilkins (1965) if the dosage he recommended is converted to mg/m^2/day. The dose of prednisone estimated in the present study is considerably lower than that recommended by Blizzard and Wilkins (1957). The mean optimal dose for growth of dexamethasone is 0.23 mg/m^2/day in this study and is lower than the dosage range recommended by Hubble (1965) which converts to approximately 0.55–1.4 mg/m^2/day.

Fine dosage adjustment is more crucial when potent synthetic glucocorticoids are used. Also, differences in the absorption of the preparations of various manufacturers have recently been documented for prednisone (Sullivan et al., 1975) and quite likely occur with the other glucocorticoids as well. This and other aspects of bioavailability could be responsible for some of the differences in individual sensitivity to glucocorticoid treatment.

The ideal of physiological replacement in congenital adrenal hyperplasia is far from being realized. In the normal individual cortisol is secreted episodically, with maximal secretion in the early morning near the time of awakening (4–8 a.m.) and minimal secretion in the late evening hours (Hellman et al., 1970; Krieger et al., 1971; Weitzman et al., 1971). A regimen of unequally split glucocorticoid doses, with the largest administered at night to suppress the early morning peak of adrenocorticotropic hormone, may seem advantageous in treating this disease. However, such a schedule may also suppress the peripheral effects of the nighttime peak secretion of growth hormone (Rudman et al., 1972). In addition, several daily doses of medication lead to a number of peak serum concentrations of glucocorticoid spaced throughout the day, in contrast to the cluster of secretory peaks over a period of less than 6 hr found in the normal (Hellman et al., 1970).

This retrospective study has limitations. Some patients were followed for years at other institutions before referral to the clinics in this study and inclusion in this treatment program. Compliance was assessed only by history and excretion of urinary 17-ketosteroids. No estimation was made of the effect of doubled or greater dosage during intercurrent illness.

These patients were among the first to be treated with glucocorticoids at a time when suppression of virilization was a predominant concern. Their final heights were decreased. The recognition that glucocorticoids may have more growth-suppressive than anti-inflammatory effects and that there is striking individual sensitivity to glucocorticoid dosage emphasizes the importance of maintaining growth velocity within the normal range by careful individualization of dosage if normal height is to be achieved.

SUMMARY

From a longitudinal analysis of children with congenital adrenal hyperplasia due to 21-hydroxylase deficiency treated with glucocorticoids, it was found that girls treated before (early-treated) or after 2 years of age (late-treated) reached a mean final height of 149 cm (2 S.D. below the normal mean), which is not significantly different from untreated girls, who reached a mean height of 146 cm (2.5 S.D. below the mean). Early-treated boys reached a mean final height of 164.7 cm (1.8 S.D. below the normal mean); late-treated boys reached 158.3 cm (2.8 S.D. below the mean); and untreated boys reached 153.5 cm (3.5 S.D. below the mean). In early-treated girls and late-treated boys and girls, pubertal growth spurts were diminished. Although much individual variation was noted, average doses most closely associated with optimal growth were estimated to be as follows (in $mg/m^2/24$ hr): cortisone acetate (oral), 22; cortisone acetate (intramuscular), 13.9; hydrocortisone, 18.4; prednisone, 3.7; 6α-methylprednisolone, 2.4; and dexamethasone, 0.23. The last three analogues were significantly more potent in their growth-suppressive effects than in their anti-inflammatory effects.

REFERENCES

Blizzard, R. M., and L. Wilkins. 1957. Present concepts of steroid therapy in virilizing adrenal hyperplasia. Arch. Intern. Med. 100:729–738.
Brook, C. G. D., M. Zachman, A. Prader, and G. Murset. 1974. Experience with long-term therapy in congenital adrenal hyperplasia. J. Pediatr. 85:12–19.
Greulich, W. W., and S. I. Pyle. 1959. Radiographic Atlas of Skeletal Development of the Hand and Wrist. Stanford University Press, Stanford, California.

260   Styne et al.

Grumbach, M. M., and L. Wilkins. 1956. The pathogenesis and treatment of virilizing adrenal hyperplasia. Pediatr. 17:418–427.

Hamill, P. V. V., F. E. Johnston, and S. Lemeshow. 1973. Height and weight of youths 12–17 years, United States. *In* Vital and Health Statistics, Series 11, No. 124, Department of Health, Education, and Welfare Publication No. (HSM) 73-1606.

Haynes, R. C., and J. Larner. 1975. Adrenocorticotropic hormone; adrenocortical steroids and their synthetic analogues; inhibitors of adrenocortical steroid biosynthesis. *In* L. S. Goodman and A. Gilman (eds.), Pharmacologic Basis of Therapeutics, Ed. 5. Macmillan Publishing Co., Inc., New York.

Hellman, L. F., J. C. Nakada, E. D. Weitzman, J. Kream, H. Roffwarg, S. Ellman, D. K. Fukushima, and T. F. Gallagher. 1970. Cortisol is secreted episodically by normal man. J. Clin. Endocrinol. Metab. 30:411–422.

Hubble, D. 1965. Retardation of skeletal maturation and linear growth in the treatment of the simple virilizing form of congenital adrenal hyperplasia. Aust. Paediatr. J. 1:84–92.

Kenny, F. M., C. Preeyasombat, C. J. Migeon, B. Lawrence, and C. Richards. 1966. Cortisol production rate. II. Normal infants, children and adults. Pediatrics 37:34–42.

Krieger, D. T., W. Allen, F. Rizzo, and H. D. Krieger. 1971. Characterization of the normal temporal pattern of plasma corticosteroid levels. J. Clin. Endocrinol. Metab. 32:266–284.

Laron, Z., and A. Pertzelan. 1968. The comparative effects of 6α-fluoroprednisolone, 6α-methylprednisolone and hydrocortisone on linear growth of children with virilizing congenital adrenal hyperplasia and Addison's disease. J. Pediatr. 73:774–782.

Migeon, C. J. 1968. Updating the treatment of congenital adrenal hyperplasia. J. Pediatr. 73:805–806.

Raiti, S., and G. H. Newns. 1970. The management of congenital adrenal hyperplasia. Br. J. Hosp. Med. 4:509–512.

Raiti, S., and G. H. Newns. 1971. Linear growth in treated congenital adrenal hyperplasia. Arch. Dis. Child. 46:376–378.

Rudman, D., D. Freides, J. H. Patterson, and D. L. Gibbas. 1973. Diurnal variation in the responsiveness of human subjects to growth hormone. J. Clin. Invest. 52:912–918.

Simmons, K. 1944. Physical Growth and Development. *In* the Brush Foundation Study of Child Growth and Development, Monograph 37. Society for Research in Child Development, National Research Council, Washington, D.C.

Smart, J. V. 1970. Elements of Medical Statistics, Ed. 2, pp. 73–78. Staples Press, London.

Sperling, M. A., F. M. Kenny, J. L. Schutt-Aine, and A. L. Drash. 1971. Linear growth and growth hormonal responsiveness in treated congenital adrenal hyperplasia. Am. J. Dis. Child. 122:408–413.

Sullivan, T. J., E. Sakmar, K. S. Albert, D. C. Blair, and J. G. Wagner. 1975. *In* vitro and in vivo availability of commercial prednisone tablets. J. Pharm. Sci. 64:1723–1725.

Tanner, J. M., R. H. Whitehouse, and M. Takaishi. 1966. Standards from birth to maturity for height, weight, height velocity, and weight velocity: British children, 1965. II. Arch. Dis. Child. 41:613–634.

Van der Veer, A. L. J., and A. J. Moolenaar. 1970. Some aspects of steroid therapy in congenital adrenal hyperplasia. J. Endocrinol. 48:lxxvii.

Weitzman, E. D., D. Fukushima, C. Nogeiro, H. Rowffwarg, T. F. Gallagher, and L. Hellman. 1971. Twenty-four-hour pattern of the episodic secretion of cortisol in normal subjects. J. Clin. Endocrinol. Metab. 33:14–22.

Wilkins, L. 1965. The Diagnosis and Treatment of Endocrine Disorders in Childhood and Adolescence, Ed. 3, p. 364. Charles C Thomas, Springfield, Illinois.

Wilkins, L., A. M. Bongiovanni, G. W. Clayton, M. M. Grumbach, and J. J. Van Wyk. 1954. The present status of the treatment of virilizing congenital adrenal hyperplasia with cortisone: experience of 3½ years. In Modern Problems in Pediatrics, Vol. 1, Suppl. and Annales Paed. pp. 329–345. S. Karger, New York.

Wilkins, L., A. M. Bongiovanni, G. W. Clayton, M. M. Grumbach, and J. J. Van Wyk. 1955. Virilizing adrenal hyperplasia: its treatment with cortisone and the nature of the steroid abnormalities. Ciba Found. Coll. Endocrinol. 8:460–481.

Wilkins, L., J. F. Crigler, S. H. Silverman, L. I. Gardner, and C. J. Migeon. 1952a. Further studies on the treatment of congenital adrenal hyperplasia with cortisone I and II. J. Clin. Endocrinol. Metab. 12:257–295.

Wilkins, L., J. F. Crigler, S. H. Silverman, L. I. Gardner, and C. J. Migeon. 1952b. Further studies on the treatment of congenital adrenal hyperplasia with cortisone III. J. Clin. Endocrinol. Metab. 12:1015–1030.

Wilkins, L., R. A. Lewis, R. Klein, L. I. Gardner, J. F. Crigler, E. Rosenberg, and C. J. Migeon. 1951. Treatment of congenital adrenal hyperplasia with cortisone. J. Clin. Endocrinol. 11:1–25.

Zacharias, L., W. M. Rand, and R. J. Wurtman. 1976. A prospective study of sexual development and growth in American girls: The statistics of menarche. Obstet. Gynecol. Survey 31:325–337.

Linear Growth and Suppressive Effects of Hydrocortisone and 9α-Fluorohydrocortisone in Long-term Therapy in Congenital Adrenal Hyperplasia

Raphael Rappaport and Jean-Marie Limal

Cortisone and hydrocortisone have generally been used to treat children affected with congenital adrenal hyperplasia (CAH) since the leading work of Wilkins et al. (1950) and Bartter, Forbes, and Leaf (1950). The object of this treatment is to suppress excessive adrenal androgen production and to compensate for the deficient cortisol production. Many pediatric endocrinology groups now have long-term experience in treating CAH, and partial or comprehensive evaluations of corticoid treatment have been published (Bergstrand, 1966; Brook et al., 1974; Laron and Pertzelan, 1968; Raiti and Newns, 1971; Rappaport et al., 1973; Rappaport, Cornu, and Royer, 1968; Sperling et al., 1971). These evaluations suggest that CAH is frequently overtreated, resulting in prepubertal growth retardation. Overtreatment is possible because the parameters used to assess adequacy of adrenal cortex suppression—urinary excretion of 17-ketosteroids and pregnanetriol—are poor indicators of overdosage. Evaluation of the results has generally been difficult because of methodological difficulties, differences in steroids used, and variations in patient compliance.

The present study involves a group of patients treated with oral hydrocortisone and evaluated regularly, who have been dealt with in two previous publications. The first (Rappaport, Cornu, and Royer, 1968) focused on infancy and demonstrated frequent overdosage with severe side effects on linear growth. The

This work was supported by the Institut National de la Santé et la Recherches Médicale, France, and by a grant from the Medical School (Conseil Scientifique de l'U.E.R. Necker, Enfants Malades, Paris, France, 1974).

second (Rappaport et al., 1973) showed that a normal growth rate was achieved in prepubertal children by limiting the dosage to 15–36 mg/m^2/24 hr (with a recommended dosage of less than 30 mg/m^2/24 hr). The purpose of the present investigation was 1) to assess the long-term effect of early overdosage with hydrocortisone, 2) to evaluate the use of hydrocortisone in late diagnosed cases, and 3) to describe the effects of 9α-fluorohydrocortisone (9α-FF) when this therapy was started in salt losers who had received no mineralocorticoids since the age of 2 or 3 years.

MATERIAL AND METHODS

Twenty-two children with congenital adrenal hyperplasia due to a 21-hydroxylation defect were studied. All patients received oral hydrocortisone with approximately two-thirds of the daily dose given in the evening. Dosage was adjusted by following the urinary pregnanetriol excretion. Our methods for assessing linear growth and bone maturation were published previously (Rappaport et al., 1973). Treatment was instituted after infancy in three children. One child, B. T., was followed for 12 years, until she had practically attained her final height at age 16 years. Changes in predicted final height were evaluated for each significant phase of the treatment, according to Bayley and Pinneau tables (Greulich and Pyle, 1959). Another child (S. B.) was a normal boy, erroneously diagnosed and treated with hydrocortisone and mineralocorticoids as a CAH patient. Eleven children were salt losers. They had been treated with the combined hydrocortisone-deoxycorticosterone regimen until the age of 2 or 3 years. Thereafter, they were maintained on hydrocortisone alone until the present study. The plasma 17-hydroxyprogesterone (17-OHP) and the urinary pregnanetriol excretion were measured before and 6 months after the reintroduction of 9α-FF (0.1 mg/24 hr, 0.05 mg b.i.d.).

RESULTS AND DISCUSSION

Effect of Early Hydrocortisone Overdosage on Linear Growth

Two groups of patients have been distinguished on the basis of the dosage of oral hydrocortisone received before the age of 18 months (Figure 1). Six children received hydrocortisone dosages of 30 mg/m^2/24 hr or less. In practice, they received 10 mg of hydrocortisone/24 hr during the first 6 months, and urinary pregnanetriol excretions remained within the normal range. Their growth curves were normal, and their mean heights remained close to the normal mean value when last measured. Another group of eight children received high doses of hydrocortisone (greater than 30 mg/m^2/24 hr) during the first 18 months. Their mean heights were significantly less than normal ($p < 0.001$) during the prepubertal period. In three cases (not shown on the figure), there has been no catch-up growth during puberty. It is unlikely that these children will attain a

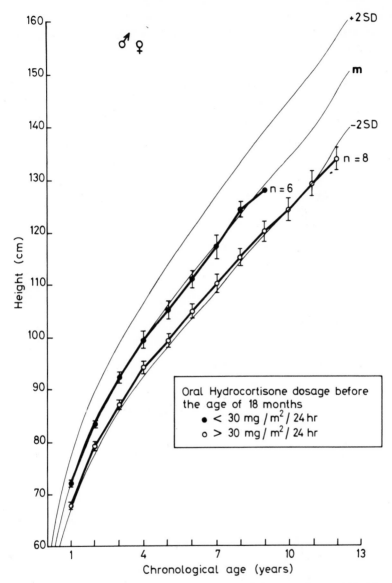

Figure 1. Mean growth curves for patients treated with hydrocortisone, divided into two groups on the basis of oral hydrocortisone dosages given before the age of 18 months.

normal final stature. After the age of 2 years, both groups of children received doses of oral hydrocortisone between 14 and 29 mg/m^2/24 hr. They showed good responsiveness, as demonstrated by the urinary pregnanetriol excretions, except for some salt losers who have shown only borderline suppression during the past 2 years (see under "Effect of 9α-Fluorohydrocortisone on Urinary

Pregnanetriol and Plasma 17-Hydroxyprogesterone"). This study shows that early overdosage is not followed by a complete catch-up growth even when the recommended average dose of hydrocortisone (25 mg/m²/24 hr) is used after the age of 18 months.

Growth processes are exquisitely sensitive to hydrocortisone, as shown in a normal child (Figure 2). Early overdosage provoked a retarded growth. Catch-up growth was seen when the daily dosage of hydrocortisone approached 20 mg/m²/24 hr. It is possible, but not proved by this single and unusual observation, that short stature (−1.5 S.D.) may result from the deleterious effect of hydrocortisone. This steroid acts at several levels: it reduces somatomedin

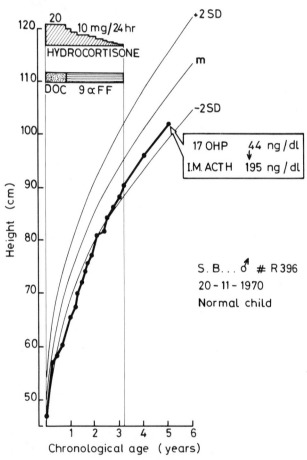

Figure 2. Normal child erroneously diagnosed and treated as a case of congenital adrenal hyperplasia who received more than 50 mg/m²/24 hr of hydrocortisone during the 1st year of life.

generation and it diminishes the effect of circulating somatomedin on proteo-glycan synthesis in cartilage (Daughaday, Herington, and Phillips, 1975). How-ever, a normal growth hormone response to arginine-insulin stimulation was reported with the range of hydrocortisone dosages used in this disease (Rappa-port et al., 1973), but plasma somatomedin activity was not measured at that time. It is also interesting that these patients showed increased plasma insulin responses to arginine infusion in relation to the dosage of hydrocortisone (Rappaport and Prevot, 1975). Mosier (1971) has shown that cortisone in rats

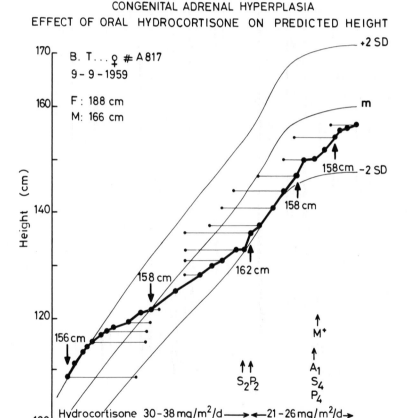

Figure 3. Growth curve and bone ages in a late diagnosed child with congenital adrenal hyperplasia. *Arrows* indicate the predicted final heights according to Bayley and Pinneau tables. *F* and *M* indicate father's and mother's heights. *P*, pubic hair stage; *A*, axillary hair stage; *M*, menses; *S*, size of breast.

permanently damages growth mechanisms and prevents catch-up growth. Alterations in chondrocyte structures have been observed (Dearden and Mosier, 1972). It is likely, but there is no direct evidence, that in some of the treated children growth mechanisms were similarly impaired at the hormone regulation level or in the epiphyseal cartilage, or in both.

Hydrocortisone Treatment in Late Diagnosed Cases

In children diagnosed after infancy, a rapid growth and bone maturation is observed. In such cases, higher doses of hydrocortisone—up to 45 mg/m^2/24

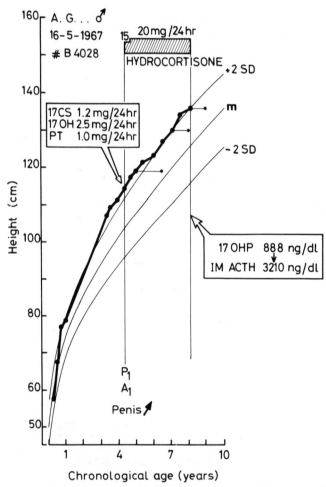

Figure 4. Late onset of virilization in a boy with enlarged penis as the unique clinical feature. *P*, pubic hair stage; *A*, axillary hair stage; 17-CS, 17-ketosteroids; 17-OH, 17-hydrocorticoids; PT, pregnanetriol.

hr—have been given. This treatment blocked bone maturation almost completely, but allowed slow linear growth over a period of several years. Height increments expressed per year of bone age maturation in two cases (B. T., represented in Figure 3, and another child) were 12 and 10 cm, respectively. The child B. T. was treated with "suppressive" doses of hydrocortisone (from age 4

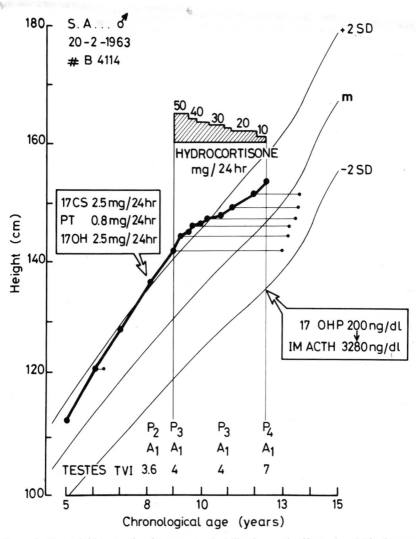

Figure 5. Natural history of a late onset of virilization and effect of variable doses of hydrocortisone on linear growth and bone maturation. *P*, pubic hair stage; *A*, axillary hair stage; 17-CS, 17-ketosteroids; PT, pregnanetriol; 17-OH, 17-hydroxysteroids.

until 11½ years) and followed until cessation of growth. As shown in Figure 3, the predicted final height according to Bayley and Pinneau tables varied between 156 and 162 cm. B. T. attained a height of 156.5 cm, demonstrating the difficulty in predicting precisely adult height in children with such gross abnormalities of bone maturation. The study of Brook et al. (1974) showed that the growth prognosis of late treated children was not improved by treatment. It is our impression that more potent corticoids or higher dosages—with the risk of severe side effects—should be avoided. Hydrocortisone remains the drug of choice in these cases with a dosage less than 40 mg/m^2/24 hr.

The delayed onset of symptoms in affected males may reflect a partial enzymatic defect. When urinary ketosteroids and urinary pregnanetriol are within the normal range or moderately increased, augmented plasma 17-OHP makes the diagnosis.

Case A. G. (Figure 4) was a cousin of a child with salt-losing CAH. This patient's only clinical sign at the age of 4½ years was an enlarged penis (60 mm stretched length) with normal testes. Urinary 17-ketosteroids were normal, and pregnanetriol was moderately increased. The child was treated with hydrocortisone, in spite of normal height and bone age. While on treatment, his basal plasma 17-OHP was 950 ng/100 ml and reached 3,250 ng/100 ml after adrenocorticotropic hormone (ACTH) stimulation (normal baseline = 54 ± 38 (S.D.) ng/100 ml, and 178 ± 102 ng/100 ml after 0.25 mg of I.M. ACTH).

Case S. A. (Figure 5) had normal bone age and height at the age of 6 years. Between 6 and 9 years of age, the bone age progressed dramatically by 6½ years. When first seen, his 17-ketosteroids and pregnanetriol were moderately increased. He was treated with the previously proposed hydrocortisone schedule. On this regimen, he recently showed a plasma 17-OHP of 200 ng/100 ml, which increased to 3,150 ng/100 ml on ACTH stimulation. It is remarkable that a daily dosage of 7 mg/m^2/24 hr for the last year allowed a normal rate of growth with normal urinary excretions of pregnanetriol. As seen in the two cases above, investigation of mild virilization in boys by measuring plasma 17-OHP should permit early diagnosis and treatment.

Effect of 9α-Fluorohydrocortisone on
Urinary Pregnanetriol and Plasma 17-Hydroxyprogesterone

Urinary pregnanetriol excretions may fluctuate in some hydrocortisone-treated children, especially in older children. Even in compliant patients it was difficult to correlate these fluctuations with precise situations, except that these patients were former salt losers. Their mineralocorticoid treatment had been interrupted at the age of 2 or 3 years, and they thereafter were receiving only hydrocortisone (19–25 mg/m^2/24 hr). Some of these children subsequently presented with severe salt depletion after episodes of vomiting or diarrhea. It was decided to resume the mineralocorticoid treatment in all salt losers (8 cases) by giving 0.1 mg of 9α-FF (0.05 mg b.i.d.). They were studied before and 6 months after the onset of 9α-FF therapy. Hydrocortisone dosages were not changed during that period. After 4 days in the hospital on a controlled sodium diet (5 mEq/kg/24 hr), plasma 17-OHP, aldosterone, and renin activity were measured at 8 a.m. Only the 17-OHP results are presented in this report. On hydrocortisone and 9α-FF, the mean (± 1 SEM) plasma 17-OHP value was 4,191 ± 2,173 ng/ml, which was significantly less than the value of 12,580 ± 1,481 ng/100 ml obtained during the previous period with hydrocortisone treatment only ($p <$ 0.01). A simultaneous decrease in urinary pregnanetriol excretions was observed, but the limited number of data obtained preclude a statistical evaluation.

First, these data suggest that replacement doses of 9α-FF were capable of suppressing endogenous ACTH release. Previous studies by Kley, Geisthövel, and Krüskemper (1973) have shown that a higher dosage of 9α-FF (a single dose of 0.9 mg in adults) could suppress the metyrapone-stimulated 11-deoxycortisol secretion. These authors claimed that this major mineralocorticoid also had significant glucocorticoid activity. The present study also points to such a dual activity of 9α-FF. Second, these studies suggest that in salt losers the combination of hydrocortisone and 9α-FF achieves better control of the disease and correction of a borderline electrolyte balance. It should be mentioned that these patients generally presented with augmented plasma renin activity, which indicated a failure to compensate for the salt-losing tendency (Limal, Bayard, and Rappaport, unpublished data). Further studies are required to assess the efficacy of treating all infants with a salt-losing syndrome with continuous mineralocorticoids. Cases with limited aldosterone response to either ACTH stimulation or a sodium restricted diet or augmented plasma renin activity with a normal sodium diet should benefit from 9αFF treatment. It is the impression of these authors that patients with a salt-losing tendency achieved better control of their disease and eliminated mild salt-losing crises when a potent mineralocorticoid was added to their hydrocortisone regimen.

REFERENCES

Bartter, F. C., A. P. Forbes, and A. Leaf. 1950. Congenital adrenal hyperplasia associated with the adrenogenital syndrome: an attempt to correct its disordered hormonal pattern. J. Clin. Invest. 29:797.

Bergstrand, C. G. 1966. Growth in congenital adrenal hyperplasia. Acta Paediatr. Scand. 55:463–472.

Brooks, C. G. D., M. Zachmann, A. Prader, and G. Murset. 1974. Experience with long term therapy in congenital adrenal hyperplasia. J. Pediatr. 85:12–19.

Daughaday, W. H., A. C. Herington, and L. S. Phillips. 1975. The regulation of growth by endocrines. Ann. Rev. Physiol. 37:211–244.

Dearden, L. C., and H. D. Mosier. 1972. Long-term recovery of chondrocytes in the tibial epiphyseal plate in rats after cortisone treatment. Clin. Orthop. 87:322–331.

Greulich, W. W., and S. I. Pyle. 1959. Radiographic Atlas of Skeletal Development of the Hand and Wrist, Ed. 2, pp. 231–251. Stanford University Press, Stanford, California.

Kley, H. K., W. Geisthövel, and H. L. Krüskempet. 1973. Effect of 9αfluoro-hydrocortisone on the hypothalamo-pituitary-adrenal axis. Acta Endocrinol. 73:417–426.

Laron, Z., and A. Pertzelan. 1968. The comparative effect of 6α-fluoropredniso-lone, 6α-methylprednisolone and hydrocortisone on linear growth of children with congenital adrenal virilism and Addison's disease. J. Pediatr. 73:774–782.

Limal, J. M., F. Bayard, and R. Rappaport. 1974. Plasma aldosterone and effect of ACTH in congenital adrenal hyperplasia, 21-OH deficiency. Pediat. Res. 9:681 (abstr.).

Mosier, H. D. 1971. Failure of compensatory (catch-up) growth in the rat. Pediatr. Res. 5:59–63.

Raiti, S., and G. H. Newns. 1971. Linear growth in treated congenital adrenal hyperplasia. Arch. Dis. Child. 46:376–378.

Rappaport, R., E. Bouthreuil, C. Marti-Henneberg, and A. Basmaciogullari. 1973. Linear growth rate, bone maturation and growth hormone secretion in prepubertal children with congenital adrenal hyperplasia. Acta Pediatr. Scand. 62:513–519.

Rappaport, R., G. Cornu, and P. Royer. 1968. Statural growth in congenital adrenal hyperplasia treated with hydrocortisone. J. Pediatr. 73:760–766.

Rappaport, R., and C. Prevot. 1975. Effect of glucose and arginine on insulin secretion in children on long-term treatment with oral hydrocortisone. In Diabetes in Juveniles. Modern Problems in Paediatrics, Vol 12, pp. 263–272. Karger, Basel.

Sperling, M. A., F. M. Kenny, J. C. Schutt-Aine, and A. L. Drash. 1971. Linear growth and growth hormonal responsiveness in treated congenital adrenal hyperplasia. Am. J. Dis. Child. 122:406–413.

Wilkins, L., R. W. Lewis, R. Klein, and E. Rosemberg. 1950. The suppression of androgen secretion in a case of congenital adrenal hyperplasia. Bull. Johns Hopkins Hosp. 86:249–252.

Long-term Follow-up of Patients with Congenital Adrenal Hyperplasia in Houston

Rebecca T. Kirkland, Bruce S. Keenan, and George W. Clayton

In this clinic, 34 children with the 21-hydroxylase form of congenital adrenal hyperplasia (CAH) have been followed until they attained mature height. These children, who have had the benefits of available replacement therapy, were evaluated to determine patterns of linear growth, complications of therapy, and social development. From this study, it is hoped that recommendations for guidelines of therapy will be generated.

PATIENTS

Mature height is that height which is maintained for at least 1 year concomitant with a skeletal age of 18 years or greater. The 34 children were divided into two groups. The 25 children in group A were followed in our clinics for 10 years or more, and therapy was begun on or before 5 years of age. Group B consisted of nine children who did not meet one or the other of these criteria. The mean age at diagnosis and initiation of treatment was 1.3 years (range 2 days–5.1 years) in the A group. In the B group, the mean age at diagnosis was 6.0 years (2 weeks–14.1 years). The age at the initial visit to this clinic was 2.9 years (2 days–11.9 years). The mean age at the initial visit to the clinic of the nine patients in the B group was 11.6 years (6–17.8 years). The mean period of follow-up in this clinic was 15.8 (10–20) years and 5.7 (1.3–16) years in groups A and B, respectively. A majority of group A patients had an advanced bone age at the time of their initial visit. In each group, those who had electrolyte disturbances with hyponatremia and hyperkalemia were designated as salt losers. In group A, 10 males were salt losers, 7 females were salt losers, and the female pseudohermaphrodite (FP) reared as a male was a salt loser. All seven in the non-salt-loser group were females. In group B, the two males were salt losers, as were one female and one FP. Four females and one FP were non-salt-losers.

THERAPY

In general, treatment of CAH has been based on the levels of urinary steroids excreted and on measurements of cortisol secretion rates in children. In addition, the effort is made to find a dose of medication which will allow normal growth velocity and bone maturation in each child. The 34 children were treated by a regimen according to Wilkins, Blizzard, and Migeon (1965). The initial therapy in infants consisted of intramuscular cortisone acetate (25 mg every 3rd day). Two deoxycorticosterone acetate (DOCA) pellets of 125 mg each were implanted subcutaneously in the infant if electrolyte imbalance was present. Subsequently, one pellet was implanted at 6–7-month intervals. Sodium chloride in the form of table salt (2.5–6 g) was added to the total daily formula. This was gradually discontinued by 3–6 months of age. Later therapy consisted of oral medications, usually starting between 3–6 years of age with either oral hydrocortisone (10–50 mg/m^2/day) or the equivalent in oral cortisone acetate. These medications were given three or four times daily. Prednisone was substituted for cortisone at maturity. In the salt losers, oral 9α-fluorohydrocortisone (0.05–0.2 mg/day) was given in the place of the pellets at 2½–3 years of age. If hypertension developed, the mineralocorticoid was discontinued.

The objectives of glucocorticoid replacement therapy were to maintain normal growth velocities and to keep adrenocorticotropic hormone (ACTH) suppressed, as evidenced by low or normal 24-hr excretion of 17-ketosteroids and pregnanetriol. The wide dose range of 10–50 mg/m^2/day was based on the individual patient's growth and degree of suppression of ACTH, as reflected in the urinary steroid excretion. Close monitoring necessitated three to four visits to the clinic per year to enable correlation of linear growth and weight with measurement of urinary steroid excretion.

In group A, 17 of the 25 patients kept regular clinic appointments and were seen at least three times a year for adjustment of medications. Reinduction of suppression by 3 days of intramuscular steroids was required only when urinary 17-ketosteroids and pregnanetriol were elevated. The noncompliant patients missed clinic appointments and did not have the benefit of adjustment of medication when growth velocity increased and urinary steroid excretion was elevated. The number of compliant patients was influenced by the mileage required to travel to the clinic. The distance required for patients from the southwest United States to reach Houston, which is equivalent to that from Brussels to Bern or from Paris to Zurich, necessitated 9–10 hr of driving for 1 hr in the clinic and resulted in noncompliance.

Overtreatment with glucocorticoids results in decreased growth and osseous maturation; undertreatment results in acceleration of growth by allowing increasing adrenal androgens, which virilize the patient and cause disproportionate advance in bone maturation with early cessation of growth and ultimately short stature. This clinic has assumed that all patients will go out of control at some point in childhood. Because of this likelihood, it is felt that selection of a dose

which permits growth along the 50th percentile will be associated with inter-
mittent periods of excessive androgen secretion resulting in inappropriate
advances in bone age. The frequency of visits (three to four per year) minimizes
the length of time during which escape from suppression occurs undetected. A
dose which allows normal 17-ketosteroid excretion may suppress growth, and no
short-term test to assess this problem is available.

RESULTS

In the A group of 25 patients, 17 or 64% of them were considered to be well
controlled or compliant. As seen in Figure 1, the compliant patients achieved a
significantly greater mean final height than either the noncompliant or group B
patients. The mean heights of the noncompliant group and Group B, the late
treated group, were not significantly different. Therefore, these two groups were
considered as one.

Figure 2 demonstrates that the mean height of the compliant group of males,
females, and female pseudohermaphrodite(s) was 166.6 cm (65.6 inches) and of
the noncompliant group was 155.95 cm (61.4 inches).

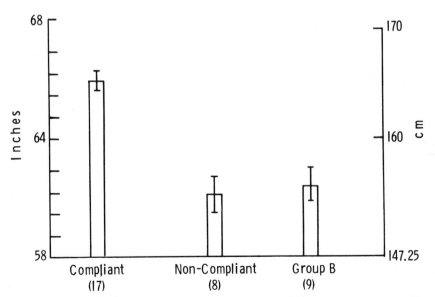

Figure 1. Mean height ± standard error (S.E.) in group A, consisting of compliant (n = 17)
and noncompliant (n = 8) patients, and in group B (n = 9) patients.

MATURE HEIGHT IN 34 PATIENTS

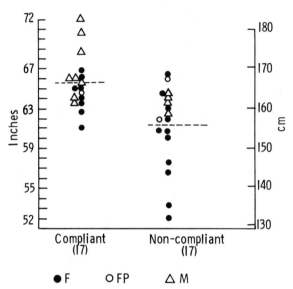

Figure 2. Mature height in 34 patients. Compliant patients (*n* = 17) are shown on the *left* and noncompliant (*n* = 17) on the *right,* with the *broken line* representing the mean height. Males, △; females, •; female pseudohermaphrodites reared as males, ○).

In order to compare the mature heights of these patients with a comparable population of Caucasians, Mexican-Americans, and American Negroes, each child's height was compared with the midparental height by the paired *t* test. Midparental height was the average of the heights of the father and mother. Figure 3 shows three columns, with the patients represented on the *left* side of each column and the mid-parent height on the *right.* The first column demonstrates the heights of compliant females and the female pseudohermaphrodite reared as a male (*left*) connected to the midparental heights (*right*). The mean height of the compliant female was 164.9 cm, and the mean midparental height was 175.3 cm ($p < 0.005$). In the middle column, the heights of compliant males (*left*) were compared with the midparental heights. The mean height of the compliant male was 170.4 cm and was not significantly different from the mean midparental height of 168.9 cm. In the right column, the heights of noncompliant males, females, and FP were compared with the midparental heights. The mean height of the noncompliant group was 156.0 cm, and the mean midparental height was 178.6 cm.

One would expect that males would actually exceed midparental height and approach or be taller than the height of their fathers. Three of the eight

HEIGHT OF PATIENT vs. MID-PARENT HEIGHT

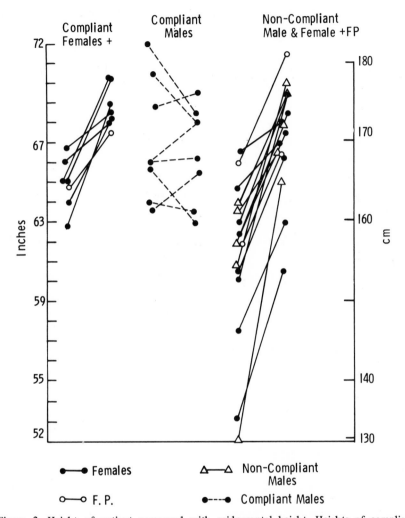

Figure 3. Height of patient compared with midparental height. Heights of compliant females and a female pseudohermaphrodite are connected to the corresponding midparental heights in the *left* column; heights of compliant males are connected by *broken lines* to the corresponding midparental heights in the *middle column;* heights of noncompliant males, females, and female pseudohermaphrodites reared as males are connected by *solid lines* to the corresponding midparental heights in the *right column.*

compliant males achieved a final height greater than paternal height, and thus, as a group, growth was possibly less than their genetic potential. The females in both groups did not approach midparental height. One would expect that a female would be less than midparental height, but equal to or greater than maternal height. In Figure 4, the heights of the females were compared with

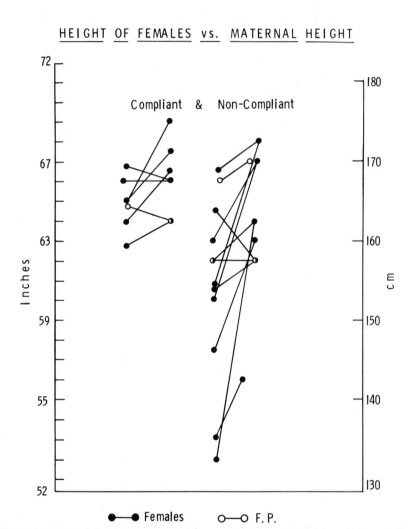

Figure 4. Height of females compared with maternal height. The heights of the compliant females and the female pseudohermaphrodite are connected to the corresponding maternal heights by *solid lines* in the *left column,* and the heights of the noncompliant females and the female pseudohermaphrodite are connected to the corresponding maternal heights by *solid lines* in the *right column.*

their maternal heights, and the paired t test was applied. The mean height of the compliant females was 164.9 cm, with a mean maternal height of 168.0 cm ($p >$ 0.05). The mean height of the noncompliant females was 154.0 cm, with a mean maternal height of 163.2 cm ($p < 0.005$). Four of six compliant females were shorter than the maternal height, but this was not statistically significant with this small sample.

The mean final height of the compliant males was 170.4 cm ($n = 8$), for compliant females 163.7 cm ($n = 8 + 1$ FP), for the noncompliant males 161.5 cm ($n = 4$), and for the noncompliant females 153.2 cm ($n = 11 + 2$ FP). These data were compared with those of Brooks et al. (1974), who found no significant difference between an untreated and a late treated group whose therapy was begun at a mean chronological age of 4.9 years and a bone age of 9.6 years. The mean height of the noncompliant group in these studies was the same as that of the late treated group in the series of Brooks et al. (1974). However, the mean final height of the compliant group was approximately 10 cm better than that of the noncompliant group in both the males and females in our series. A typical growth curve of a child with the salt-losing form of CAH indicated that growth was less than the third percentile until age 5 years, at which time the velocity improved. The height approached a normal mean for age in later childhood. The dose/m^2 of glucocorticoid required for suppression appeared to decrease with age. In general, the non-salt-loser had better growth in early childhood than the salt loser and required a lower dose for suppression.

The complications in treated patients, listed in Table 1, existed in both the compliant and noncompliant groups. Severe morbidity and mortality were not a problem in the older children with CAH. In the compliant group, 100% of the males and females had difficulty maintaining their weight in the equivalent height percentiles during midchildhood, from 6−12 years of age. All had weights above the height percentile, and 50% had weights >2 S.D. above the height percentile. An increase in glucocorticoid dose that allowed normal growth resulted in dramatic weight gain; in some instances, a decrease in dose that allowed normal growth permitted maintenance or decrease in weight. Thus, a dissociation appeared to exist between the effects of glucocorticoid on growth and on weight gain which were dosage-dependent. Interestingly, changing from cortisone acetate or hydrocortisone to an equivalent dosage of prednisone was associated with easier weight control. Obesity became a problem for the noncompliant patient only after control of the CAH was instituted. A 5 1/2-year-old female was at the 25th percentile for height and the 10th percentile for weight when she was initially treated with 4 mg of Medrol. She did not grow, so she was then given a 20 mg total dose of hydrocortisone (25 mg/m^2) with improvement in growth velocity. During the next 6 years, while her dose was constant and she maintained a normal growth velocity, she had an inappropriate increase in weight to the 90th percentile. During these 6 years, her 17-ketosteroid excretion and rate of bone maturation were normal. The effect of glucocorticoids on fat

Table 1. Complications in treated patients

I. Compliant
   A. Obesity
   B. Bone problems
      1. Idiopathic avascular necrosis of epiphyses
      2. Short stature
   C. Hypertension
II. Noncompliant and later treated
   A. Voluntary noncompliance in adolescence
   B. Uncooperative parents
   C. Virilism
      1. Short stature and dwarfism
      2. Sexual precocity
      3. Masculine habitus and masculine behavior of females
      4. Menstrual problems
         a. Amenorrhea
         b. Menorrhagia
         c. Stein-Leventhal syndrome
      5. Testicular problems
         a. Nodules
         b. Small testes with aspermia
III. Compliant and noncompliant
   A. Menstrual irregularity
   B. Postural hypotension

distribution, increase in appetite, and fluid retention may have played a role in the weight gain.

Bone problems, which were idiopathic avascular necrosis of epiphyses, occurred in two males. One had Legg-Perthes disease with a markedly retarded bone age and short stature. He had normal growth hormone release to insulin-arginine stimulation. The other had Osgood-Schlatter's disease. The effect of glucocorticoids on linear growth and bone maturation was probably a result of inhibition of the peripheral effect of growth hormone and of possible changes in cartilage structure.

The hypertension secondary to mineralocorticoid therapy resulted in removal of DOCA pellets and reduction or discontinuation of oral mineralocorticoid in some salt losers. The patients subsequently were normotensive.

The problems in the noncompliant patient were related to the lack of suppression of ACTH and thus to an excess of adrenal androgens. This would result from voluntary discontinuation of medication during adolescence and from lack of cooperation of parents who for one reason or another failed to bring the child back to the clinic. The effect was the same in that the child would go out of control.

The resultant virilization caused several problems. Short stature and dwarfism with height less than 147.3 cm occurred more often in females who entered puberty shortly following initiation of therapy. Sexual precocity followed the initiation of therapy in three patients. The masculine habitus and masculine behavior of females were less a problem for the patient herself than for the family.

The menstrual problems of amenorrhea and menorrhagia occurred in five of nine noncompliant females. The Stein-Leventhal syndrome occurred in two girls who were diagnosed as having CAH at an older age. Testicular problems occurred in two noncompliant males.

Both the compliant and noncompliant females experienced irregular menses which improved with adrenal suppression. Postural hypotension occurred in the older males who had increased physical activity. In these individuals, large doses of glucocorticoids were required for suppression of 17-ketosteroids and improvement of symptoms. Decreased physical activity resulted in a Cushingoid appearance. Therefore, the possibility of an altered metabolic clearance rate or absorption has been considered.

Finally, the effects on development of the constant threat of illness and of concern about medication and health led us to examine the social status of these children, who are now adolescents or adults (Table 2). The compliant individuals

Table 2. Current occupations

---

15 – School/high school
   1 Female competes in track
   1 Female excels in shot put
5 – College
   1 Male is pre-medical student
1 – Masters-Ph.D. program in marine biology
1 – Licensed practical nurse
1 – Laboratory technician
6 – High school graduates occupied as follows:
   Heavy equipment operator
   Architectural draftsman
   Pharmaceutical house salesman
   Welder
   Newspaper typesetter
3 – Lost to follow-up
7 – Married
   1 Male with CAH is father of child by artificial insemination
   1 Male with CAH is father of naturally conceived child
   1 Female with CAH and Stein-Leventhal syndrome had 2 children
   1 Female with CAH had 1 child

---

accepted their defect and adjusted well to their school, work, and marriages. As a group, they appeared to be goal-oriented. The noncompliant appeared to have more difficulty adjusting to their situation. The noncompliant pattern seemed to result in and also to result from adjustment and environmental difficulties.

SUMMARY

In summary, although a majority of the well controlled patients grew poorly in early childhood, their later growth and ultimate height were good. The poor growth in early childhood may be caused by several factors, including salt loss, illness, and doses of glucocorticoid and mineralocorticoid. The effects of these three factors on growth all decrease with age.

Catch-up growth appears to be related to decreased glucocorticoid dose/m^2 at an older age. The problem of obesity appears to be dosage-dependent, but in a range which permits good control of the CAH by established criteria. With adequate control, CAH appears to be compatible with normal social and sexual adaptation and career development. In conclusion, adequate control and therapy beginning in early childhood appear to give the best opportunity for optimal growth and development.

REFERENCES

Brooks, C. G. D., M. Zachmann, A. Prader, and G. Mürset. 1974. Experience with long-term therapy in congenital adrenal hyperplasia. J. Pediatr. 85:12–19.
Wilkins, L., R. M. Blizzard, and C. J. Migeon. 1965. The Diagnosis and Treatment of Endocrine Disorders in Childhood and Adolescence, Ed. 3. Charles C. Thomas, Springfield, Illinois.

Diagnosis and Management of Congenital Adrenal Hyperplasia

Derek Gupta, Klaus Rager, Werner Klemm, and Andrea Attanasio

The descriptions of ambiguous genitalia by de Crecchio in 1865 first paved the way for the recognition of congenital adrenal hyperplasia (CAH) as a disorder. CAH is a genetic defect in one of the enzymes in the biosynthetic pathway leading to cortisol. Increased amounts of the precursors of cortisol are produced as a consequence of the enzymatic block. In addition, because in most instances the biosynthesis of androgens is not blocked, large amounts of adrenal androgens are produced, causing virilization. Effective therapy for this condition was possible after Wilkins and his collaborators (1962, 1965) successfully demonstrated that the administration of glucocorticoids could arrest or correct the symptoms related to CAH.

The prime objectives of therapy for patients in the pediatric age group are the maintenance of normal growth rate and bone age velocity during childhood and prevention of premature-pubertal virilization. The periodic determination of 24-hr urinary levels of 17-oxosteroids and pregnanetriol (the principal metabolite of 17-OHP) was considered to be the main biochemical control in the treatment of CAH due to 21-hydroxylase defect, the most common form (Bongiovanni and Root, 1963).

However, now that radioimmunoassay is an established methodology, the availability of specific assays for the serum concentrations of 17-OHP, progesterone, deoxycorticosterone (DOC), 11-deoxycortisol, cortisol, and testosterone has stimulated renewed interest in understanding the role of these compounds in the diagnosis and management of patients with CAH.

PATIENTS

The 31 patients reported here comprise all patients available in University Children's Hospital, Tübingen, Germany, together with a number of cases referred to us by outside hospitals. Among them were 20 girls and 10 boys. One patient was genetically a girl, but had been raised as a boy. All patients had 21-hydroxylation defect; 12 (9 girls and 3 boys) had the salt-losing form of the disorder; and the remainder had CAH with simple virilization. Six patients were

283

initially evaluated with the use of steroid studies using radioimmunoassay techniques. Serum samples from other patients at the time of original diagnosis were not available.

All patients were maintained on glucocorticoid therapy (cortisol or prednisone), and medication was not interrupted during investigation. Oral salt-retaining hormone (9α-fluorocortisol) was prescribed in cases with the salt-losing form of CAH. Clinical control of patients was arbitrarily described as "good," "poor," and "inconsistent," according to the following clinical criteria: 1) height velocity, 2) skeletal age maturation, and 3) clinical signs of virilization. The term "inconsistent" meant that the patient sometimes showed good clinical control, while at other times his clinical control seemed to be poor.

Estimation of individual 11-deoxy-17-oxosteroids, as well as of pregnanetriol and pregnanetriolone, was carried out by gas-liquid chromatography (Gupta, 1970; Gupta and Marshall, 1971). The radioimmunoassay for simultaneous estimations of 17-OHP, progesterone, 11-deoxycortisol, deoxycorticosterone, and cortisol was developed in this laboratory (Klemm and Gupta, 1975; Rager, Klemm, and Gupta, 1975). Testosterone was estimated by radioimmunoassay according to a technique detailed elsewhere (Attanasio and Gupta, 1975).

Blood for steroid estimations was drawn in most instances between 8 and 10 a.m. Blood and 24-hr urine samples were obtained as closely together as possible.

Bone age was evaluated according to the standards of Greulich and Pyle (1959), and height velocity was compared to the standards of Tanner, Whitehouse, and Takaishi (1966).

PROBLEMS OF DIAGNOSIS

Serum progesterone and 17-OHP levels in CAH due to a 21-hydroxylase defect have been found to be highly elevated prior to therapy, as would be predicted from the physiology of the disease (Barnes and Atherden, 1972; Franks, 1974; Lippe et al., 1974; Strott, Yoshimi, and Lipsett, 1969). A very high serum level of these two steroids should clearly differentiate a 21-hydroxylase deficiency from an 11β-hydroxylase or a 3β-hydroxysteroid dehydrogenase deficiency. Similarly, a high level of serum 11-deoxycortisol can point toward an 11β-hydroxylase deficiency.

However, it is not easy to differentially diagnose a CAH patient from a subject suffering from other disorders with only the absolute determination of serum concentration of the above steroids. There are inherent difficulties in the diagnosis even when proper laboratory studies are obtained. Normal pregnanetriol values were found until 14 months of age in a reported case (Shackleton, Mitchell, and Farquhar, 1972). These studies were unable to discern any significant differences in absolute steroid values between salt-losing and non-salt-losing patients when the patients were already treated with steroids. To distinguish patients who were incorrectly diagnosed and mistakenly given steroid therapy from true CAH patients, two types of steroid ratios, arbitrarily called 21-oxygenation index (F and B pathways), were applied. The former was the ratio between progesterone plus 17-OHP and 11-deoxycortisol plus cortisol, whereas the latter was the ratio between progesterone and deoxycorticosterone. Among the patients with simple virilization, the 21-oxygenation index (F pathway) was not significantly different from that of patients with the salt-losing syndrome, but both varied significantly ($p < 0.01$) from subjects without any adrenocortical enzyme defects (Figure 1). When the 21-oxygenation index (B pathway) was considered, the values for the normal controls and CAH patients with simple virilization did not differ significantly, but both showed significant ($p < 0.01$) differences compared to the value for salt-losing patients.

Another interesting diagnostic tool could be the use of exogenous adrenocorticotropic hormone (ACTH) in a situation in which steroids have already been

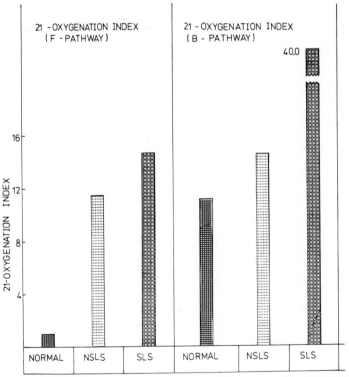

Figure 1. 21-Oxygenation index in normal, non-salt-losing type of CAH (NSLS), and salt-losing type (SLS) of the disorder. F pathway, ratio of progesterone plus 17-OHP to 11-deoxycortisol plus cortisol; B pathway, ratio of progesterone to deoxycorticosterone.

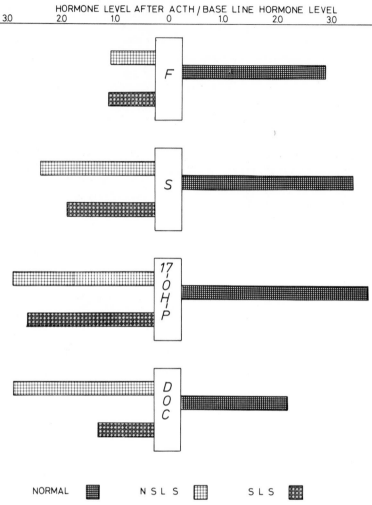

Figure 2. Ratio of post-ACTH to pre-ACTH hormone levels for cortisol (F), 11-deoxy-cortisol (S), 17-OHP, and deoxycorticosterone in normal, non-salt-losing (NSLS), and salt-losing patients (SLS).

misused as therapy. Figure 2 demonstrates the ratios between post- and pre-ACTH serum concentrations of four steroid hormones measured in patients with 21-hydroxylase defect and in subjects without any true adrenocortical abnormality but given steroids as therapy. The ratios for cortisol, 11-deoxycortisol, and 17-OHP for the CAH patients were significantly less when compared to the control subjects without any adrenocortical dysfunction. The value for deoxycorticosterone, on the other hand, clearly differentiated the salt-losing patients from the non-salt-losing and control subjects. The lower response to exogenous ACTH in CAH subjects may well be a consequence of the degree of endogenous stimulation of the adrenal cortex, because the maximally stimulated gland could not respond normally to more ACTH.

STEROID VALUES: BEFORE AND DURING MANAGEMENT

Figures 3 and 4 summarize graphically two typical cases in which steroids were serially estimated before therapy was introduced and sequentially estimated during the continuation of treatment. Figure 3 gives the data of a boy whose chronological age was 5.42 years and whose bone age was 12.50 years at the time of diagnosis. The pretherapy values of all the steroids studied were highly elevated, but started declining as soon as therapy was initiated. According to the clinical criteria, the control of the subject was good, but the serum levels of steroids became elevated toward the end of the study, indicating that the dosage of medication was perhaps not adequate at this stage to keep the steroid values well within the control levels.

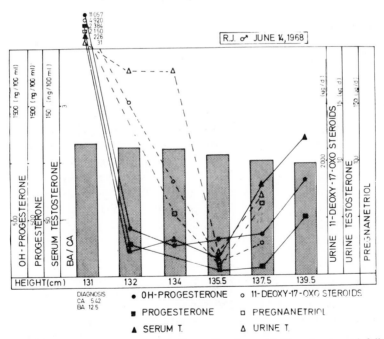

Figure 3. Urinary and serum concentrations of various steroids prior to and following therapy in an adequately controlled patient. The *bars* indicate the bone age (BA) to chronological age (CA) ratio. Height has been given below each *bar*.

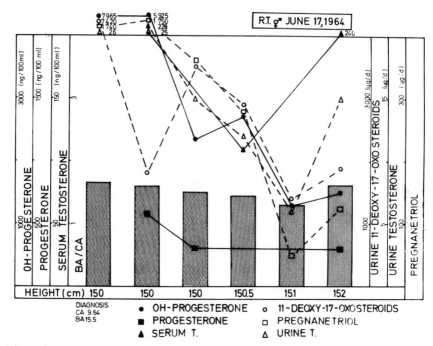

Figure 4. Urinary and serum concentrations of various steroids prior to and following therapy in a patient whose gender was wrongly assigned and whose clinical control was inadequate. The *bars* indicate the bone age (BA) to chronological age (CA) ratio. Height has been given below each *bar*.

Figure 4 gives the data of a child in whom gender assignment was wrong; although genetically a girl, he was raised as a boy. His chronological age was 9.64 and bone age 15.5 at the time of initial diagnosis. The enormously elevated levels of serum steroids declined with the start of therapy, although not so promptly as in the previous case. Toward the end of the present serial study, the levels of serum steroid concentration increased; the ratio of bone age to chronological age also registered elevation at this stage. This patient had bilateral ovariectomies. Cooperation with clinical management was poor. He was put into the category of inconsistent control.

CLINICAL CONTROL AND STEROID VALUES

The mean serum 17-hydroxyprogesterone level for normal children was 98 ± 44.2 ng/100 ml (S.D.). Under ACTH treatment, the normal serum concentration rose to a mean level of 386 ± 104 ng/100 ml. Figure 5 demonstrates the serum concentrations of 17-hydroxyprogesterone in the CAH patients under treatment. The patients were classified as good, poor, or inconsistent, according to the previously described clinical criteria. It is interesting to note that, even when the patient was judged to be in good clinical control, the serum concentration of 17-OHP in the majority of the cases was not within the normal range. The majority of these values for the well controlled patients lay just below the + 1 S.D. value of the ACTH-stimulated level in normal children.

The 17-OHP serum concentrations of patients in poor or inconsistent clinical control lay above this upper limit in the majority of cases. It is also interesting that the majority of the patients in poor and inconsistent control were boys more than 5 years old with the non-salt-losing form of CAH. This suggests that late diagnosis among boys with non-salt-losing CAH makes good control more difficult. These later treated subjects in many cases had severe loss of their developmental potential, which may also be reflected in the analysis of serum concentrations of steroids.

In contrast to 17-hydroxyprogesterone levels, patients in good control in most cases had urinary pregnanetriol levels within 2 S.D. of the normal level (Figure 6). The patients in inconsistent control also had values close to normal levels. The patients in poor control revealed elevated pregnanetriol levels, as did subjects older than 5 years.

When the serum concentration of 17-OHP and urinary levels of pregnanetriol were examined together in relation to the clinical control of patients, there were

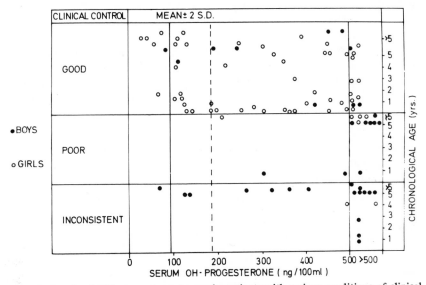

Figure 5. Levels of 17-hydroxyprogesterone in patients with various conditions of clinical management according to the criteria detailed under "Patients." The mean ± 2 S.D. for the normal children has been given on the left side, while the limit of 500 ng/100 ml roughly coincides with the + 1 S.D. of ACTH-stimulated value in normal children.

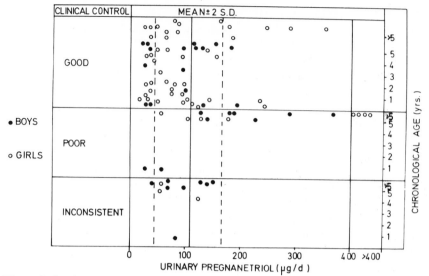

Figure 6. Levels of urinary pregnanetriol in patients with various conditions of clinical management according to the criteria detailed under "Patients."

no instances in which low 17-OHP was observed simultaneously with elevated pregnanetriol values. However, the contrary, in which pregnanetriol was low but serum concentration of 17-OHP was elevated, has been observed to occur in many instances.

Why serum 17-hydroxyprogesterone levels did not provide results as consistent as those of urinary pregnanetriol is uncertain. But it is possible that the existing diurnal variation of 17-OHP in CAH patients, in contrast to the speculation of Strott, Yoshimi, and Lipsett (1969), may be one of the causes for such discrepancies. In some cases, the time lag for the collection of blood and urine samples could also be another reason.

Serum concentrations of testosterone, however, fluctuated more often during sequential studies, and to establish a relationship between serum level and clinical control of the patients was difficult. As has been shown in Figures 3 and 4, prior to therapy both patients had highly elevated serum testosterone concentration, which declined to prepubertal range during therapy. This suppression was temporary, however. Figure 7 shows serum testosterone concentration plotted against the ratio of bone age to chronological age in CAH patients under treatment. The testosterone levels in most cases remained at a much higher level than the prepubertal range. Almost all the girl patients had serum levels higher than that for a pubertal stage 5 girl (Tanner, 1962) when their bone age to chronological age ratios were well within normal range. In one instance, a girl patient showed a serum testosterone concentration equal to that of a stage 5 boy, although her bone age to chronological age ratio was only 0.75.

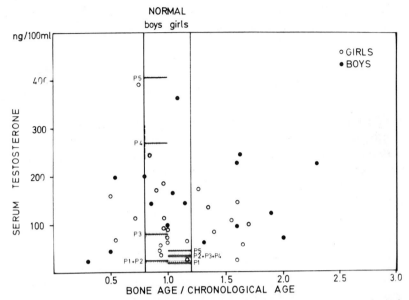

Figure 7. Distribution of serum testosterone in relation to the bone age to chronological age ratio. Concentrations of serum testosterone at pubertal stages P1 to P5 (Tanner, 1962) in boys and girls are also provided. The *shaded areas* indicate ± 1 S.D.

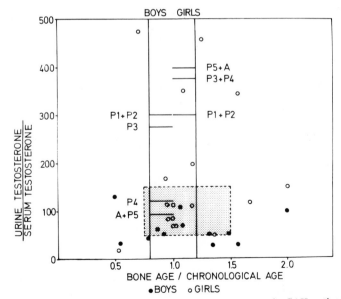

Figure 8. The ratio of urine testosterone to serum testosterone in CAH patients plotted against the bone age to chronological age ratio in the same subjects. P1 to P5 denote pubertal stages (Tanner, 1962) in boys and girls; A, adult. The *shaded area* denotes the mean ± 1 S.D.

When the serum testosterone was related to urine testosterone and plotted against the bone age in chronological age ratio, a similar pattern of low values emerged corresponding to pubertal stages 4 and 5 for boys (Figure 8). In agreement with previous observations of the serum concentration of 17-OHP and urinary pregnanetriol levels, testosterone values revealed that, although in a clinically well controlled patient the urinary level of testosterone declined to well within normal range, the serum testosterone concentration remained far above the normal threshold for the corresponding pubertal stage.

With serum testosterone values, it was, therefore, not possible to select a testosterone threshold to differentiate between adequate and inadequate adrenal suppression in prepubertal and midpubertal children, as suggested by some investigators (Solomon and Schoen, 1975). A maximal permissible threshold for serum testosterone in relation to adequate clinical control should be set at a higher level.

CORRELATION BETWEEN STEROIDS

Because of these apparent discrepancies between serum concentration and urine levels of the steroids estimated, the relationship between serum 17-OHP and

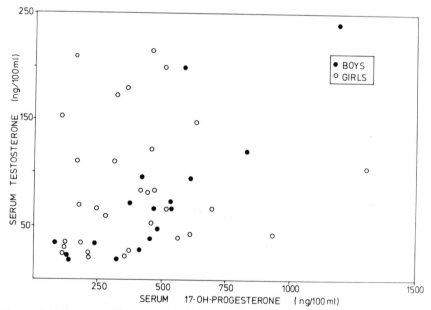

Figure 9. Relationship between serum testosterone concentration and serum 17-OHP concentration in CAH patients.

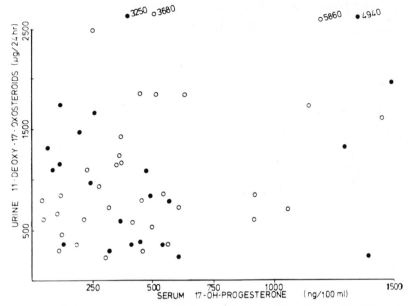

Figure 10. Relationship between urine 11-deoxy-17-oxosteroids and serum 17-OHP concentration in CAH patients.

serum testosterone was investigated. Figure 9 demonstrates such a comparison between 48 sets of estimations. When all children were considered, a poor correlation was obtained, giving a coefficient of only 0.13. A higher correlation coefficient of 0.33 was found when only the boys were considered.

On the other hand, urinary 11-deoxy-17-oxosteroids, i.e., the total of individually estimated androsterone, etiocholanolone, and dehydroepiandrosterone, showed a slightly better relationship with a correlation coefficient of 0.25 when all children were considered (Figure 10). Calculated only for the girls, this value was, however, much higher ($r = 0.41$).

The serum concentration of progesterone had better correlation ($r = 0.63$), although, in many instances, when serum 17-OH-progesterone values were found to be 50–100 times those of normal children, serum progesterone values were only 12–20 times those of normal subjects. These data confirm previous observations of Strott, Yoshimi, and Lipsett (1969).

The increase in serum concentration of progesterone probably reflects the inability of the 17α-hydroxylase to convert all the precursors presented to it. Likewise, with urine values there were many instances in which high urinary 11-deoxy-17-oxosteroids were associated with low serum concentrations of 17-OHP and vice versa.

BONE AGE DEVELOPMENT AND STEROID VALUES

To assess serum concentrations of 17-OHP or urinary levels of 11-deoxy-17-oxo-steroids and the biochemical control of CAH, the change in serum concentrations of 17-OHP (Figure 11) and urinary levels of 11-deoxy-17-oxosteroids (Figure 12) was related to the change in the bone age to chronological age ratio. Because in CAH there is often a wide discrepancy between chronological age and bone age, the ratio should allow for the variations in rates of maturation during therapy. In most instances, a decrease in serum concentration was associated with a decrease in the bone to chronological age ratio, although in several cases a sharp decline in the former value was associated with only a slight decrease in the ratio. There were also a few instances in which the increment in serum concentration of 17-OHP was related either to an increase or decrease in the

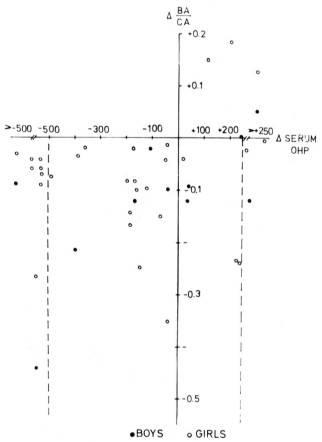

Figure 11. Changes in serum 17-OHP concentrations in CAH patients during therapy related to the changes in the bone age to chronological age (BA/CA) ratios in the same subjects.

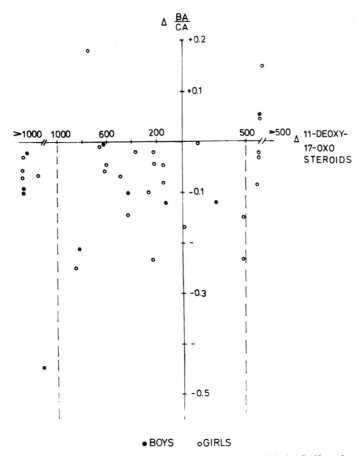

● BOYS   oGIRLS

Figure 12. Changes in urinary level of 11-deoxy-17-oxosteroids in CAH patients during therapy related to the changes in the bone age to chronological age (BA/CA) ratios in the same subjects.

ratio of bone age to chronological age; however, there was no instance in which a decrease in serum 17-OHP concentration was related to an increase in the ratio. The change in the urinary level of 11-deoxy-17-oxosteroids showed a similar pattern when examined in relation to the change in the bone age to chronological age ratio (Figure 12).

HEIGHT VELOCITY IN RELATION TO THERAPY AND BONE AGE VELOCITY

In the treatment of CAH, regulation of glucocorticoid dosage is based on two major criteria—height velocity and bone age maturation. Blizzard and Wilkins

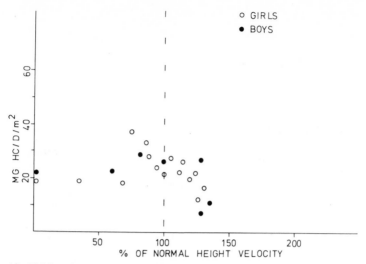

Figure 13. Height velocity in CAH patients shown as the percentage of height velocity seen in normal children (Tanner, Whitehouse, and Takaishi, 1966) in relation to the dosage of medication given in mg/m²/day during the 1st year of treatment. Each point represents one individual. HC, cortisol.

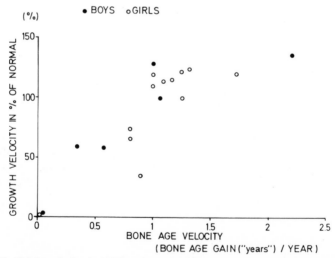

Figure 14. Height velocity in CAH patients shown as the percentage of height velocity seen in normal children (Tanner, Whitehouse, and Takaishi, 1966) in relation to the bone age velocity of the same subjects. Each point represents one individual.

(1957) reported normal growth for patients receiving adequate steroid replacement. Visser (1966) reported much greater growth suppression in patients treated with prednisone as opposed to cortisol. Using methylprednisolone and α-methylprednisolone, Laron and Pertzelan (1968) observed greater growth retardation than with cortisol. Digman, Maranan, and Staub (1962), on the other hand, could not differentiate the effects produced by cortisol and depomethylprednisolone. Most children in our hospital were treated with cortisol. Figure 13 illustrates height velocity as the percentage of normal height velocity (Tanner, Whitehouse, and Takaishi, 1966) in relation to the amount of cortisol given to the patient $(mg/m^2/day)$ during the 1st year of treatment. In order to avoid introducing a bias by using some subjects more than once, only one point representing each child has been used. It can be seen that in most instances the amount of therapy used was 20 $mg/m^2/day$. Of the nine patients who had greater velocity than the normal controls, four had definitely lower dosages of medication. The two patients who registered no height velocity were late diagnosed when their growth rate virtually stopped. Figure 14 summarizes graphically the findings when height velocity was related to bone age velocity (bone age gain measured in "years"/year) in the same group of patients. The two patients who failed to grow occupy the extreme left corner of the graph. Of the remaining 16 patients, 9 showed overall improvement of bone age velocity in relation to height velocity during therapy. In two subjects for whom treatment was started late, it was not possible to reduce the bone age velocity below normal. In the other five patients, the bone age velocity declined below normal but perhaps not without compromising their height velocity.

CONCLUSION

The following conclusions can be made:

1. Estimations of serum 17-OHP, progesterone, and deoxycorticosterone clearly help in the diagnosis of CAH.
2. When prior administration of steroids has made diagnosis more complicated, the 21-oxygenation index and exogenous administration of ACTH are clearly of value.
3. During therapy, patients with CAH should be checked at fixed intervals according to the established clinical criteria.
4. For biochemical criteria of good control, the older methods of measuring 24-hr urine levels of 11-deoxy-17-oxosteroids and pregnanetriol seem to provide more reliable information.
5. For patients with adequate control, each laboratory should have its own established threshold of serum 17-OHP and progesterone levels.
6. Serum testosterone concentration provides poor correlation with adequate clinical control.

ACKNOWLEDGMENT

The authors gratefully acknowledge the scientific assistance of Mr. T. Chow in measuring serum hormones.

REFERENCES

Attanasio, A., and D. Gupta. 1975. Simultaneous radioimmunoassay of estrogens and androgens in plasma of prepubertal children. *In* D. Gupta (ed.), Radioimmunoassay of Steroid Hormones, pp. 91–100. Verlag Chemie, Weinheim.

Barnes, N., and S. Atherden. 1972. Diagnosis of congenital adrenal hyperplasia by measurement of plasma 17-hydroxyprogesterone. Arch. Dis. Child. 47: 62–65.

Blizzard, R., and L. Wilkins. 1957. Present concepts of steroid therapy in virilizing adrenal hyperplasia. Arch. Intern. Med. 100:729–738.

Bongiovanni, A., and A. Root. 1963. Adrenogenital syndrome. N. Engl. J. Med. 268:1283–1289.

Digman, J., L. Maranan, and M. Staub. 1962. Treatment of adrenogenital syndrome. J. Am. Med. Assoc. 180:1017–1020.

Franks, R. C. 1974. Plasma 17-hydroxyprogesterone, 21-deoxycortisol and cortisol in congenital adrenal hyperplasia. J. Clin. Endocrinol. 39:1099–1102.

Greulich, W. W., and S. I. Pyle. 1959. Radiographic Atlas of Skeletal Development of the Hand and Wrist, Ed. 2. Stanford University Press, Stanford, California.

Gupta, D. 1970. A longitudinal study of the urinary excretion of individual steroids in children during adolescent growth. Steroidologia 1:267–294.

Gupta, D., and W. A. Marshall. 1971. A longitudinal study of the urinary excretion of individual steroids in children from 3 to 7 yr old. Acta Endocrinol. (Kbh) 68:141–163.

Klemm, W., and D. Gupta. 1975. A routine method for the radioimmunoassay of plasma cortisol without chromatography. *In* D. Gupta (ed.), Radioimmunoassay of Steroid Hormones, pp. 143–151. Verlag Chemie, Weinheim.

Laron, Z., and A. Pertzelan. 1968. The comparative effect of 6-alphafluoroprednisolone, 6-alpha-methylprednisolone, and hydrocortisone on linear growth of children with congenital adrenal virilism and Addison's disease. J. Pediatr. 73:774–782.

Lippe, B. M., S. H. La Franchi, N. Lavin, A. Parlow, J. Coyotupa, and S. Kaplan. 1974. Serum 17α-hydroxyprogesterone, progesterone, estradiol and testosterone in the diagnosis and management of congenital adrenal hyperplasia. J. Pediatr. 85:782–787.

Rager, K., W. Klemm, and D. Gupta. 1975. Simultaneous radioimmunoassay of plasma 17-hydroxyprogesterone, 11-deoxycortisol, deoxycorticosterone and cortisol. *In* D. Gupta (ed.), Radioimmunoassay of Steroid Hormones, pp. 127–133. Verlag Chemie, Weinheim.

Shackleton, C., F. Mitchell, and J. Farquhar. 1972. Difficulties in the diagnosis of the adrenogenital syndrome in infancy. Pediatrics 49:198.

Solomon, I. L., and E. J. Schoen. 1975. Blood testosterone values in patients with congenital adrenal hyperplasia. J. Clin. Endocrinol. 40:355–362.

Strott, C. A., T. Yoshimi, and M. B. Lipsett. 1969. Plasma progesterone and

17-hydroxyprogesterone in normal men and children with congenital adrenal hyperplasia. J. Clin. Invest. 48:930–939.

Tanner, J. M. 1962. Growth at Adolescence, Ed. 2. Blackwell Scientific Publications, Oxford.

Tanner, J. M., R. H. Whitehouse, and M. Takaishi. 1966. Standards from birth to maturity for height, weight, height-velocity and weight-velocity. British Children. Arch. Dis. Child. 41:613.

Visser, H. 1966. Growth of children with congenital adrenal hyperplasia. *In* J. J. van der Werften Bosch and A. Hoak (eds.), Somatic Growth of the Child, p. 248. Leiden.

Wilkins, L. 1962. Adrenal disorders. II. Congenital virilizing adrenal hyperplasia. Arch. Dis. Child. 37:231.

Wilkins, L. 1965. The Diagnosis and Treatment of Endocrine Disorders in Childhood and Adolescence, Ed. 3. Charles C. Thomas, Springfield, Illinois.

Growth and
Glucocorticoid Excess

H. David Mosier, Jr.

The following chapter is a description of some experiments which have a bearing on the problem of the effects of glucocorticoid excess on growth both during the period of exposure to high levels of steroid and during subsequent recovery.

It has been noted that catch-up growth may not occur in certain cases of Cushing's syndrome even after levels of cortisol are restored to normal. An example was seen in a case previously reported (Mosier, Smith, and Shultz, 1972). A girl with Cushing's syndrome beginning at age 8 years, at which time the patient had normal height, did not grow for 4 years, until both adrenals were removed. Subsequently, she resumed a normal growth rate, but did not undergo catch-up acceleration. This author has also reported studies on rat models comparing growth recovery after a fast, cortisone injections, or propylthiouracil feeding (Mosier, 1971). The treatments were given at around 40 days of age. Under certain experimental conditions, there was catch-up acceleration after the fast; cortisone treatment was followed by resumption of normal growth rate, but no catch-up acceleration; propylthiouracil feeding was followed by only partial catch-up growth.

Studies of radioimmunoassayable growth hormone in plasma during treatment and recovery in the fast and cortisone models have shown a significant occurrence of sporadic high values in both cortisone and fast recovery periods, indicating that the presence of elevated plasma growth hormone values cannot per se ensure catch-up recovery (Mosier and Jansons, 1976).

Cartilage sulfating ability in vitro has been examined in these experimental models in order to show whether or not cartilage has a functional disturbance which might account for failure of catch-up growth in the cortisone model. Previously, it has been shown that ultrastructural disturbances occur in the cortisone, fast, and propylthiouracil models (Dearden and Mosier, 1972, 1974a, 1974b).

With increasing age, controls followed a linear regression in sulfating ability. Hypophysectomized rats maintained a fairly constant low level which ultimately approximated the control line. During treatment, fasted rats took up sulfate at the hypox level, but during recovery uptake surged above control values, then declined toward the control level. Cortisone treatment resulted in a depression of sulfate uptake; during recovery the rats recovered normal sulfate uptake at 1

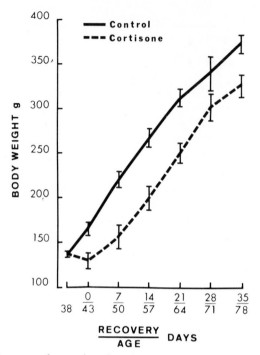

Figure 1. Growth curves of controls and cortisone-treated rats. (Reprinted from Mosier, H. D., Jr., R. A. Jansons, R. R. Hill, and L. C. Dearden. 1975. Endocrinology 99:580–589. By permission of the author and publisher.)

week, but at 2 weeks sulfate uptake appeared to be still increasing. The propylthiouracil results appeared about comparable to the cortisone results.

A more detailed study of the cortisone model was undertaken (Mosier et al., 1976). Figure 1 shows the body weight growth curve of controls and cortisone-treated rats that received injections of cortisone acetate in a dose of 5 mg/rat/day for 5 days. Numbers at the bottom of the chart show recovery days on the top row and the age of the rat on the bottom row. The usual patterns— resumption of normal growth rate, but failure of catch-up growth—can be seen.

Figure 2 shows the in vitro sulfation by rib cartilage, expressed as ^{35}S uptake per wet weight of cartilage. These results were remarkably reproducible between experiments. In this study, extended well into recovery, increased cartilage sulfation persisted to the 5th week of recovery.

Growth hormone levels in serum showed a pattern like that previously reported (Mosier and Jansons, 1976); however, this study differed in that the

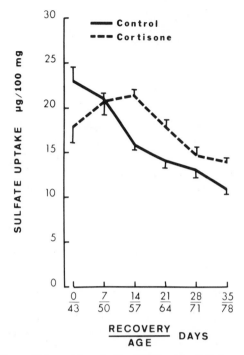

Figure 2. In vitro sulfate uptake of rib cartilage of controls and cortisone-treated rats. (Reprinted from Mosier, H. D., Jr., R. A. Jansons, R. R. Hill, and L. C. Dearden. 1976. Endocrinology 99:580–589. By permission of the author and publisher.)

rats were submitted to various environmental stresses known to depress serum growth hormone levels in the rat. In spite of this, random occurrences of high values still occurred.

Pituitary radioimmunoassayable growth hormone content and concentration were both increased by cortisone treatment, but during recovery they dropped below control values. Pituitary content showed a persistent decrease. On the other hand, pituitary concentration recovered to the normal value by about the 4th week of recovery.

Somatomedin levels in serum determined by bioassay in the porcine rib cartilage method showed a drop during treatment and slow recovery toward control values by the 4th week.

These studies also compared the sulfating ability of parabiosed and non-parabiosed controls and cortisone-treated rats at two points in recovery. At 31 days of recovery, cartilage of controls parabiosed to the cortisone-treated rats takes up sulfate at a significantly greater rate than that of nonparabiosed controls, indicating that a humoral factor appears in vivo to cause the increased sulfating ability shown by the cartilage in vitro.

SUMMARY

During recovery after glucocorticoid excess, catch-up growth may fail to occur. Compensatory changes occur in pituitary and plasma growth hormone concentration and in serum somatomedin concentration, but these do not correlate with failure of catch-up growth. Cartilage sulfation is enhanced during recovery. This may be the effect of a humoral factor, the identity of which is unknown, or the result of direct effect of the glucocorticoid treatment on chondrocytes.

REFERENCES

Dearden, L. C., and H. D. Mosier, Jr. 1972. Long-term recovery of chondrocytes in the tibial epiphyseal plate in rats after cortisone treatment. Clin. Orthop. 87:322–331.

Dearden, L. C., and H. D. Mosier, Jr. 1974a. Growth retardation and subsequent recovery of the rat tibia, a histochemical, light, and electron microscopic study. I. After propylthiouracil treatment. Growth 38:253–275.

Dearden, L. C., and H. D. Mosier, Jr. 1974b. Growth retardation and subsequent recovery of the rat tibia, a histochemical, light, and electron microscopic study. II. After fasting. Growth 38:277–294.

Mosier, H. D., Jr. 1971. Failure of compensatory (catch-up) growth in the rat. Pediatr. Res. 5:59–63.

Mosier, H. D., Jr., and R. A. Jansons. 1976. Growth hormone during catch-up growth and failure of catch-up growth in rats. Endocrinology 98:226–231.

Mosier, H. D., Jr., R. A. Jansons, R. R. Hill, and L. C. Dearden. 1976. Cartilage sulfation and serum somatomedin in rats during and after cortisone-induced growth arrest. Endocrinology 99:580–589.

Mosier, H. D., Jr., F. G. Smith, Jr., and M. A. Shultz. 1972. Failure of catch-up growth after Cushing's syndrome in childhood. Am. J. Dis. Child. 124:251–253.

Various Aspects of Adrenal Hyperplasia in Adult Subjects

Peter Göbel and F. Heni

At the beginning of this work on adult patients with adrenal hyperplasia, it was shown that patients with 21-hydroxylase deficiency had a characteristic paper chromatogram of urinary 17-ketosteroids (Göbel, Heni, and d'Addabbo, 1958). Figure 1 shows the chromatogram of patient F. H.; large amounts of metabolites of 21-deoxycortisol and 11β-hydroxyandrostenedione can be seen. Patient F. H. (Figure 2) is a 37-year-old XX individual with short stature, virilism, clitoral hypertrophy, and primary amenorrhea. The 21-hydroxylase deficiency is rarely diagnosed in adult subjects, and in the past 20 years this laboratory has observed only three subjects with this disorder. Figure 3 shows the values of the urinary 17-ketosteroids (Porter-Silber chromogens (PSC), dehydroepiandrosterone, (DHA), pregnanetriol, and pregnanediol) in the three cases. In all cases, elevated levels are evident when compared to the normal levels, except in the PSC. Unfortunately, the first two patients were lost to follow-up.

For 20 years, the third patient (S. D.) was treated daily with 25 mg of cortisone. In addition, during the last 5 years she was given cyclic treatment with cyproterone acetate and estradiol. This treatment decreased facial hair growth and acne. She is now 38 years old and is a chemical engineer. Recent laboratory determinations showed normal plasma testosterone (207 pg/ml), adrenocorticotropic hormone (ACTH) (68 pg/ml), and aldosterone (8.2 ng/100 ml). However, her urinary pregnanetriol remained somewhat elevated (3.3 mg/24 hr).

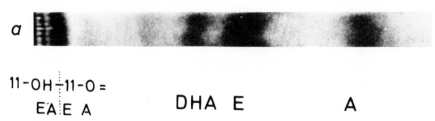

Figure 1. Paper chromatograms of individual urinary 17-ketosteroids in 21-hydroxylase deficiency (patient F. H.).

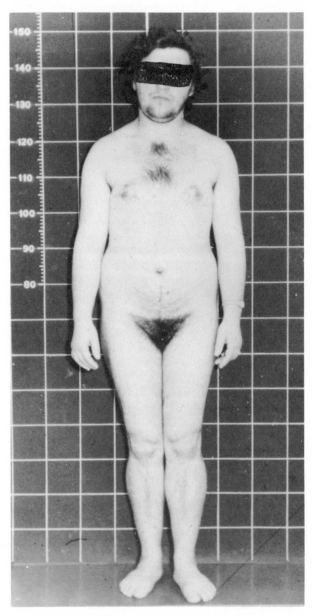

Figure 2. A 37-year-old chromosomal female (F. H.) with 21-hydroxylase deficiency.

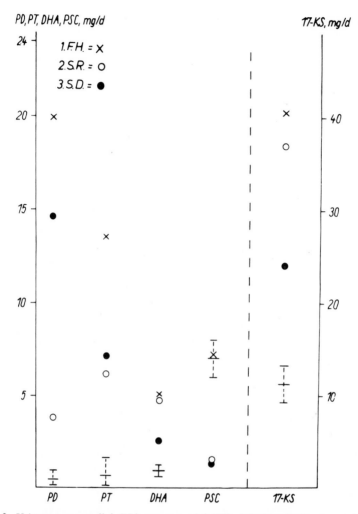

Figure 3. Urinary pregnanediol (PD), pregnanetriol (PT), dehydroepiandrosterone (DHA), Porter-Silber (1950) chromogens (PSC), and 17-ketosteroids (17-KS) in three cases of 21-hydroxylase deficiency diagnosed in adults. The *vertical bars* indicate ranges for normal persons.

According to another type of paper chromatogram, it is apparent that only DHA is elevated in a series of hirsute women. These patients showed varying degrees of virilization, clitoral hypertrophy, and amenorrhea.

In Figure 4, the symbols for patients 4 and 5 indicate an elevation of 17-ketosteroid and DHA excretion. Cases 6, 8, and 10 show only increased DHA excretion. This graph also indicates that cases 4, 5, and 7 have an increase of

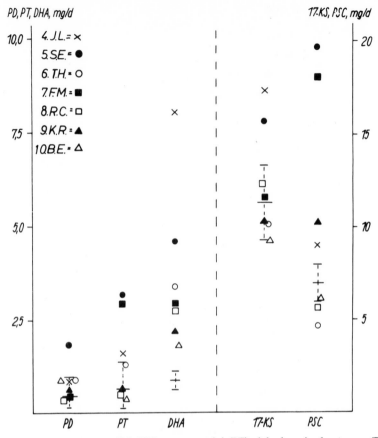

Figure 4. Urinary pregnanediol (PD), pregnanetriol (PT), dehydroepiandrosterone (DHA), 17-ketosteroids (17-KS), and Porter-Silber chromogens (PSC) in seven females with hirsutism. The *vertical bars* indicate the normal range.

pregnanetriol and PSC, in addition to elevated DHA. Patient F. M. (case 7) is shown in Figure 5 when she was 29 years of age. She presented a typical picture of hypercorticoidism with truncal obesity, hirsutism, menstrual irregularity, and hypertension (blood pressure, 170/100 mm Hg). The left adrenal gland was removed, and its histology showed adrenal hyperplasia with widening of the zona fasciculata. Steroid treatment for 15 years was not successful. X-ray treatment of the pituitary was ineffective, and for this reason the patient was treated with 0.5 g of aminoglutethimide daily and her blood pressure returned to normal. Table 1 illustrates the decrease of most urinary androgens under therapy with aminoglutethimide.

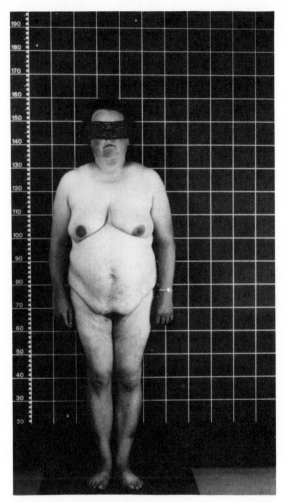

Figure 5. A 29-year-old female (F. M.) with hypercorticoidism.

Figure 6 presents a chromosomal male with 17-hydroxylase deficiency, hypertension, and pseudohermaphroditism. This patient was the first report in the literature of 17-hydroxylase deficiency in a male subject (Göbel, 1974; Göbel and Faber, 1970; Göbel et al., 1967; Göbel and Kling, 1969). The gynecological examination showed underdeveloped labia but otherwise normal female external genitalia with a blind vagina. The exploratory laparotomy showed a gonad resembling a testicle on each side in the process vaginalis and no uterus. Histologically, Leydig cell hyperplasia and small tubules without germinal elements were found.

Table 1. Individual urinary 17-ketosteroids (mg/24 hr) in patient F. M. during aminoglutethimide therapy

Date	Days	Androsterone	Etiocholanolone	DHA	11-0-Androsterone	11-0-Etiocholanolone	11-Hydroxyandrosterone	11-Hydroxyetiocholanolone
25/7/75	14	2.64	3.07	0.35	0.33	1.0	0.78	0.43
25/8/75	45	1.40	2.07	0.0	0.21	1.73	0.32	0.46
23/9/75	74	0.67	2.09	0.0	0.16	1.1	0.41	0.53

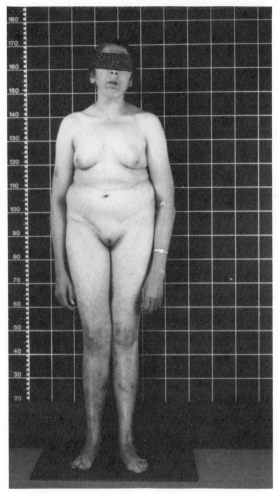

Figure 6. A 34-year-old XY patient (F. G.) with pseudohermaphroditism and hypertension as a consequence of 17-hydroxylase deficiency.

The clinical and biochemical data are presented in Figure 7. Blood pressure was elevated (220/150 mm Hg). There was a hypokalemic, hypochloremic, metabolic alkalosis and hypernatremia. The most striking feature of the urinary steroid pattern was the preponderance of corticosterone and 11-deoxycorticosterone metabolites. The secretory rates of these two steroids were abnormally high. Furthermore, plasma ACTH was markedly elevated (507.5 pg/ml). Aldosterone excretion was clearly below the normal level, although the urinary pregnanediol level was increased and pregnanetriol was not detectable. The 17-ketosteroids were also diminished.

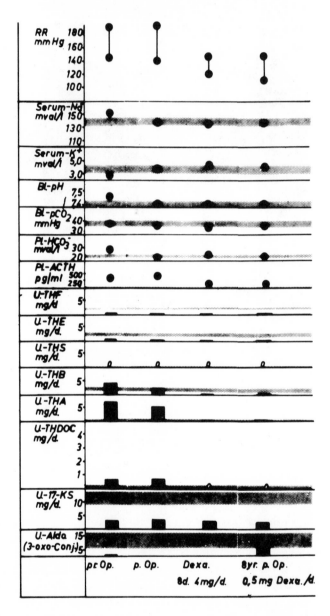

Figure 7. 17-Hydroxylase deficiency (F. G.), clinical and biochemical data.

After total resection of the left adrenal gland and partial resection of the right gland, there was no change in the clinical picture. Histologically, the adrenals showed bilateral hyperplasia with multiple nodular formations. Dexamethasone administration resulted in almost complete suppression of the abnormal excretion of urinary tetrahydrocorticosterone and tetrahydrodeoxycorticosterone, with a marked drop in plasma ACTH. Blood pressure decreased, electrolytes and acid base status returned to normal, along with plasma renin and urinary aldosterone. With adrenal suppression and substitution (0.5 mg of dexamethasone daily), the patient has been well and active for 8 years. Similar cases have been described in the meantime by New (1970), Mantero et al. (1971), and Bricaire et al. (1972).

ACKNOWLEDGMENTS

The authors would like to express their personal thanks to Mrs. A. Show and Mr. T. Wiehr for their excellent technical assistance.

REFERENCES

Bricaire, H., J. P. Luton, P. Laudat, J. C. Legrand, G. Turpin, P. Corcol, and M. Lemmer. 1972. A new male pseudohermaphroditism associated with hypertension due to a block of 17-hydroxylation. J. Clin. Endocrinol. Metab. 35: 67–72.

Göbel, P. 1974. 17-Hydroxylation deficiency with mineralocorticoid and testicular feminization syndrome. *In* Birth Defects Original Articles Series, Vol. X, pp. 301–303. Williams and Wilkins, Baltimore.

Göbel, P., and K. Faber. 1970. Endogener männlicher und induzierter weiblicher pseudohermaphroditismus. *In* Symp. Deutsch. Ges. Endokrin. Vol. 16, pp. 278–279. Springer-Verlag, New York.

Göbel, P., F. Heni, and A. d'Addabbo. 1958. Eine methode zur papierchromatographischen trennung und quantitativkolorimetrischen bestimmung der 17-ketosteroide im urin. Hoppe Seylers Z. Physiol. Chem. 311:201–212.

Göbel, P., D. Klaus, H. Siebner, U. Schmidt, J. Schürholz, and M. Minssen. 1967. Syndrom des 17α-hydroxylasemangels mit testikulärer feminisierung und multiplen missbildungen. Therapiewoche 17:2031–2033.

Göbel, P., and U. Kling. 1969. Nicht-aldosteronbedingter mineralo-corticoidismus. Verh. Dtsch. Ges. Inn. Med. 75:785–789.

Mantero, F., B. Busnardo, A. Riondel, R. Veyrat, and M. Austoni. 1971. Hypertension artérielle, alcalose hypokalémique et pseudohermaphroditisme mâle par déficit en 17-hydroxylase. Schweiz. Med. Wochenschr. 101:38–43.

New, M. I. 1970. Male pseudohermaphroditism due to 17α-hydroxylase deficiency. J. Clin. Invest. 49:1930–1941.

Porter, C. C., and R. H. Silber. 1950. A quantitative color reaction for cortisone and related 17,21-dihydroxy-20-ketosteroids. J. Biol. Chem. 1985:201–207.

Dysmorphism in Congenital Adrenal Hyperplasia

Thomas A. Good and Elaine E. Kohler

It is the purpose of this chapter to ask several questions. Can infants and children with congenital adrenal hyperplasia (CAH) be readily recognized by their facial and physical appearance? Can primary physicians be helped to be aware of CAH by emphasis on these features, so that a CAH child may be more readily recognized at 1–3 weeks of age and proper testing can be instituted for diagnosis of CAH? Certainly, in an infant with a diagnosis of diarrhea and gastroenteritis, pseudotumor cerebri, or pyloric stenosis (all of which are common misdiagnoses which can lead to death of the infant), a characteristic facial appearance would be useful. This is particularly true in the male infant, in whom genital changes are not very apparent.

The second problem relates to connective tissue neoplasia and CAH. In these studies, connective tissue neoplasia has been observed in 3 of 17 children with CAH. These authors are unaware of previous reports of this problem. Hypothetically, the aberrant androgen-rich state of the patient could support growth of neoplastic connective tissue cells.

All 17 patients reported here had 21-hydroxylase deficiency based on increased urinary pregnanetriol and 17-ketosteroid excretion (Table 1). Five males were non-salt-losers, and the rest of the children were salt-losers.

Of nine males, there were two deaths from adrenal crises. A 5-year-old non-salt-losing male (S. L.) died from a glucocorticoid-withdrawal adrenal crisis. The other death from adrenal crisis was in an undiagnosed newborn male. It is not uncommon that the first-born infant dies, if he is a male and the subsequent female children are recognized as having CAH (B. H., W. H., and T. H.; see Table 1). One additional death was from a malignancy, but two other tumors have also been observed in these children.

NEOPLASIA AND CAH

The first of these three boys with CAH was diagnosed at birth (C. W.; see Table 1). At age 5, he was noted to have a mass in his lower abdomen. The tumor

This study was supported in part by the Jeannette McKelvey Foundation, Milwaukee, Wisconsin.

Table 1. Case material of CAH patients

Patient	Sex	Type	PT[a]/17-KS (mg/24 hr)	Status	FU age (years:months)	BA/CA/Height (years:months)	IVP/Heart	Facies
S. L.	M	NSL	26/28	D	5:0	6:6/3:0 > 99%	N N	+
J. R.	M	NSL	44/10	L,T	7:7	13:6/6:1 > 99%	N N	++
B. M.	M	NSL	21/10	L	12:7	12:6/7:0 > 99%	N	++
B. M.	M-XYY	NSL	63/21	L,T	13:1	13:0/5:10 > 99%	N N	+++
G. M.	M-XY	NSL	28/16	L	2	2:6/2:0 80%	N N	+
J. B.	M	SL	12/4	L	4:1	6:0/4:0 75%	N N	+
C. W.	M	SL	1/3	D,T	5:0	25%	N N	+
V. C.	M	SL	10/4	L	9:4	6:0/9:4 < 3%	Ab Ab	++
B. H.	M	SL		D	7 days			
L. R.	F	SL	67/45	L	18:5	16:0/13:0 < 3%	N N	++
D. B.	F-XX	SL	1/2	L	5:10	2:6/4:1 < 3%	N N	+
L. R.	F	SL	1/9	L	3:10	2:6/3:2 30%	N N	+
D. B.	F	SL	16/9	L	13:3	11:0/11:6 25%	N N	
K. B.	F	SL	0.4/5	L	8:2	6:10/8:2 15%	N N	+
W. H.	F-XX	SL	5/	L	4:6	0:1/0:1 < 3%	N Ab	+
T. H.	F-XX	SL	7/8	L	5:6	13:8/4:5 10%	N N	+
M. B.	F	SL	12/5	L	3:5	1:8/2:4 10%	N N	++

[a]The abbreviations used are as follows: PT, pregnanetriol; 17-KS, 17-ketosteroids; FU, follow-up; BA, bone age; CA, chronological age; IVP, intravenous pyelogram; NSL, non-salt-losing; D, deceased; N, normal; L, living; T, tumor; SL, salt-losing; Ab, abnormal.

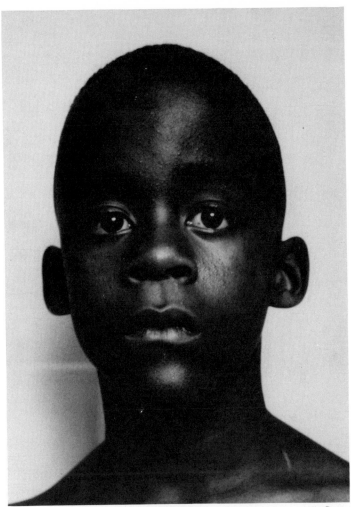

Figure 1. Facial appearance of a 7-year-old non-salt-losing black male with late diagnosed CAH. Note the dome-shaped head, pointed chin, and simplified ears.

appeared as a bluish perirectal perineal mass which was diagnosed on biopsy as an embryoma. The tumor was severely malignant, morphologically, with many mitotic figures. The child died from chest metastases about 2 1/2 months after the diagnosis was made. Autopsy was refused. The second child was found to have an osteogenic sarcoma of the distal end of the left femoral metaphysis (B. M.; see Table 1). The tumor contained disorganzied new bone formation, very few mitotic figures, and was invading the periosteum. Following leg amputation,

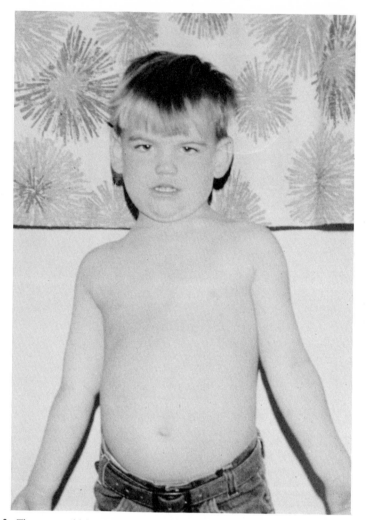

Figure 2. Three-year-old boy with salt-losing CAH. Note the prominent forehead, pointed chin, delayed inner canthal development, and increased carrying angles for a boy.

the diagnosis of CAH was made by dexamethasone suppression of extremely high urinary pregnanetriol and 17-ketosteroids excretion, and he was subsequently controlled with cortisone therapy. This case has been reported in detail by Mallin and Walker (1972). These authors commented on the fact that, even though the boy was only 7 years of age when the diagnosis of osteogenic sarcoma was made, his bone age was advanced to 13 years. They related the problem of neoplasia primarily to his chromosomal abnormality (XYY), because no cases of osteogenic sarcoma had been associated with CAH. One wonders whether or not his survival (presently of 7 years) might be related to the suppressive effect of the corticosteroid on the aberrant adrenal androgenic hormones which could have supported a bone tumor like this. This boy is mentally retarded, has a prominent chin, and marked calvarial facial disproportionment. However, two other siblings (male and female) with non-salt-losing CAH have also been diagnosed with normal chromosomes. These siblings are

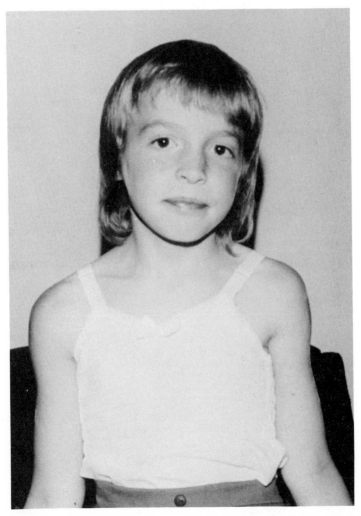

Figure 3. Six-year-old girl with salt-losing CAH displaying characteristic facies plus delayed inner canthal development.

more eumorphic. This indicates that B. M.'s dysmorphism may be more closely related to the chromosomal anomaly than to his hormonal imbalance.

The third boy was diagnosed as having CAH at 6 years of age with sexual precocity and a bone age of 11 years, with very high pregnanetriol and 17-keto-steroid excretions, which were suppressible by dexamethasone. This boy had complained of abdominal pains for several years. He was found to have a large spinal astrocytoma, classified as an astrocytoma type II, extending from T_3 to L_2. This tumor was almost entirely removed and the site irradiated. He has done well since that time, with adequate control of his CAH.

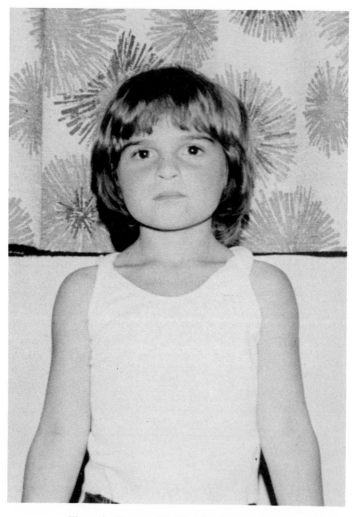

Figure 4. Six-year-old girl with salt-losing CAH.

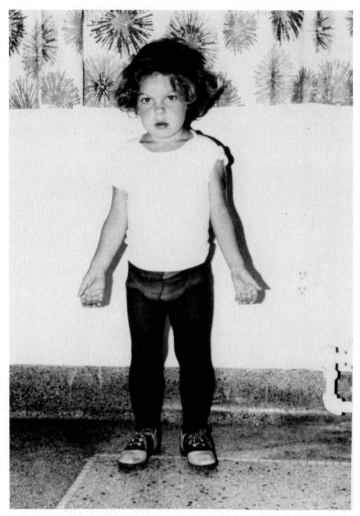

Figure 5. Three-year-old girl with salt-losing CAH. Note similarity to boy in Figure 2.

DYSMORPHISM IN CAH

A fitting definition of dysmorphism is the condition in which children with the same disease resemble each other more than they resemble other members of their immediate family (parents, siblings, and grandparents). The semblances determined by minor genetic code can be altered significantly enough by a major abnormality in the genetic code to result in a characteristic appearance. This is seen most easily in the chromosomal anomalies and the lysosomal enzyme deficiency diseases such as Hunter's or Hurler's disease and neurolipid storage disorders.

Children with non-salt-losing CAH have a characteristic dome-shaped head with a high forehead. There is a prominence at the tip of the chin, and calvarial-facial disproportionment is evident even in different racial cases. The patient in Figure 1 is rather typical of the children who are non-salt-losers diagnosed late. His facial appearance probably represents the effect of androgens upon the growth of the skull, the mandible, and apparently androgen-sensitive

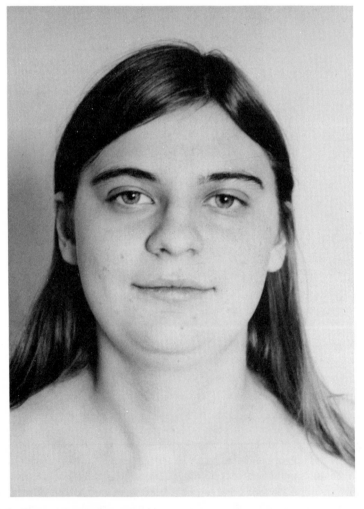

Figure 6. Sixteen-year-old girl with salt-losing CAH. Note the characteristic facies and small mandible.

fibrous tissue at the tip of the chin and the cartilagenous tissue of the nose. He also has simplification of his ears.

A boy with salt-losing CAH who was diagnosed in the neonatal period is depicted in Figure 2. He has prominence of his forehead, epicanthal folds, and a pointed chin. This boy, as in many males with CAH, has an increased carrying angle of his elbows. A girl who also has a pointed chin and a rounded head is shown in Figure 3. She is a salt-loser. The prominence of the calvaria and forehead are not as great as found in a non-salt-loser. She has a normal carrying

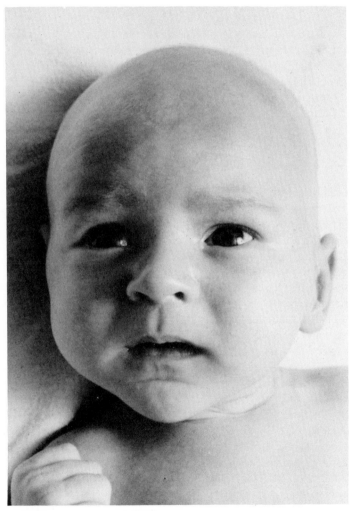

Figure 7. Facial appearance of a 1-month-old male infant with salt-losing CAH. Note similarity to previous cases.

angle for a young girl. Figure 4 presents a girl from a completely different ethnic group who again has the characteristic rounding of the mandible, pointing of the chin, rounding of the calvaria, and straight arms. Carrying angles in girls may be reduced in CAH.

The 3-year-old girl shown in Figure 5 has the same disorder, and again the rather characteristic facial appearance is noted. A delay in inner canthal development can also be seen in this child. This delay remains in some of these children until a much later age (see Figure 3). Perhaps this is related to the corticosteroid treatment, but some children with CAH have more prominent epicanthal folds than other infants early in the neonatal period, indicating a congenital mechanism.

A 16-year-old who was diagnosed as having salt-losing CAH in the neonatal period is shown in Figure 6. She also shows the characteristic facial appearance with the prominent chin tip and relative calvarial-facial disproportionment, less obvious than in the non-salt-losing patients, but still evident.

The 1-month-old baby in Figure 7 also shows the characteristic pointing of the chin. He has rounding of the calvaria and a prominent nose tip. Infants of different racial origin also have the same appearance of the face.

DERMATOGLYPHICS AND HAND GROWTH IN CAH

A 9-year-old boy, with facies similar to those described above (Figure 8), has a retracted fourth knuckle and shortened hands, with some broadening of the thumbs. The palmar dermatoglyphics of this youngster are shown in Figure 9A. There is an absence of the C area triradii. It is of some interest, however, that the hand print of this boy's father is very similar to the boy's, and, additionally, his mother's hand print (Figure 9B) resembles that of the father and the boy. The correlation between a parent and a child is about 0.5 for the hand prints on a quantitative dermatoglyphic analysis (Holt, 1968), but between parent and parent the correlation is usually less than 0.1. In this instance, the parents of a patient with an expressed recessive trait (CAH) both have hand prints which are almost identical with those of the child.

Because abnormal dermatoglyphics have been associated with neoplasia (Wertelecki et al., 1973), in this investigation quantitative dermatoglyphics were performed in a total of 11 children in 10 families. One of the characteristic dermatoglyphic features frequently seen in the families of CAH patients is an increased frequency of radially directed whorls on the hypothenar areas and double triradii. These are not very specific findings and are common dermatoglyphic variants. Abnormality in numbers of hypothenar triradii has been reported in hypothyroidism (Delabre et al., 1970). Another characteristic noted in the dermatoglyphics of these youngsters is a transverse A line with terminus high on the hypothenar area. Eighteen of 22 (male and female) palm prints had a

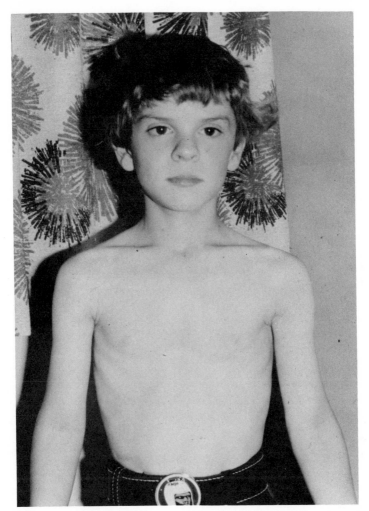

Figure 8. Nine-year-old male with salt-losing CAH. Note the small face and mandible with pointed chin.

transverse A line. This probably is explained by the fact that they had disturbance of linear hand growth in utero.

Because the development of the dermal ridges is subsequent to the organogenesis of the adrenal gland, the aberrant adrenal metabolism may influence the growth and the conformation of the dermatoglyphics of the propositus, which would influence the development of the dermal ridges and flexion creases.

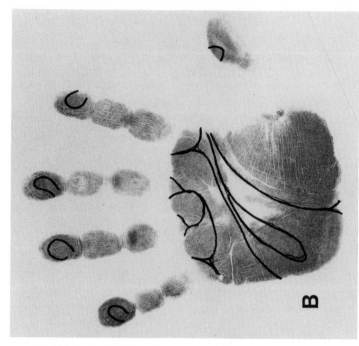

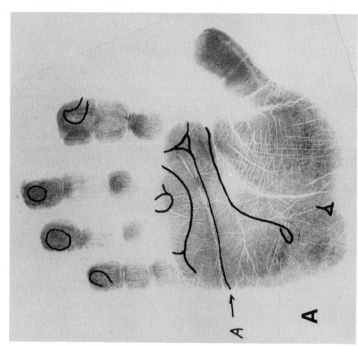

Figure 9. *A*, palm print of a 9-year-old boy with salt losing CAH. Note the absence of C triradii, the radically directed hypothenar whorl, and the transverse A line. *B*, palm print of the mother, which resembles those of the father and child.

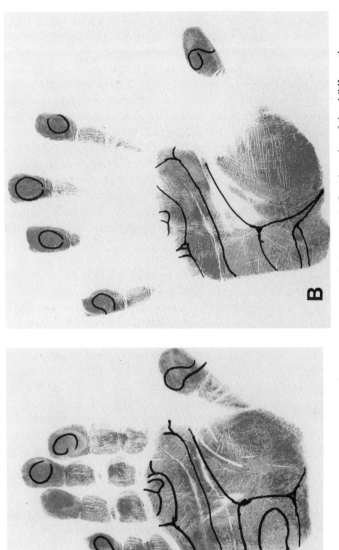

Figure 10. *A*, palm print of 3 1/2-year-old salt-losing CAH patient. Note the Sydney crease. *B*, palm print of the child's mother.

The Sydney crease is a flexion crease and results rather late in utero, developing from about the 16th–18th week up to the time of birth (Holt, 1968). The flexion creases provide some idea of the relative intrauterine growth of the hand. Although Sydney creases are relatively common and are seen in about 9% of the population, they are more frequent in hypothyroidism and leukemia. In children with CAH, it was found that 36% of 22 palm prints of 11 children had Sydney creases. This probably reflects a disturbance in hand growth and correlates with the transversing A line phenomena. The A line usually is much more oblique in a normal hand. The palm print from another child with adrenal hyperplasia shows some characteristics associated with Down's syndrome (Plato, Gereghino, and Steinberg, 1973) (Figure 10A). She has ulnar-directed whorls on the hypothenar area and associated distal triradius of the major T line and double triradii. This child's mother has prints which are very similar to those of her daughter (Figure 10B), which suggests that the genetics of palmar dermatoglyphics in some instances may not be significantly altered by intrauterine androgens.

In Down's syndrome, generalized biochemical and somatic abnormalities are present at conception and thereafter in most of the cells. Dermal ridge development is so profoundly influenced that the palm prints of mongoloid children can be readily distinguished. Although a characteristic palm print in children with CAH was not found, by using statistical quantitative methods it may be possible to show that dermatoglyphics in CAH patients are different from the general population. These patients have a very high incidence of transversing A lines, an increase in the Sydney flexion creases, and occasionally the so-called pseudopseudosimian creases. Simian creases have not been noted. A C line disturbance in the C area was observed, suggesting that there was an increased absence of C triradii. The radial-directed terminus of C line was not predominant. There were no consistent hypothenar patterns, but there seemed to be an increase of ulnar-directed loops, as seen in Down's syndrome. There appears to be an increase in ulnar whorling. This was true in the little boy who had the astrocytoma (see under "Neoplasia and CAH"), and was mentioned in the brother of the boy with the osteogenic sarcoma. Therefore, because there have been some associations between dermatoglyphics and cancer, these dermatoglyphic patterns should be followed up and carefully quantitated in patients with CAH.

SUMMARY AND SUGGESTIONS

Because effective treatment of these infants was developed only 25 years ago, a new population with problems related to CAH will undoubtedly be seen. An increased incidence of neoplasia may be one of these problems. Dermatoglyphics and flexion creases seem altered, similar to those reported for leukemic children and children with hypothyroidism. Hence, a patient registry could be useful in examining the possibility of increased incidence of connective tissue tumors in CAH and establishing dermatoglyphic differences from the general population.

ACKNOWLEDGMENTS

The authors wish to express appreciation to Drs. S. Mallin, F. Walker, and A. Pequet for the privilege of reviewing their cases.

REFERENCES

Delabre, M., D. Gnamey, T. Zettwoog, and G. Fontaine. 1970. Etude des dermatoglyphes dans le myxoedema congenital. Lille Med. 15:1055—1058.

Holt, S. B. 1968. The Genetics of Dermal Ridges. Charles C. Thomas, Publishers, Springfield, Illinois.

Mallin, S. R., and F. A. Walker. 1972. Effects of XYY karyotype in one of two brothers with congenital adrenal hyperplasia. Clin. Genet. 3:490—494.

Plato, C. C., J. J. Gereghino, and F. S. Steinberg. 1973. Palmar dermatoglyphics of Down's syndrome: revisited. Pediatr. 7:111—118.

Wertelecki, W., C. C. Plato, J. F. Fraumeni, and J. D. Niswander. 1973. Dermatoglyphics in leukemia. Pediatr. Res. 7:620—626.

Evidence for Cortisol Secretion by Testicular Masses in Congenital Adrenal Hyperplasia

Nezam Radfar, Jerry Kolins, and Frederic C. Bartter

The occurrence of bilateral testicular tumors in patients with congenital adrenal hyperplasia has been known for many years (Allibone, Baar, and Cant, 1947; Burke, Gilbert, and Uehling, 1973; Cohen, 1946; Fore et al., 1972; Gardner, Sniffen, and Zygmuntowicz, 1950; Hedinger, 1954; Landling and Gold, 1951; Larson and Regerger, 1954; Prader, 1953; Sobel, Sniffen, and Talbot, 1951; Thelander, 1946; Wilkins, Fleischmann, and Howard, 1940). There has not been agreement, however, on the origin of these tumors. Although some authors have called them "ectopic adrenal tissues" (Wilkins, Fleischmann, and Howard, 1940), others (Landling and Gold, 1951) have believed that they represent Leydig cells. This confusion results from the great similarity between the histopathological picture of adrenal rests and that of Leydig cells. Only with the advent of new biochemical methods for determination of steroid hormones in recent years has it been possible to study these testicular tumors in more detail and to show that, regardless of their histological appearance, some behave like adrenal tissue, i.e., they can be stimulated by adrenocorticotropic hormone (ACTH) and suppressed by dexamethasone (Glen and Boyce, 1963; Schoen, DiRaimond, and Dominguez, 1961).

The purpose of this chapter is to present a patient with congenital adrenal hyperplasia and bilateral testicular tumors which were secreting cortisol, although they resembled Leydig cells morphologically.

CASE REPORT

A 19-year-old man with salt-losing congenital adrenal hyperplasia (CAH) resulting from 21-hydroxylase deficiency was admitted to the National Institutes of Health for evaluation of bilateral testicular enlargement. Twelve months prior to admission, he had noted bilateral testicular swelling and tenderness but had not

331

sought medical attention. He was otherwise asymptomatic. His medications included hydrocortisone (25 mg p.o./day) and deoxycorticosterone trimethyl-acetate (12.5 mg I.M./month).

The diagnosis of congenital adrenal hyperplasia had been made shortly after birth, because an older brother had died at the age of 2 years from salt loss and dehydration, shown at autopsy to be a result of untreated congenital adrenal hyperplasia. Of five siblings, two boys and two girls were afflicted with the disorder. This patient had been maintained in good health with cortisol, deoxy-corticosterone, and salt replacement. At the chronological age of 10, his height age was 10 years and his bone age 8½–9 years. At the age of 14 years 5 months, his height age was 13½ and his bone age 15 years. The pubertal period was unremarkable except that his father thought that the patient's testes were larger than usual for his age when he was 14.

On physical examination, the patient appeared to be a normal, virilized, muscular young adult in no distress. His height was 167 cm, his weight 54.85 kg, his blood pressure 112/64 mm Hg, his pulse 84 beats/min. His examination was unremarkable except for testicular enlargement (the left testis measured 8.0 X 4.0 cm, the right 7.8 X 4.0 cm). Both testes were firm and tender and showed nodular swellings. The epididymes and spermatic cords appeared normal.

Routine laboratory studies showed normal results as follows: hematocrit, 43.1%; hemoglobin, 15 g%; white blood cell count, 10,600/mm^3 with normal differential; sodium, 138; potassium, 4.0; chloride, 102; and carbon dioxide content, 23 mEq/liter. Blood urea nitrogen, creatinine, chest x-ray, and intra-venous pyelogram were all normal.

STUDY DESIGN

The patient was evaluated during three periods, according to the following protocol:

1. Basal. Hydrocortisone was administered in the patient's usual daily dose (10 mg at 0800 hr; 5 mg at 1500 hr; 10 mg at 2200 hr). Twenty-four-hr urines were collected for measurement of 17-ketosteroids (17-KS) and pregnanetriol. Testic-ular length was measured in centimeters. Left testicular open biopsy was per-formed under general anesthesia.

2. Complete adrenocorticotropic hormone (ACTH) suppression. Dexametha-sone (0.5 mg/6 hr) was administered for 2 days in addition to the patient's usual daily hydrocortisone. Twenty-four-hr urinary 17-KS and pregnanetriol were measured daily. Testicular length was measured as noted above.

3. Adrenal stimulation with ACTH. While the patient was receiving hydro-cortisone (25 mg/day), ACTH (Acthar, Armour) was administered intramuscu-larly (40 U./12 hr) to fully stimulate adrenal tissues. After 2 days of stimulation with ACTH, heparinized samples were obtained simultaneously from a right forearm vein and left spermatic vein under fluoroscopy. The plasma was frozen

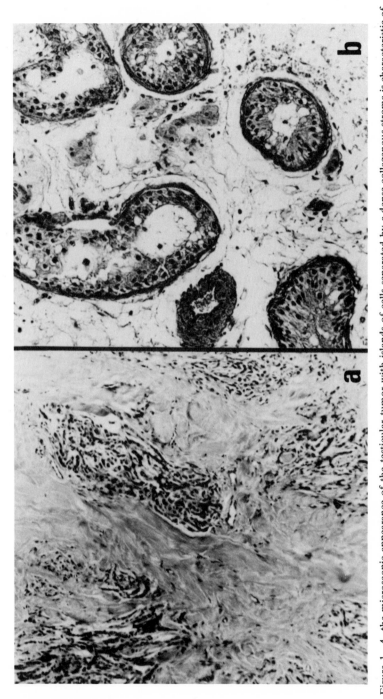

Figure 1. *A*, the microscopic appearance of the testicular tumor with islands of cells separated by a dense collagenous stroma is characteristic of Leydig cell tumor. ×60. *B*, nontumorous portion of the testis contains seminiferous tubules with spermatocytic arrest. Normal-appearing Leydig cells are within the interstitium. ×170.

at −20°C until assayed. Plasma cortisol and testosterone concentrations were determined by radioimmunoassay as previously described (Dufau et al., 1972; Loriaux, Guy, and Lipsett, 1973).

RESULTS

Testicular Biopsy

At operation, multiple nodules protruded from the superior and middle portions of the testis. The tissue was rubbery firm, yellow in color, and had a reticular pattern.

On microscopic examination, there was hyalinization of the tumor stroma (Figure 1A), which correlated with the reticular pattern seen at gross inspection. The tumor was composed of homogeneous round cells with eosinophilic cytoplasm and finely stippled nuclei. Cell boundaries were indistinct; Reinke's crystalloids were not identified. Seminiferous tubules were absent from the tumor mass and were compressed at the periphery of the lesion. These tubules showed a maturation arrest, with only spermatocytes within tubular lumina. An extremely rare tubule contained spermatozoa. Normal Leydig cells which

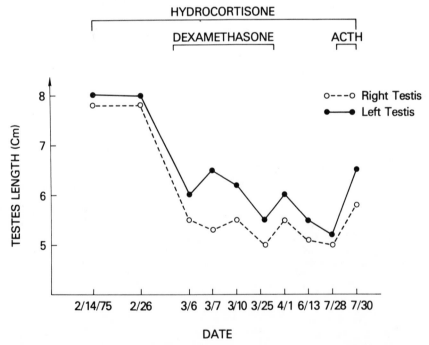

Figure 2. The changes in the length of the right and left testes during basal period, after dexamethasone administration, and after stimulation with ACTH.

contained Reinke's crystalloids were identified in the interstitial tissue of the nontumorous portion of the testis (Figure 1*B*).

Testicular Size

The changes in testicular length during ACTH suppression and adrenal stimulation with ACTH are summarized in Figure 2. Prior to suppression with dexamethasone, the testicular sizes were 8.0 X 4.0 cm (left) and 7.8 X 4.0 cm (right). A marked decrease in testicular size was evident by the 2nd day of dexamethasone. Administration of ACTH for 2 days resulted in an increase in testicular size and a recurrence of both pain and tenderness in the testes.

Spermatic Vein Sampling

After 2 days of stimulation with ACTH, the concentration of cortisol in the spermatic vein (14.5 μg/dl) was about 3 times that in the peripheral vein (5.2 μg/dl). Simultaneous values for testosterone in the spermatic vein (3,411 ng/dl) were 7.8 times those in a peripheral vein (437 ng/dl).

Urinary Steroid Metabolites

Basal urinary excretion of 17-KS and pregnanetriol were 33.0 and 18.5 mg/24 hr, respectively. Following ACTH suppression for 6 days, the excretion of 17-KS and pregnanetriol had decreased to 12.3 (37% of basal) and 4.3 (23% of basal) mg/24 hr, respectively.

DISCUSSION

The rare occurrence of bilateral testicular nodules in patients with congenital adrenal hyperplasia has been appreciated for many years. There has been, however, no agreement about the nature of such nodules. Whereas some authors have called them adrenal rests, others have believed that they are composed of Leydig cells. This confusion results from the similarity in the histological appearance of these two types of cells. According to many authors, the two basic characteristics of Leydig cell tumors are intratesticular location and the presence of Reinke's crystalloids.

These criteria, however, are not always absolute. For example, although adrenal rests had not been thought to be located in the substance of the testes, Wilkins, Fleischmann, and Howard (1940) reported a case in which the testes were completely replaced by the aberrant adrenal tissue. Similar cases have also been reported by others (Allibone, Baar, and Cant, 1947; Cohen, 1946; Gardner, Sniffen, and Zygmuntowicz, 1950; Thelander, 1946). In addition, although the presence of Reinke's crystalloids is thought to be pathognomonic for Leydig cells (Reinke, 1896), these crystalloids are present in only 40% of testicular nodules which morphologically resemble Leydig cell tumors (Mostofi and Price, 1973). As a third example, Savard (1960) reported a case of "Leydig cell tumor" in which 11β-hydroxylase activity was shown in vitro, a finding which has not been reported for normal Leydig cells. This suggests that the testicular tumor in Savard's patient contained adrenal rest cells.

The difficulty involved in differentiating adrenal rest cells from Leydig cells makes the endocrine evaluation of such tumors mandatory. There are only a few cases in which endocrine studies have been performed to separate these two tissues by their functional properties. Although Dominguez (1961) demonstrated 11β-hydroxylase activity in vitro in the testis of a patient with the adrenogenital syndrome, and Hamwi et al. (1963) isolated radioactively labeled cortisone and cortisol by incubating such a testicular tumor in a medium containing 4-[^{14}C] progesterone, Fore et al. (1972) were the first to show cortisol secretion into the testicular venous effluent in the syndrome. Our patient, therefore, represents the second in whom the ability of the testicular tumor to secrete cortisol is documented in vivo.

As the functional evaluation was not performed in many of the previously reported cases of testicular tumors found in CAH, it is not known how many of the cases of "Leydig cell tumors" could have been adrenal rest tumors. Regardless of the morphology of their cells, these testicular tumors appear to be ACTH-dependent, because it has been shown that ACTH suppression reduced testicular size in such cases (Burke, Gilbert, and Uehling, 1973; Gardner et al., 1950; Glen and Boyce, 1963; Kaplan, 1966; Linguette et al., 1970). In this patient, testicular volume decreased rapidly during treatment with dexamethasone and subsequently increased during treatment with ACTH.

The appearance of testicular tumors in this patient during a time when he was treated with cortisol suggests either that the dosage was not adequate for optimal suppression of ACTH or that he did not take his medication. The dangers of inadequate therapy in males are 2-fold in regard to spermatogenesis and fertility: 1) the tumor can destroy the seminiferous tubules by compression, and 2) the great contribution of adrenal androgen from hyperplastic adrenal tissues to plasma testosterone may result in suppression of plasma luteinizing hormone with subsequent reduction in intratesticular testosterone concentration. It has been shown that high intratesticular testosterone is required for adequate spermatogenesis (Steinberger and Steinberger, 1969). The low testosterone concentration in this patient may, therefore, have contributed to his oligospermia. The details of pituitary-gonadal feedback regulation, as well as the oligospermia, are the subject of an as-yet unpublished paper, which will appear in the *Journal of Clinical Endocrinology and Metabolism*.

SUMMARY

This chapter has presented a study of a young man with bilateral testicular tumors in association with salt-losing congenital adrenal hyperplasia with secretion of cortisol directly from the testes, a condition reported only once previously. These studies emphasize the importance of functional evaluation of such testicular tumors for the diagnostic work-up and for adequate treatment.

ACKNOWLEDGMENTS

The authors wish to express their appreciation to Dr. Nasser Javadpour for performing an open testicular biopsy, to Dr. John Doppman for spermatic vein sampling, and to Miss Kathy Telfar for secretarial assistance.

REFERENCES

Allibone, E. C., H. S. Baar, and W. H. P. Cant. 1947. Interrenal syndrome in childhood. Arch. Dis. Child. 22:210–225.

Barkte, A. R., E. Steele, N. Musto, and B. W. Caldwell. 1973. Fluctuations in plasma testosterone levels in adult male rats and mice. Endocrinol. 92: 1223–1228.

Burke, E. F., E. Gilbert, and D. T. Uehling. 1973. Adrenal rest tumors of the testes. J. Urol. 109:649–652.

Cohen, H. 1946. Hyperplasia of the adrenal cortex associated with bilateral testicular tumors. Am. J. Pathol. 22:157–173.

Dominguez, O. V. 1961. Biosynthesis of steroids by testicular tumors complicating congenital adrenocortical hyperplasia. J. Clin. Endocrinol. Metab. 21: 663–674.

Dufau, M. L., K. J. Catt, T. Tsuruhara, and D. Ryan. 1972. Radioimmunoassay of plasma testosterone. Clin. Chim. Acta 37:109–116.

Fore, W. W., T. Bledsoe, M. D. Weber, R. Akers, and T. Brooks. 1972. Cortisol production by testicular tumors in adrenogenital syndrome. Arch. Intern. Med. 130:59–63.

Gardner, L. I., R. C. Sniffen, and A. S. Zygmuntowicz. 1950. Followup studies in a boy with mixed adrenal cortical disease. Pediatrics 5:808–823.

Glen, J. F., and W. H. Boyce. 1963. Adrenogenitalism with testicular adrenal rests simulating interstitial cell tumor. J. Urol. 89:457–463.

Hamwi, G. J., G. Gwinip, J. H. Mostow, and P. K. Besch. 1963. Activation of testicular adrenal rest tissue by prolonged excessive ACTH production. J. Clin. Endocrinol. Metab. 23:861–869.

Hedinger, C. 1954. Beidseitige Hodentumoren und Kongenitales Adrenogenitales syndrom (Leydig-Zellen oder Nebennierenrindingewebe?) Schweiz Zeitschr. Allgemeine Pathol. 17:743–750.

Kaplan, M. 1966. Congenital adrenal hyperplasia with large testicles. Apropos of a further case. Ann. Pediatr. (Paris) 13:607–610.

Landling, B. H., and E. Gold. 1951. The occurrence and significance of Leydig cell proliferation in familial adrenal cortical hyperplasia. J. Clin. Endocrinol. Metab. 11:1436–1453.

Larson, C. P., and C. C. Regerger. 1954. Macrogenitosomia precox with adrenal hyperplasia and bilateral heterotropic adrenal cortical tissue of the testes. Western J. Surg. 62:602–606.

Linguette, M., A. Dupont, P. Fossati, M. Decouix, and R. Mesmacque. 1970. Tumeur testiculaire bilatérale chez un sujet porteur d'une hyperplasie congénitale des surrenales. Lille Med. 15:936–938.

Loriaux, D. L., R. Guy, and M. B. Lipsett. 1973. A simple, quick, solid-phase method for radioimmunoassay of plasma estradiol in late pregnancy and of plasma cortisol. J. Clin. Endocrinol. Metab. 36:788–790.

Mostofi, F. K., and E. B. Price. 1973. Tumors of the male genital system: atlas of tumor pathology. Fascicle 8:86.

Prader, V. A. 1953. Die Cortisondauerbehandlung des Kongenitalen Adrenogenitalen Syndroms. Helv. Paediatr. Acta 8:386–423.

Reinke, F. 1896. Beritrage zur histolgiedes menshen. I. Ueber Krystalloidbildurgen inden interstitiellen zellen des menschlichen Hoders. Arch. Mikrobiol. Anat. 47:34–38.

Savard, K. 1960. Biosynthesis of steroids by testicular tumors complicating congenital adrenocortical hyperplasia. J. Clin. Invest. 39:534–553.

Schoen, E. J., V. DiRaimond, and O. U. Dominguez. 1961. Bilateral testicular tumors complicating congenital adrenocortical hyperplasia. J. Clin. Endocrinol. Metab. 21:518–532.

Sobel, E. H., R. C. Sniffen, and N. B. Talbot. 1951. Testis V. Use of testicular biopsies in the differential diagnosis of precocious puberty. Pediatrics 8: 701–716.

Steinberger, E., and A. Steinberger. 1969. The spermatogenic function of the testis in the gonads. In E. W. McKerns (ed.), The Gonads, p. 715. Appleton-Century-Crofts, New York.

Thelander, H. D. 1946. Congenital adrenal cortical insufficiency associated with macrogenitosomia: followup and terminal report. J. Pediatr. 29:213–221.

Wilkins, L., W. Fleischmann, and J. E. Howard. 1940. Macrogenitosomia praecox associated with adrenogenic tissue of the adrenal and death from cortico adrenal insufficiency. Endocrinology 26:385–395.

Congenital Adrenal Hyperplasia
Mortality Experience

Robert J. Winter[1] and Georgeanna Jones Klingensmith[2]

Prior to the introduction of cortisol and 11-deoxycorticosterone acetate (DOCA) as therapy for congenital adrenal hyperplasia (CAH), the clinical course in the salt-losing form of the disease was invariably a fatal one. Although mortality in the simple virilizing form of CAH was less common, virilization remained unrestrained. Cortisone therapy promptly reversed this trend. Replacement of steroids in CAH during childhood traditionally follows the guidelines found in Table 1.

Mortality in CAH during the first decade of therapy was approximately 8% (Cleveland, Green, and Wilkins, 1962). A review of the mortality experience in CAH during the first 25 years of cortisone therapy is presented here, either as the experience with CAH at the Johns Hopkins Clinic or as the cumulative data of eight endocrine clinics in the United States. Despite the limitations of a retrospective, multiclinic mortality study, the data suggest that some children with CAH, usually infants, die during a stressful illness despite traditionally appropriate management of their adrenal replacement.

Table 2 gives the cumulative statistics from 1950–1975 from the Pediatric Endocrine Clinic at the Johns Hopkins Hospital. A total of 195 patients with adrenal hyperplasia were diagnosed and treated during this 25-year period. The majority were Caucasians, female, with CAH of the non-salt-losing variety. Current information is available on 148 of these patients. Seventeen patients have died since 1950, representing 8.7% of the total population and 11.5% of the group currently being followed. In the past decade, only 2.3% have died. Eight of the 17 patients were salt-losers and 9 were not. Therapy was presumed inadequate in six patients, adequate in nine, and unknown in three (Table 3).

Data over the past decade have also been collated from several clinics. A total of 584 patients from eight clinics is represented in Table 4. Nine of these patients have died for a percentage mortality of 1.5%, a rate in the last decade

---

[1] Recipient of Trainee Grant 5T01 AM 05219-14 from the United States Public Health Service.

[2] Recipient of a grant from the Stetler Research Fund for Women Physicians.

Table 1. Recommended steroid replacement in adrenal hyperplasia

	Daily Maintenance	During stress
Glucocorticoids (as cortisol)		
Oral dose	25 mg/m^2/day	2–3 times maintenance dose
Parenteral dose	12.5 mg/m^2/day	2–3 times maintenance dose
Mineralocorticoids		
Oral dose		
(as 9α-fluorocortisol)	0.05–0.10 mg/day	0.05–0.10 mg/day
Parenteral dose		
(as DOCA I.M.)	1.0–2.0 mg/day	1.0–2.0 mg/day
Subcutaneous DOCA pellets	Two 125-mg pellets every 9–12 months	See text (recommendation 2)

Abstracted from Migeon (1974) and Gutai and Migeon (1975).

which is significantly lower than that of 8.7% for the past 25 years. Seven of the nine patients who died were known salt-losers. Cause of death in these nine individuals varied. One patient fell from a window and died immediately; another, for whom no record is available, died at age 33. The remaining seven patients had salt-losing adrenal hyperplasia. At least four died as a result of inadequate therapy during times of stress. Assessment of the adequacy of this therapy is by necessity somewhat subjective. Nevertheless, two patients died with a documented infection while receiving only oral steroids in maintenance or less than maintenance doses. In both cases, inadequate understanding or compliance by the parents accounted for the deaths. Another patient died in an outlying hospital during surgery in the absence of steroid replacement. In the fourth patient, presented in detail below, the relationship of CAH therapy to death is much less clear.

Table 2. Mortality experience in congenital adrenal hyperplasia at the Johns Hopkins Clinic (1950–1975)

Total ($n = 195$)		Deceased ($n = 17, 8.7\%$)
50 (25.6%)	Genetic male	1 (5.9%)
145 (74.4%)	Genetic female	16 (94.1%)
188 (96.4%)	Caucasian	15 (88.2%)
7 (3.6%)	Black	2 (11.8%)
83 (42.6%)	Salt-losing	8 (47.0%)
108 (55.4%)	Non-salt-losing	8 (47.0%)
4 (2.1%)	Hypertensive	1 (6.0%)

Table 3. Causes of death due to congenital adrenal hyperplasia at the Johns Hopkins Clinic (1950–1975)

Cause of death ($n = 17$)	
Presumably inadequate therapy	6
Presumably adequate therapy	8
CAH-related	5
Crib death	1
Wilson's disease	1
Breast carcinoma	1
Unknown	3

The patient was the product of a 38-week, uncomplicated gestation in a 22-year-old mother, who had suffered a first trimester abortion 2 years previously. Ambiguous genitalia were noted at birth. Symptoms of adrenal insufficiency began on the 6th day. Laboratory studies, including serum sodium of 127 mEq/liter, potassium of 8.0 mEq/liter, and 17-ketosteroids of 2.2, 2.8, and 3.0 mg/24 hr, all were consistent with congenital virilizing adrenal hyperplasia of the salt-losing variety. The baby was begun on parenteral administration of maintenance glucocorticoids, and DOCA pellets were implanted.

Table 4. Combined experience in congenital adrenal hyperplasia from eight United States clinics

Clinic	Current follow-up	Deaths Salt-loss/ non-salt-loss	Percentage of mortality
Johns Hopkins, Baltimore	134	2/1	2.3%
Children's Hospital, Philadelphia	101	1/0	1.0%
Columbia Hospital, New York City	50	0/1	2.0%
University of California, San Francisco	30	0/0	0 %
University of Virginia, Charlottesville	30.	1/0	3.3%
Northwestern University, Chicago	74	1/0	1.4%
Children's Hospital, Pittsburgh	90	2/0	2.2%
Children's Hospital, Boston	75	0/0	0 %
Totals	584	7/2	1.5%

She was maintained on parenteral cortisone acetate (12.5 mg/m^2/day) until the age of 19 months, when oral hydrocortisone was begun at a dose of 30 mg/m^2/day. Two DOCA pellets were reimplanted at 10 months of age. Growth and development were normal, and urinary ketosteroid levels were persistently suppressed.

At the age of 20 months, the patient vomited twice during the night, and 15 mg of cortisone acetate was given intramuscularly the next morning. That afternoon the child was examined, and bilateral otitis media was diagnosed. She had a temperature of 40.8°C and received Bicillin (long-acting penicillin) and Gantrisin (sulfisoxazole). Serum sodium was 135 mEq/liter and serum potassium 4.8 mEq/liter. DOCA pellets were still palpable. Surface area was 0.5 m^2.

The following day the child remained slightly febrile vomited twice, but otherwise ate and behaved normally. She received 15 mg of cortisone acetate I.M. that morning and appeared well at that time. The parents remained in phone contact with the physician throughout the duration of the illness. During the night, she had four diarrheal stools. At 6:30 a.m., she was found moribund with labored respirations. She died on the way to the hospital. Permission for an autopsy was refused.

Cause of death in this child is unclear. She received greater than twice maintenance parenteral glucocorticoid during this illness. Nevertheless, on the basis of borderline electrolyte values and the lapse of time since DOCA pellet implantation, one may question whether additional mineralocorticoid was indicated as well. However, the course of her illness and her sudden deterioration remain poorly understood.

Three additional deaths occurred despite appropriate therapy. One died at home during a mild viral illness after receiving a 3-fold increase parenterally of maintenance cortisone acetate the night before. DOCA pellets were palpable in situ at the time of death. Autopsy was inconclusive. Another child died in the hospital, 18 hr after admission, again despite presumably appropriate increases in glucocorticoid and mineralocorticoid therapy. Normal blood pressure and pulse were recorded in this febrile child only 10 min before cardiorespiratory arrest.

Table 5. Age at death

	No. of deaths	Age range	age <2 years (%)
Johns Hopkins' experience (1950–1975)			
Total deaths	17	1 month–45 years	41%
CAH-related deaths	11	1 month–7 years	55%
Combined clinics' experience (1965–1975)			
Total deaths	9	6 months–33 years	56%
CAH-related deaths	7	6 months–5 years	71%

The third child died at home 3 days after hospital discharge. She had been uneventfully and appropriately treated for *Hemophilus influenza* meningitis. Cerebrospinal fluid cultures were sterile before discharge and at autopsy, and she received maintenance steroid doses at home. Two DOCA pellets had been implanted 5 months previously. Her only symptoms before death were lethargy and mild fever. She was found dead in bed a few hours after breakfast. Autopsy revealed no identifiable cause of death. Thus, of the seven CAH-related deaths, all patients were salt-losers. Specific information is available for five of these patients; all were female and four of the five had DOCA pellets implanted from 5–11 months before death.

Age at time of death is presented in Table 5 (the Johns Hopkins Clinic experience from 1950–1975, combined clinic experience from 1965–1975). It is apparent that infancy and early childhood are high risk periods for individuals with adrenal hyperplasia. Tabulating CAH-related deaths only, 55–71% of the deaths occurred prior to age 2. Of the CAH-related deaths in the past decade, all had salt-losing adrenal hyperplasia and all deaths occurred in the morning hours.

Assessment of cause of death in a retrospective mortality survey cannot be convincingly objective, particularly when the therapy for a disease such as adrenal hyperplasia is a recent and evolving entity. The observations presented suggest that this therapy may well need continual evolution. Three or possibly four deaths in the past decade occurred despite traditionally acceptable therapy. Thus, therapeutic guidelines may need revision and expansion, as indicated under "Recommendations."

CONCLUSIONS

1. The mortality rate in CAH during the decade of 1965–1975 in eight United States clinics has been 1.5%. This appears to be a significant reduction from CAH mortality during the preceding 15 years (1950–1965).
2. CAH mortality appears to be more common in individuals with the salt-losing form.
3. Death was most common during infancy and early childhood.
4. Death was most common in the early morning hours.
5. Although some patients died as a result of inadequate therapy during the periods of acute stress, others died of undetermined causes while receiving traditionally appropriate therapy. Autopsies either were not performed or were inconclusive.

RECOMMENDATIONS

1. All patients with CAH should receive at least double or triple doses of maintenance glucocorticoid replacement during illness or stress.

2. Mineralocorticoid replacement is best judged by clinical criteria and by frequent electrolyte determinations, especially after subcutaneous DOCA pellets have been in place 9 months. Measurements of plasma renin may prove to be a guideline to the efficacy of the DOCA pellets.

3. Fever may be an indicator of stress, but its absence should not be a contraindication to increasing steroid replacements.

4. Parenteral therapy during stress should be considered a) when vomiting interferes with oral therapy; b) when illness is of such severity that enteric absorption of drugs may be inadequate; c) if DOCA pellets are small, non-palpable, or have been in situ for more than 9 months; or d) if infection, stress, and/or fever continue despite appropriate therapy.

5. The number of deaths occurring in the morning hours suggests more frequent administration of steroids during stress may be beneficial.

6. Hospitalization of the ill child should be contemplated early in the course of the illness, particularly for infants.

ACKNOWLEDGMENTS

The assistance of the following physicians in collating the data is greatly appreciated: Drs. John Parks, Dennis Styne, Carol Huseman, Ann Johanson, Orville C. Green, S. Pang, John Crigler, and Claude J. Migeon. The thoughtful advice of Drs. Migeon and Green has been of great help as well.

REFERENCES

Cleveland, W. W., O. C. Green, and L. Wilkins. 1962. Deaths in congenital adrenal hyperplasia. Pediatrics 29:3—17.

Gutai, J. P., and C. J. Migeon. 1975. Adrenal insufficiency during the neonatal period. Clin. Perinatol. 2:163—182.

Migeon, C. J. 1974. Hypoadrenocorticism. *In* V. C. Kelley (ed), Metabolic, Endocrine, and Genetic Disorders of Children, pp. 245—262. Harper and Row, Hagerstown, Maryland.

SURGICAL CORRECTION AND SEXUAL MATURATION

Necessity for and the Technique of Secondary Surgical Treatment of the Masculinized External Genitalia of Patients with Virilizing Adrenal Hyperplasia

Howard W. Jones, Jr., Silvia C. Garcia, and Georgeanna Jones Klingensmith

Jones and Verkauf (1970) previously reported results through 1968 of the surgical reconstruction of the masculinized external genitalia of 84 female patients with congenital virilizing adrenal hyperplasia. In that report, it was noted that approximately 18% of the patients required a secondary operation to provide a vaginal outlet satisfactory for coitus. However, in no case was there any problem with the egress of menstrual blood. The mean follow-up period after the first operation was 6 years 9 months. Although for the psychological benefit of patient and family it has been considered preferable to perform such operations before 17 months of age, several patients in the series were operated upon after this, because they were already older than 17 months when it was discovered in 1950 that cortisone was effective in reversing the otherwise progressive virilization of such patients.

In connection with a symposium commemorating the twenty-fifth anniversary of the discovery of the use of cortisone in the adrenogenital syndrome, the same 84 patients were reevaluated through 1974. This chapter reports the findings of that follow-up.

MATERIAL

The details of the initial operative procedure in the 84 patients were set forth in the report of Jones and Verkauf (1970). Briefly, all patients had incision of the urogenital sinus plus clitorectomy, according to the technique previously described (Jones and Jones, 1954; Jones and Wilkins, 1961). In most instances, the

Table 1. Eighty-four patients classified according to number of surgical procedures

	Number	Percentage
One procedure	59	70
Two procedures	20	24
Three procedures	5	6

vaginal orifice could be exteriorized satisfactorily at the initial operation, but in a few instances the vaginal exteriorization was deliberately postponed when it was considered important to achieve female-appearing external genitalia at the earliest practical time. The second stages of the elective two-stage procedures were included among the 18% of reoperations reported as of 1968.

The second follow-up of these 84 patients was carried out as of the end of 1974. In most instances, a simple review of the record was all that was necessary; others were contacted by letter or telephone. Contact could not be made with 21 patients; therefore, the 1974 follow-up was 75% complete. For those who could not be followed, the 1968 result was tabulated. The mean follow-up period was 12 years 9 months, with extremes of 7–22 years.

RESULTS

By 1969, 15 of the 84 patients, or 18%, had required a second procedure. One of these 15 required a third procedure, so that 16 secondary procedures were actually required for the 15 patients.

Through 1974, 10 more patients required secondary procedures, and 5 of the 25 patients requiring secondary procedures required a third procedure (Table 1).

Two of the secondary procedures were for excision of a painful clitoral stump. The remaining procedures were to provide a vaginal orifice adequate for coitus (Table 2).

Table 2. Surgical procedures in 84 patients

Type of surgery	No. of Procedures		
	One	Two	Three
Reconstruction	84		
Exteriorization of vagina		12	
Relaxation of orifice		11	5
Other		2	

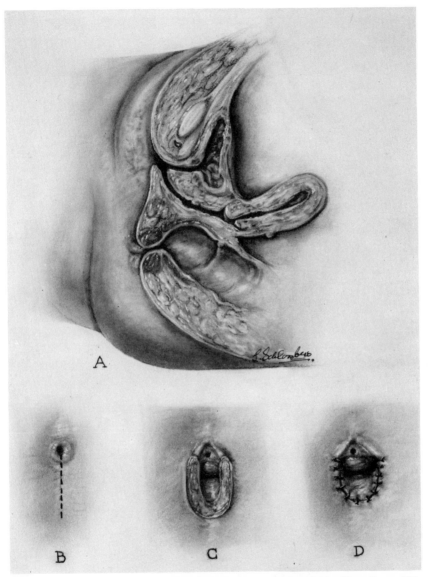

Figure 1. *A,* a sagittal view of an inadequately exteriorized vaginal orifice; *B,* a midline incision to correct the defect; *C,* the vagina, which may be freed posteriorly and laterally; *D,* interrupted sutures which join the vaginal vestibule to the skin.

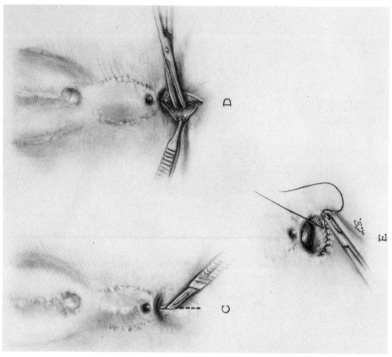

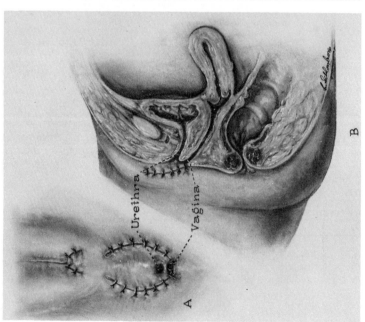

Figure 2. *A*, the situation at the primary operation showing the suture lines. Note that the vaginal orifice is adequately exteriorized but is small, and the epithelium at the orifice itself (as contrasted with the urogenital sinus epithelium exterior to the orifice which forms the vestibule) is sutured to the perineal skin. *B*, a sagittal view of the situation at the primary operation. *C*, enlargement of the contracted orifice by a posterior midline incision. *D*, freeing of the vagina posteriorly and laterally. *E*, enlargement of the orifice by suturing horizontally.

OPERATIVE TECHNIQUE
FOR SECONDARY OPERATIONS AT VAGINAL OUTLET

The problems at the vaginal orifice are basically of two kinds, although the operative procedure required for both is more or less the same.

The first problem arises from failure to adequately exteriorize the vaginal orifice at the first operation. This may result either from the fact that in some instances of marked external deformity the vagina communicates with the urogenital sinus deep in the perineum and, therefore, primary exteriorization is technically difficult, or from simple failure at the first operative procedure to carry the original midline incision far enough posteriorly to expose the vaginal orifice.

Fortunately, secondary exteriorization when the child is older is easier and facilitated by the feminization at puberty. In fact, it seems advisable not to attempt secondary exteriorization, especially that which is due to deep communication, until pubertal feminization has been well established.

In either circumstance, exteriorization can be accomplished by a midline incision of adequate length—2 or 3 cm is usually sufficient—to expose the orifice. Suture of the urogenital sinus epithelium immediately peripheral to the orifice (vulvar vestibule) to the skin completes the procedure (Figure 1).

A second problem at the vaginal outlet arises from linear contraction of the original incision between the epithelium of the urogenital sinus and the perineal skin. This may result in a contraction of the orifice if the original suture line is just at the orifice, i.e., at the hymenal ring, where there is already a natural constriction.

In most instances, at the primary operation vaginal orifice exteriorization can be accomplished without actually invading the orifice per se. The exteriorization is best accomplished by using the epithelium immediately surrounding the orifice, i.e., the epithelium of the vestibule, to suture to the skin. As noted above, when the original midline incision involves the orifice itself (hymen), contraction of the orifice tends to occur by simple linear contraction of the scar.

The correction of this problem is very simple and can often be performed on an outpatient basis. A vertical midline incision repaired horizontally should solve the problem, although it is interesting that it was necessary to repeat the procedure on five patients (Figure 2).

SUMMARY

Among 84 patients with virilizing adrenal hyperplasia who were operated upon for deformed genitalia and followed for 7–22 years (mean 12 years, 9 months), 25 (30%) required secondary operations. For the most part, the secondary procedures were to provide a vaginal orifice adequate for coitus. The difficulties were due to either failure to adequately exteriorize the orifice at the first operation or to contraction of the outlet due to scar. Simple operative procedures correct these difficulties.

REFERENCES

Jones, H. W., Jr., and G. E. S. Jones. 1954. The gynecological aspects of adrenal hyperplasia and allied disorders. Am. J. Obstet. Gynecol. 58:1330–1365.
Jones, H. W., Jr., and L. Wilkins. 1961. Gynecological operations in 94 patients with intersexuality. Am. J. Obstet. Gynecol. 82:1142–1150.
Jones, H. W., Jr., and B. S. Verkauf. 1970. Surgical treatment in congenital adrenal hyperplasia—age at operation and other prognostic factors. Obstet. Gynecol. 36:1–10.

Linear Growth, Age of Menarche, and Pregnancy Rates in Females with Steroid-treated Congenital Adrenal Hyperplasia at the Johns Hopkins Hospital

Georgeanna Jones Klingensmith,[1] *Silvia C. Garcia,*
Howard W. Jones, Jr., and Claude J. Migeon[2]

After cortisone therapy was demonstrated to suppress adrenal androgens in patients with congenital adrenal hyperplasia (CAH), the hope arose that women patients, if treated from an early age, would grow and develop normally. The female patients treated at the Johns Hopkins Hospital during the past 25 years have been reviewed to determine whether glucocorticoid therapy has been successful in allowing optimal linear growth and normal sexual development.

PATIENT POPULATION

The patient population (Table 1) consisted of 84 females, 10 years or older, divided into four groups: 1) eight patients were first treated after the age of 20 and are now 33–57 years old; 2) 20 patients were initially treated with glucocorticoids between the ages of 6 and 20 and are now 11–40 years old; 3) 14 girls were initially treated between 1 and 6 years of age; and 4) 42 girls began cortisone before 1 year of age and are now 10–26 years of age.

Supported in part by Research Grants R01-HD-06-284, AM-00180, and HD-08926 from the National Institutes of Health, United States Public Health Service and Clinical Research Centers Grant 5-M01-RR-0052 of the Division of Research Resources, National Institutes of Health, United States Public Health Service.

[1] Recipient of a grant from the Stetler Research Fund for Women Physicians.

[2] Recipient of Research Career Award 5-K06-AM-21855-10 from the National Institutes of Health, United States Public Health Service.

Table 1. Patient population of 84 females with virilizing CAH due to either 21-hydroxylase or 11β-hydroxylase enzyme deficiency

Onset of therapy	Age at study	No. of patients
>20 years	33–57 years	8
6–20 years	11–40 years	20
1–6 years	10–26 years	14
0–1 years	10–25 years	42

RESULTS AND DISCUSSION

Table 2 indicates the adult height of these patients. All but three patients who began treatment after the age of 6 had bony fusion at the onset of treatment. If these three patients are excluded, the mean final height $\pm$ 1 S.D. for female patients treated after the age of 6 was 150.9 $\pm$ 4.3 cm. Patients first treated between 1 and 6 years of age achieved a mean final height of 156.2 $\pm$ 5.2 cm, and the patients treated prior to 1 year of age who completed their linear growth had a mean final height of 158.2 $\pm$ 7.2 cm. The latter two groups were both significantly taller than the first group at the $p < 0.01$ level. Although 158.2 $\pm$ 7.2 is not significantly greater than 156.2 $\pm$ 5.2, one-fourth of the girls in the earliest treated group were taller than the tallest patient in the group initially treated between 1 and 6 years. There was a noticeable range in height in each group, but especially in the latter group. Because this group contained salt losers as well as patients with the simple virilizing disorder, it seemed that salt loss might affect final height. To examine this possibility, the patients treated prior to 1 year of age were divided into simple virilizing patients and salt losers. There was, however, no significant difference in their mean final heights (Table 2).

The standard deviation score (S.D.S.) for the mean adult height of 158.2 $\pm$ 7.2 was −0.68. This was essentially identical with that found by Brook et al. (1974) in studying the patients at the University of Zurich. An S.D.S. of −0.68 (Figure 1) corresponded roughly to the 25th percentile for normal adult women.

Table 2. Mean final height of study patients

Onset of therapy	Height (cm)
6–20 years ($n = 17$)	150.9 $\pm$ 4.3
1–6 years ($n = 11$)	156.0 $\pm$ 5.2
0–1 years ($n = 24$)	158.2 $\pm$ 7.2
Simple virilizing ($n = 9$)	157.3 $\pm$ 6.4
Salt losers ($n = 15$)	158.3 $\pm$ 7.7

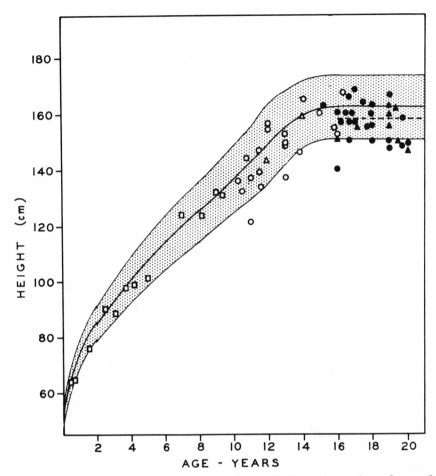

Figure 1. Heights of female patients begun on glucocorticoid treatment prior to 6 years of age. *Solid symbols* denote final heights. *Squares* represent patients now less than 10 years of age; *circles* represent patients over 10 years of age who were initially treated prior to 1 year of age; and *triangles* denote patients over 10 years of age who were initially treated between 1 and 6 years of age. The *dashed line* indicates the mean final height of patients initially treated prior to 1 year of age.

The present heights of patients who were treated prior to 6 years of age, including the youngest female patients, have been plotted in Figure 1. Although their mean height was not at the 50th percentile, it did approximate the 25th percentile and thus was well within the normal range.

Thus, it was found that height is definitely increased by glucocorticoid therapy and does not seem to be affected by salt loss. The earlier therapy is begun, the greater the effect on height.

The timing of menarche was then examined. Menarche did not occur in any of these patients prior to the initiation of the therapy. In 12 patients treated between 1 and 6 years of age, the mean age for menarche was 13.6 years, and in 16 patients treated prior to 1 year of age, the mean was 13.9 years. There was no difference between these two numbers; therefore, the mean age of menarche for patients treated prior to 6 years was 13.77 years, with a range of 12—19 1/2. Two standard deviations for our population would include patients 10—17 1/2 years of age.

The mean was significantly delayed ($p < 0.01$) when compared to a population of normal North American girls whose mean age at menarche was 12.9 years (Frisch and Revelle, 1971). In addition, the calculated mean age could not reflect the percentage of girls who had not yet attained their menarche. If the percentage of patients menstruating by a given birthday is determined, 50% were menstruating by age 15, and 100% menstruated by age 20, if one patient who discontinued her therapy and was amenorrheal at age 25 years is excluded. Therefore, menstruation is obviously delayed when compared with the general population.

The mean urinary 17-ketosteroid (17-KS) excretion measured within 2 months of menarche was available for 41 patients, with a range of 1.4—12.5 mg/24 hr. It is of significant interest that all patients with a 17-KS excretion greater than 6.2 mg/24 hr had menstrual irregularities, consisting of secondary amenorrhea, oligomenorrhea, or persistent anovulatory basal body temperature charts. This is important to remember when discussing the possible etiologies for the menstrual delay encountered in these patients.

To elucidate the reasons for menstrual delay and menstrual irregularities, the 26 patients who were treated prior to 1 year of age and who are now 15—25 years of age were evaluated. All of these patients had a 21-hydroxylase enzyme defect. Ten of the patients had simple virilizing CAH and 16 had the salt-losing variety. These patients were chosen so that the effect of late treatment could be excluded. They were all evaluated for age of onset of menses, menstrual regularity, urinary 17-KS excretion, glucocorticoid dosage/m^2, and degree of medication compliance.

Of the 26 patients, the 6 girls who were having regular menses all had menarche before 16 years of age. Five girls had oligomenorrhea, 4 had secondary amenorrhea, and 11 had delayed menarche, defined as absence of menses between ages 16 and 25. One of these latter girls reached menarche at 19 1/2. However, the remaining 10 patients have not yet attained menarche. Thus, 20 of 26 patients treated since infancy had menstrual disorders. Of the 20 patients with menstrual irregularities, 13 took their medications irregularly at best. These patients had urinary 17-KS levels of >20 mg/24 hr. Five of these girls had not had their steroid dosage increased with their adolescent growth spurt and therefore were prescribed inadequate therapy, i.e., their glucocorticoid dose was less than the calculated adrenal replacement dose (Kenny, Preeyasombat, and

Migeon, 1966) in the face of 17-KS excretion of 7.5–25 mg/24 hr. Three of these girls were also in the group which complied erratically. The one patient who attained menarche at 19 1/2 had typical constitutional delay, with a familial history for delayed menses and a bone age of 13 years 9 months at the chronological age of 17, during the peak of her pubertal growth spurt. It could not be determined whether this delay was secondary to excessive circulating levels of steroids while she was an infant. She was never clinically Cushingoid. She had a normal bone age at 3 years of age and was given low replacement steroids since that age. Another patient is now 18, with a bone age of 16 and a 17-KS excretion level of 3.5 mg/24 hr. The etiology of her delayed menses was unclear, but she did have markedly elevated 17-hydroxyprogesterone values and a male habitus. In three of the patients, 17-KS values were not available. Thus, of 17 patients with menstrual irregularities, 88% were not taking adequate gluco-corticoid replacement, and of the 11 patients with delayed menarche, 9 had elevated 17-KS excretion.

The relationship of menstrual delay to salt loss was also investigated. Forty percent of the girls with simple virilizing CAH and 44% of the salt losers had not had their menarche by age 16. This difference was not significant. Likewise, there was no difference in the percentage of patients with delayed menses secondary to poor compliance. Twenty percent of the patients with simple virilizing CAH and 25% of the salt losers had discontinued their medications for periods of at least 6 months.

The five patients with menstrual irregularities who had not had appropriate increases in their steroids during their adolescent growth spurt stimulated an interest in the 11–15-year-old girls in our clinic, especially because none of them were menarchal. Nine patients 11–15 years old, all having begun therapy as infants, were followed. Three of the nine were receiving appropriate replacement steroids. They were 12–12 1/2 years of age and had a mean 17-KS excretion of 6.2 mg/24 hr. All had breast development, pubic hair, and some estrogen effect on the vaginal mucosa. Six girls were on inadequate steroids for their body size. Three were 11–12 years of age, and 3 were 12–13 1/2 years of age. The three younger girls had mean 17-KS excretion of 4.3 whereas the older girls had 17-KS excretion of 9.8–14.5 mg/24 hr. This would suggest that in 10–14-year-old patients the glucocorticoid therapy must be monitored carefully to insure appropriate increases as body size increases and to avoid an unacceptable increase in 17-KS excretion as adrenarche occurs.

Thus, in patients in this study, the mean age of menarche was later than normal, but 94% of patients with delayed menses or secondary amenorrhea were receiving inadequate therapy.

Lastly, the fertility of our female patients was studied (Table 3). In the first three of the four groups listed in Table 3, only the married patients were sexually active. None of the four patients treated after the age of 20 was able to conceive. All of them had either anovulatory basal body temperature

Table 3. Pregnancy rate for sexually active patients

Onset of therapy	Married	Pregnant	Pregnancy rate (%)
>20 years	4	0	0
6–20 years	11	7	64
1–6 years	3	1	33
0–1 years	4	2	50

charts or absent corpora lutea at surgery. Seven of 11 patients, or 64% of the patients initially treated between 6 and 20 years of age, had at least one pregnancy. Among the four patients with infertility, one did not take her medications and one was married at 35, was markedly obese, and had mildly elevated 17-KS. The other two patients had no infertility evaluation. Of the three married patients initially treated between 1 and 6 years of age, one had a normal pregnancy and two had infertility for 1 year and 7 years. The woman with infertility for 7 years had extensive evaluation, demonstrating some response to clomid but only occasional spontaneous ovulation. The other patient had not been evaluated. In the youngest group, there were no patients who were married; however, four reported sexual intercourse of varying frequency. Two of these girls took their medications irregularly at best, never menstruated, and did not become pregnant. The two girls who did become pregnant were menstruating regularly before pregnancy.

The mean age at pregnancy was 26.3 years, with a range of 20–31 years, if the two unmarried patients are excluded (Table 4). The mean number of cycles required for conception was six, with a range of 1–12 months, which is normal for this age group (Whitelaw, 1960). The average cortisone acetate dose for four women during six pregnancies was 35.8 mg/m^2/24 hr, with a range of 30–56 mg/m^2/24 hr. The mean prednisone dose was 6.4 mg/m^2/24 hr, with a range of 6.1–6.9 mg/m^2/24 hr, for three women during five pregnancies. The range for 17-KS excretion at the onset of pregnancy was 2.5–5.3 mg/24 hr (Table 4). It is noteworthy that these 17-KS values were less than 6 mg/24 hr, the level above which menstrual abnormalities occurred. All women were maintained during pregnancy on their prepregnancy dosage of steroids.

Table 4. Fertility statistics

	Mean	Range
Age (years)	26.3	20–31
Time required to conceive (months)	5.7	1–12
Cortisone dose (mg/m^2/24 hr)	35.8	30–56
Prednisone dose (mg/m^2/24 hr)	6.4	6.1–6.9
17-KS (mg/24 hr)		2.5–5.3

Table 5. Pregnancy outcome

Onset of therapy	No. of pregnancies	No. of children	Viable outcome (%)
>20 years	0		
6–20 years	12	8	67
1–6 years	1	1	100
0–1 years	2	0[a]	

[a]Electively terminated.

Evaluation of pregnancy outcome demonstrated that the seven fertile women in the group of patients first treated between 6 and 20 years of age had 12 pregnancies producing eight healthy children (Table 5). The four unsuccessful pregnancies occurred in four women. There were one spontaneous first trimester abortion, two spontaneous second trimester abortions, and one term infant born with a meningomylocoel and multiple skeletal anomalies. The mother of this infant also had systemic lupus erythematosis and was on high dose salicylates, as well as twice the maintenance dosage of glucocorticoids. The infant's anomalies were thought to be due to the maternal salicylates. The one patient initially treated between 1 and 6 years of age who did become pregnant delivered a normal term infant. The two patients treated since infancy were not married at the time of their pregnancy and elected to have the pregnancy interrupted in the first trimester. Eight of the nine living children were term babies and are doing well. All eight were delivered by cesarean section without complications. One infant was a 3 pound 14 ounce preterm baby and was delivered vaginally. The child had mild residual cerebral palsy.

Thus, although fertility is certainly possible, the patients seem to fall into two groups: those with normal fertility and those with infertility secondary to anovulatory cycles. The etiology of the anovulation is unclear at this time.

In summary, patients in this study demonstrate that height is improved with glucocorticoid therapy. Sexual maturation should occur within the normal time span if steroid therapy is adequate, and fertility is possible for the majority of patients.

REFERENCES

Brook, C. G. D., M. Zachman, A. Prader, and G. Mürset. 1974. Experience with long-term therapy in congenital adrenal hyperplasia. J. Pediatr. 35:12–19.

Frisch, R., and R. Revelle. 1971. Height and weight at menarche and a hypothesis of menarche. Arch. Dis. Child. 46:695–701.

Kenny, F. M., C. Preeyasombat, and C. J. Migeon. 1966. Cortisol production rate. II. Normal infants, children and adults. Pediatrics 37:34–42.

Whitelaw, M. G. 1960. Statistical evaluation of female fertility. Fertil. Steril. 11:428–436.

Disordered Puberty in Treated Congenital Adrenal Hyperplasia

Lenore S. Levine, Sigrun Korth-Schutz, Paul Saenger, William J. Sweeney, III, Carl G. Beling, and Maria I. New

After 25 years of treatment of congenital adrenal hyperplasia, data on complications which appear in adolescence in treated congenital adrenal hyperplasia (CAH) are now being collected. Although ovarian pathology has been documented and delayed menarche has been reported (Jones and Verkauf, 1971), it is generally stated that with treatment females with CAH will ovulate and become fertile (Zurbrügg, 1969). In this chapter studies in four girls with treated congenital adrenal hyperplasia who have demonstrated disordered puberty with amenorrhea and ovarian pathology are reported.

MATERIALS AND METHODS

All of the patients were admitted to the Clinical Research Center of The New York Hospital-Cornell Medical Center. Glucocorticoid administration was discontinued 2 days prior to admission in patients T. P. and K. P., on admission in patient S. M., and 1 day after admission in patient A. M. The periods of study were as follows: 1) baseline, no treatment; 2) adrenocorticotropic hormone (ACTH) (Acthar, Armour), 40 U. intravenously for 8 hr; 3) dexamethasone, 0.5 mg every 6 hr for 2 days, followed by 2 mg every 6 hr for 2 days for patient A. M.; 2 mg every 6 hr for 5 days for patient S. M.; 2 mg every 6 hr for 6 days for patients T. P. and K. P.; 4) norethindrone (Norlutin, Parke-Davis), 30 mg plus 8 mg of dexamethasone or norgestrel, 0.5 mg, and ethinyl estradiol, 0.05 mg (Ovral, Wyeth), 30 mg plus 8 mg of dexamethasone for 3 days; 5) human

This investigation was supported by Research Fellowship AM-000329 and Grant HD00072 from the National Institutes of Health, United States Public Health Service; Pediatric Clinical Research Center Award RR-47 from the Division of Research Facilities and Resources, National Institutes of Health, United States Public Health Service; Grant CRBS 278 from the National Foundation—March of Dimes; Career Scientist Award I-749 and Research Contract U-2204 from the Health Research Council of The City of New York; and by Deutsche Forschungsegemeinschaft.

chorionic gonadotropin (HCG), 5,000 U. plus 8 mg of dexamethasone intramuscularly for 3 days. Blood was drawn 2 hr after the third HCG injection.

Peripheral serum testosterone, Δ4-androstenedione, and dehydroepiandrosterone (DHEA) were determined by double isotope dilution technique (Gandy and Peterson, 1968), in patients T. P. and K. P. Ovarian and adrenal vein androgens in T. P., K. P., and S. M. and peripheral serum androgens in A. M. and S. M. were determined by radioimmunoassay (Korth-Schutz, Levine, and New, 1976). Plasma follicle-stimulating hormone (FSH) and luteinizing hormone (LH) (Saxena et al., 1968), urinary 17-ketosteroids (Peterson, 1963), and estrogen excretion (Beling, Gustasson, and Kostron, 1975) were determined by previously reported methods.

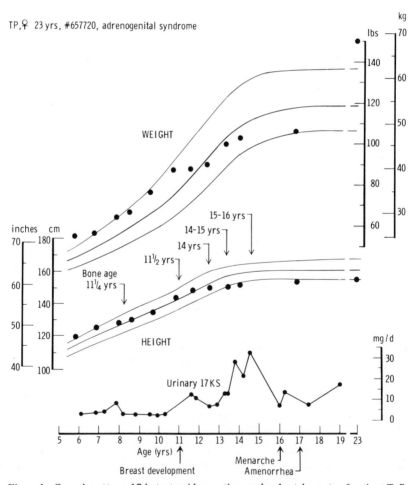

Figure 1. Growth pattern, 17-ketosteroid excretion, and pubertal events of patient T. P.

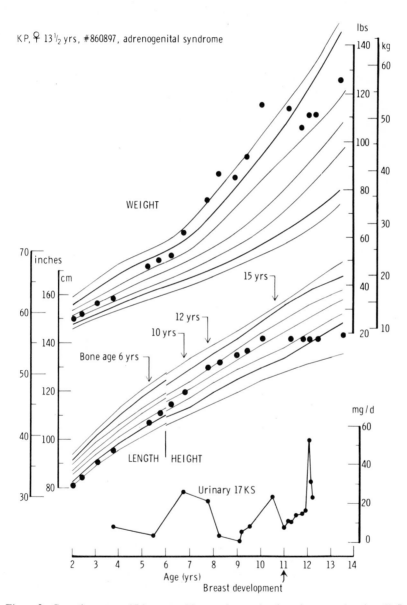

Figure 2. Growth pattern, 17-ketosteroid excretion, and pubertal events of patient K. P.

CASE REPORTS

T. P. was noted to have ambiguous genitalia at birth. During her first 3½ years of life, she was treated irregularly with extra salt and glucocorticoid, requiring several hospital admissions for dehydration and hyponatremia. At 3½ years, her height age was four years 9 months and bone age seven years 3 months. 17-Ketosteroid excretion was 22.5 mg/day. She was subsequently treated regularly with glucocorticoid replacement. At 11 years of age, breast development was noted. Between 11 and 16 years of age, ketosteroid excretion was elevated, and large doses of steroids were required to achieve ketosteroid suppression (Figure 1). At 16 years of age, menarche occurred with subsequent sporadic vaginal spotting lasting 1–2 days. Amenorrhea was noted at 17 years of age. At 17½ years of age, increased facial hair growth began. Rapid weight gain and progressive hirsutism occurred between 20 and 23 years of age. Stimulation and

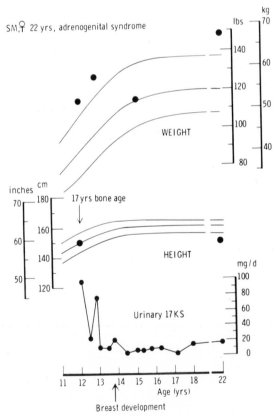

Figure 3. Growth pattern, 17-ketosteroid excretion, and pubertal events of patient S. M.

suppression tests and biopsy of the ovaries were performed when T. P. was 23 years of age, and ovarian and adrenal vein catheterization at 25 years of age.

K. P., the younger sibling of T. P., was documented to have salt-losing CAH at 2 weeks of age. She was treated with glucocorticoid and mineralocorticoid until 8 months of age and subsequently with glucocorticoid replacement alone. Ketosteroids were poorly suppressed between 6 and 8 years of age, associated with a growth spurt and bone age advancement (Figure 2). Breast budding appeared at 11 years of age, and hirsutism and acne were noted at that time. Acne and hirsutism subsequently increased, and ketosteroid excretion was markedly elevated despite repeated assertions that the medication was taken. No menarche has occurred. Stimulation and suppression tests and biopsy of the ovaries were performed at 12 years of age, and adrenal and ovarian vein catheterization was performed at 14 years of age.

S. M. (kindly referred to us by Dr. Sigurdur Gudmundsson, Iceland, at 22 years of age) was diagnosed to have CAH at birth, but remained untreated until 12 years of age. Ketosteroids suppressed with glucocorticoid treatment and breast development were noted at 14 years of age (Figure 3). Adequate ketosteroid suppression was difficult to achieve and often required doses that made her appear very Cushingoid. No spontaneous menstrual periods occurred, and only spotty vaginal bleeding followed estrogen-progesterone treatment. Ovarian biopsies were obtained at 13 and 22 years of age, and stimulation and suppression tests and ovarian vein studies were performed at 22 years of age.

A. M. was noted to have ambiguous genitalia at birth and was diagnosed to have simple virilizing 21-hydroxylase deficiency at 2 years of age. Glucocorticoid treatment was begun at 2 years, and ketosteroid suppression was satisfactorily maintained throughout childhood except for periods at 4 years and between 8 and 10 years of age. Breast development was noted at 11 years of age, and menarche occurred at 15 years of age (Figure 4). Menstrual periods occurred regularly for 7 months and then ceased. Amenorrhea has persisted for 3 years. Stimulation and suppression tests were performed at 17 years of age and ovarian biopsy at 18 years of age.

RESULTS

Plasma testosterone and Δ4-androstenedione were markedly elevated in T. P., K. P., and S. M., and to a lesser degree in A. M. DHEA was in the normal range in all the patients (Figures 5–8). ACTH infusion produced a rise in serum testosterone in T. P., but no significant rise in the other patients. Serum DHEA increased in two patients (S. M. and A. M.) with ACTH infusion, but remained unchanged in two (T. P. and K. P.). Δ4-androstenedione increased in all following ACTH infusion. Dexamethasone administration produced a marked fall in all the serum androgens, although serum testosterone in T. P. and K. P. remained elevated above the normal range for the adult female. The addition of Norlutin or Ovral

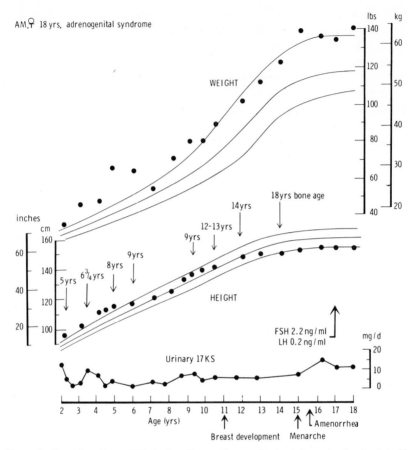

Figure 4. Growth pattern, 17-ketosteroid excretion, and pubertal events of patient A. M.

produced a further fall in all serum androgens in S. M. and A. M. and in testosterone and DHEA in T. P. and K. P. Following HCG administration, serum testosterone concentration increased in T. P. and K. P., whereas serum Δ4-androstenedione levels increased in K. P., S. M., and A. M.

Plasma FSH was initially elevated, but was subsequently in the normal range in T. P. throughout the study and was not suppressed by Norlutin administration; LH was initially normal, but subsequently was elevated above the normal level in all the periods. In K. P., FSH was below the normal range in all periods; LH was markedly elevated in the dexamethasone period. FSH was decreased in A. M. in all but the baseline period, whereas LH was decreased throughout the study. FSH was low in all periods in S. M., and LH was in the normal range.

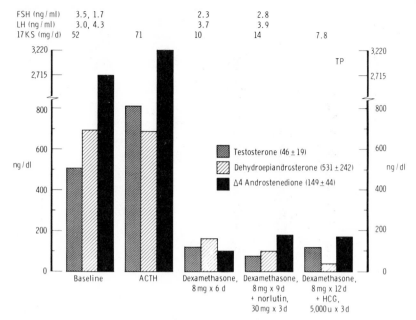

Figure 5. 17-Ketosteroid excretion, plasma gonadotropin, and serum androgen concentrations during stimulation and suppression tests in patient T. P. FSH in normal women, 1.4–2.7 ng/ml; LH in normal women, 1.4–3.6 ng/ml (Saxena et al., 1969).

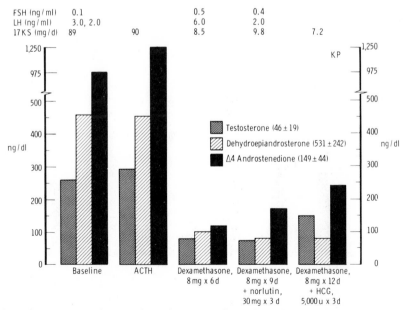

Figure 6. 17-Ketosteroid excretion, plasma gonadotropin, and serum androgen concentrations during stimulation and suppression tests in patient K. P.

367

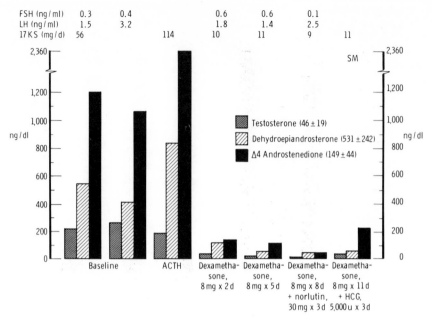

Figure 7. 17-Ketosteroid excretion, plasma gonadotropin, and serum androgen concentrations during stimulation and suppression tests in patient S. M.

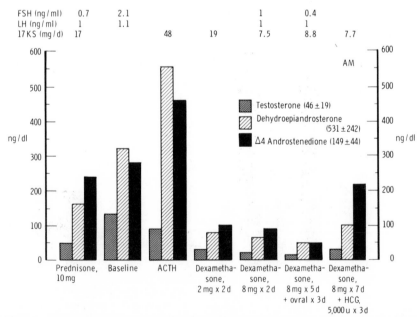

Figure 8. 17-Ketosteroid excretion, plasma gonadotropin, and serum androgen concentrations during stimulation and suppression tests in patient A. M.

17-Ketosteroid excretion was markedly elevated in T. P., K. P., and S. M. in the baseline periods and only slightly elevated in A. M. ACTH produced a further rise in 17-ketosteroid excretion in T. P., S. M., and A. M. With dexamethasone administration, 17-ketosteroid excretion decreased, but not to the level which would be expected with the dose and length of suppression. There was little change with Norlutin, Ovral, or HCG administration. T. P., K. P., and S. M. had generally more elevated androgen concentrations than did A. M. The lack of adequate suppression of testosterone in T. P. and K. P. was also revealed. Furthermore, only S. M. and A. M. demonstrated a rise in Δ4-androstenedione with HCG administration.

In patient T. P., urinary estrone was elevated and estriol was decreased in the baseline period; estradiol was normal. There was a parallel rise in estrone and estriol with ACTH and suppression of all urinary estrogens with dexamethasone. Furthermore, suppression occurred with the addition of Norlutin, and there was an increase in urinary estrogens with HCG administration (Figure 9).

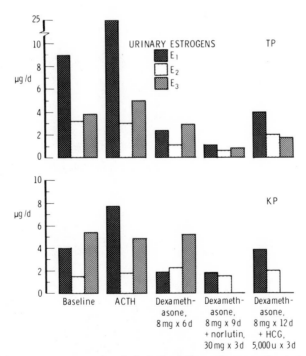

Figure 9. Urinary estrogen excretion during stimulation and suppression tests. E_1, estrone; E_2, estradiol, and E_3, estriol. The ranges of urinary estrogen levels in μg/day were as follows: days 5–8, estrone 2–7, estradiol 0–3, and estriol 5–10; ovulation peak, estrone 8–30, estradiol 2–10, and estriol 10–50; luteal maximum, estrone, 8–21, estradiol, 4–6, and estriol 8–48 (Beling, Gustasson, and Kostron, 1975).

Table 1. Peripheral, ovarian, and adrenal vein androgen concentrations in three patients with CAH and reported values for normal women

| Source | Method | Testosterone (ng/dl) | | | | | Dehydroepiandrosterone (ng/dl) | | | | |
		Peripheral	Ovary r	Ovary l	Adrenal r	Adrenal l	Peripheral	Ovary r	Ovary l	Adrenal r	Adrenal l
Patients with CAH											
T. P.	RIA[a]	27	466	3.4	39	26	38	659	63		bl
K. P.	RIA	111	93	82		78	108	324	404	bl	209
S. M.	RIA	27					50				
Reported values for normal women											
Wieland et al., 1965	DID										
Horton, Romanoff, and Walter, 1966	DID	32–62	54–95								
Rivarola et al., 1967	DID	49–59	52–206				495–1,460	716–2,511			
	DID	10–110	120–1,040				240–1,370	760–1,590			
Gandy and Peterson, 1968	DID	20–80									
Migeon, 1968	DID		Up to 200		950					254,000	
Lloyd et al., 1971	DID, GLC										
Follicular phase		27–114	83–674					840–16,750			
Luteal phase		36–94	74–2,004					340–746			
Kirschner and Jacobs, 1971	GLC	20–70	<1,000		<1,000						

[a] The following abbreviations are used: RIA, radioimmunoassay; bl, blank; DID, double isotope dilution derivative; GLC, gas-liquid chromatography.

Table 1–*Continued*

Source	Peripheral	Ovary		Adrenal		Comments
		r	l	r	l	
Patients with CAH						
T. P.	90	13,036	315		209	On prednisone (25mg/day)
K. P.	328			63	1,068	On prednisone (20 mg/day)
S. M.	206	1,200	1,001			On hydrocortisone (100 mg/day)
Reported values for normal women						
Wieland et al., 1965				0–12,000		
Horton, Romanoff, and Walter, 1966	105–144	451–1,000				Ovarian to peripheral androstenedione ratio is 6.5:1
Rivarola et al., 1967	253–264	473–3,556				
Gandy and Peterson, 1968	50–990	1,400–5,970				
Migeon, 1968	200–400	Up to 3,400		40,000		One patient
Lloyd et al., 1971						Essentially all steroids higher in ovarian than peripheral venous plasma; mean ovarian to peripheral concentration ratio: testosterone, 6.8; androstenedione, 37.9
Follicular phase	97–554	1,390–30,730				
Luteal phase	139–633	68–25,800				
Kirschner and Jacobs, 1971			<2,000–3,000		<2,000–3,000	

The urinary estrogens were in the normal range in the baseline period in K. P. ACTH produced an increase in estrone, but no increase in estradiol or estriol. Dexamethasone administration resulted in a decrease in estrone excretion, which did not change further with Norlutin or HCG administration. Estradiol changed very little with dexamethasone, Norlutin, and HCG. Estriol was suppressed to unmeasurable levels with Norlutin and did not increase with HCG.

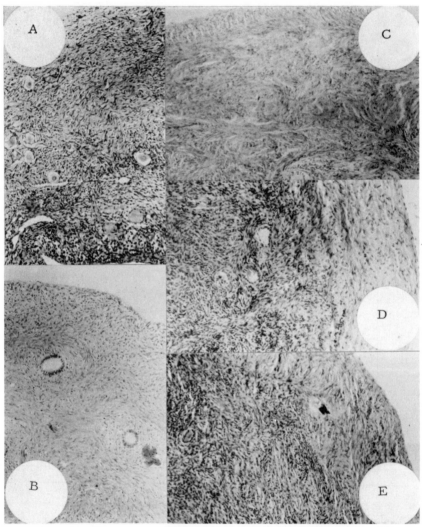

Figure 10. Ovarian histology. *A*, patient S. M. at 13 years; *B*, patient S. M. at 22 years; *C*, patient T. P. at 23 years; *D*, patient K. P. at 12 years; and *E*, patient A. M. at 18 years. Note the normal appearance of *A* at 13 years, with a decrease in follicles at 22 years, and peripheral sclerosis and decrease in follicles in *C*, *D*, and *E*. Magnification × 10.

Ovarian or adrenal vein bloods or both were obtained by selective catheterization with venography in T. P. and K. P. and during laparotomy in S. M. (Table 1). In T. P., there was a gradient between right ovarian vein and peripheral androgen concentration. The ratio of ovarian to peripheral concentrations was 17:1 for testosterone and DHEA and more than 1,400:1 for Δ4-androstenedione. In K. P., attempts at ovarian vein catheterization were unsuccessful. Left adrenal vein Δ4-androstenedione and DHEA were greater than the peripheral levels by a ratio of 3:1 and 2:1, respectively. In S. M., a gradient was present between all the ovarian vein androgen concentrations, with a ratio of ovarian to peripheral concentrations of 3–3.5:1, 6–8:1, and 5–6:1 for testosterone, DHEA, and Δ4-androstenedione, respectively. No adrenal vein bloods were obtained.

LAPAROSCOPY OR LAPAROTOMY
FINDINGS AND OVARIAN BIOPSY HISTOLOGY

Patient T. P. (Figure 10) was found to have a very small uterus and bilaterally enlarged, white, sclerotic-thickened, and smooth ovaries. Under microscopic examination, the ovaries showed peripheral sclerosis with a decrease in primordial follicles. K. P. had an infantile uterus and bilaterally enlarged white ovaries. Microscopic examination revealed peripheral sclerosis with few follicles present. A. M. had a normal uterus, bilaterally enlarged white ovaries, and no cystic components were identified. Microscopic examination showed peripheral sclerosis with a reduction in the number of primordial follicles. S. M., at age 22, was found to have a normal uterus and a large serous left ovarian cyst, with the right ovary normal in size with a hard papillomatous projection on the serosa of the ovary. Microscopic examination at age 13 gave no evidence of peripheral sclerosis. Primordial follicles were normal in number. At age 22, microscopic examination revealed right and left ovarian cyst adenofibroma, a decreased number of follicles, and endometrial currettings showed proliferative endometrium.

DISCUSSION

This chapter attempts to elucidate in these patients the mechanism for the amenorrhea present in all and the hirsutism present in two.

The association of abnormal ovaries and CAH has been documented previously. DeCrecchio (1865) described smooth, elongated ovaries with no corpora lutea in his dissection of a female with CAH. Broster et al. (1938) described several virilized girls with enlarged adrenals and either normal or small sized cystic and fibrotic ovaries. Polycystic ovaries in association with CAH have been described (Axelrod, Goldzieher, and Ross, 1965; Bergman, Sjögren, and Hakansson, 1962; Greenblatt et al., 1958), as well as other ovarian pathological changes (Abu-Haydar et al., 1954; Brown, Toyama, and Gonzales, 1970; Gabrilove,

Sharma, and Dorfman, 1965; Gold and Scommegna, 1960). Sizonenko et al. (1972) studied two females raised as boys, 6 and 4 years of age, with 11β-hydroxylase deficiency. Their ovaries were of normal size with multiple follicular cysts, and numerous primordial follicles with some fibrosis of the cortex and stroma. Progressive changes in ovarian morphology in CAH were described by Jones and Jones (1954). In infancy, the ovaries appear normal with abundant follicles. With age, the ovaries become increasingly abnormal with no signs of ovulation, less and less follicular activity, and disappearance of primordial follicles. All of the patients described here had a decrease in the number of primordial follicles, no evidence of ovulation, and, in three, peripheral sclerosis. Patient S. M. demonstrated the progression of the change, having normal appearing ovaries at 13 years of age (after treatment for 1 year) and decreased follicles at age 22 despite treatment.

Experimentally, the ovaries of adult monkeys given prolonged testosterone treatment demonstrated increased fibrous thickening of the tunica without underlying follicular cystic change (Scott and Wharton, 1959). Prepubertal rats given single injection (Barraclough, 1961) or prolonged (Bradbury, 1941; Huffman, 1941; Mazer and Mazer, 1939; Pfeiffer, 1936) androgen therapy have been made infertile. The ovaries of rats receiving single injections of testosterone propionate were small, with absent corpora, although large vesicular follicles were present (Barraclough, 1961). The infertility was postulated to be secondary to hypothalamic dysfunction, because ovulation occurred with progesterone priming and artificial hypothalamic stimulation (Barraclough and Gorski, 1961). The patients studied here demonstrated varying abnormalities in plasma gonadotropins which did not seem to respond to changes in serum and urinary steroid concentrations. Previous studies in females with CAH have demonstrated both the presence and absence of normal cyclicity (Kirkland et al., 1974), and normal luteinizing hormone-releasing factor response has been demonstrated in both prepubertal (Reiter et al., 1975) and pubertal females (Kirkland et al., 1974; Reiter et al., 1975). Urinary FSH and LH were elevated in several children by bioassay method (Stevens and Goldzieher, 1968). More detailed longitudinal studies are needed to more carefully define the hypothalamic-pituitary-gonadal axis from birth to adulthood in CAH.

The peripheral androgen concentrations are in the range reported in CAH (Gandy and Peterson, 1968; New and Levine, 1973; Rivarola et al., 1967). However, all of the patients in this study demonstrated androgen secretion which was not completely suppressed by dexamethasone, as evidenced by the urinary ketosteroid excretion in all and the serum testosterone concentration in T. P. and K. P., despite prolonged dexamethasone administration. The serum androgens in A. M. and S. M. and Δ4-androstenedione and DHEA in K. P. and T. P. in the dexamethasone period are in the range reported by others in normal females treated with glucocorticoid (Abraham, 1974; Abraham et al., 1975; Kim, Hosseinian, and Dupon, 1974; Rosenfield, Ehrlich, and Cleary, 1972). The ovarian contribution of testosterone is suggested in T. P. and K. P. by the Norlutin and HCG studies. However, the most significant ovarian vein to peripheral vein gradient demonstrated in T. P. was in Δ4-androstenedione (>1400:1) as compared to testosterone and DHEA (17:1). The results in K. P. and S. M. are within the very wide range reported in normal controls. Unfortunately, the ovarian veins could not be catheterized in K. P. The difficulty in the accurate placement of the catheter and the question of the episodic nature of adrenal and ovarian androgen secretion suggest that this technique may not provide an answer.

Previous studies in patients with congenital adrenal hyperplasia have demonstrated increased urinary excretion of estrogens (Baulieu, Peillon, and Migeon, 1967; Goldzieher, 1967; Hall and Hökfelt, 1966; Migeon, 1953; Migeon and Gardner, 1952), which increased with ACTH stimulation and decreased with glucocorticoid administration (Baulieu, Peillon, and Migeon, 1967; Goldzieher, 1967; Migeon and Gardner, 1952; Sizonenko et al., 1972). Bidlingmaier et al. (1973) observed abnormally high levels of estrone and estradiol in children with CAH and found the highest values in those in poorest control or untreated. Goldzieher's studies (1967) led him to postulate de novo secretion of adrenal estrogen in some cases. Estrone was elevated and estriol decreased in the baseline period in T. P., and in both T. P. and K. P. there was a disproportionate rise in estrone as compared to estriol following ACTH administration. This correlates with the elevated serum Δ4-androstenedione level and may reflect the conversion of Δ4-androstenedione to estrone. Barlow (1964) reported a 2–3-fold rise in estrone and estradiol excretion in normal women in the follicular phase with ACTH administration and also with dexamethasone.

In a subsequent study of patients with polycystic ovary syndrome, Barlow (1969) observed either no rise with ACTH administration in urinary estrogens or a disproportionate rise in estrone relative to estriol. One patient with "adrenal hyperplasia" demonstrated a fall in estrone and estradiol and a slight rise in estriol. An abnormal adrenal influence on ovarian estrogen production or metabolism, or both, in women with polycystic ovaries was suggested by Barlow (1969). In their estrogen response, patients in this study more closely resemble those with polycystic ovaries than the normal women studied by Barlow.

Because the importance of estrogen in modulating pituitary responsiveness to luteinizing hormone-releasing factor has been demonstrated (Keye and Jaffe, 1974; Thompson, Arfania, and Taymor, 1973; Vandenberg, Devane, and Yen, 1974; Wang and Yen, 1975), perhaps the abnormalities in estrogen production in CAH may affect gonadotropin release and ovarian function.

In summary, four postpubertal amenorrheic females with treated CAH have been evaluated. Ovarian pathology with a decreased number of follicles and peripheral sclerosis, incompletely suppressed androgen secretion, and abnormalities in gonadotropin secretion were demonstrated. The etiology of this disorder may reside in the exposure of the hypothalamus and ovary to excessive androgen in prenatal as well as postnatal life. Although initially the events of normal puberty seem to occur, later abnormalities may demonstrate a delayed effect of the abnormal hormonal milieu in early life.

ACKNOWLEDGMENTS

We are grateful to Drs. E. Kramer and J. Mouradian for their help with the ovarian pathology and to Dr. T. Sos for the catheterization studies.

REFERENCES

Abraham, G. E. 1974. Ovarian and adrenal contribution to peripheral androgens during the menstrual cycle. J. Clin. Endocrinol. Metab. 39:340–346.

Abraham, G. E., Z. H. Chakmakjian, J. E. Buster, and J. R. Marshall. 1975. Ovarian and adrenal contributions to peripheral androgens in hirsute women. Obstet. Gynecol. 46:169–173.

Abu-Haydar, N., J. C. Laidlaw, B. Nusimovich, and S. Sturgis. 1954. Hyperadrenocorticism and the Stein-Leventhal syndrome. J. Clin. Endocrinol. Metab. 14:766.

Axelrod, L. R., J. W. Goldzieher, and S. D. Ross. 1965. Concurrent 3β-hydroxysteroid dehydrogenase deficiency in adrenal and sclerocystic ovary. Acta Endocrinol. 48:392–412.

Barlow, J. J. 1964. Adrenocortical influences on estrogen metabolism in normal females. J. Clin. Endocrinol. Metab. 24:586–596.

Barlow, J. J. 1969. Abnormal estrogen responses to ACTH stimulation in the polycystic ovary syndrome. Am. J. Obstet. Gynecol. 103:585–591.

Barraclough, C. A. 1961. Production of anovulatory, sterile rats by single injections of testosterone propionate. Endocrinol. 68:62–67.

Barraclough, C. A., and R. A. Gorski. 1961. Evidence that the hypothalamus is responsible for androgen-induced sterility in the female rat. Endocrinol. 68:68–79.

Baulieu, E. E., F. Peillon, and C. J. Migeon. 1967. Adrenogenital syndrome. In A. B. Eisenstein (ed.), The Adrenal Cortex, pp. 553–637. Little, Brown and Company, Boston.

Beling, C. G., P. O. Gustasson, and H. Kostron. 1975. Metabolism of estradiol in greyhounds and in German shepherds. An investigation with a special reference to hip dysplasias. Acta Radio. (Diag.) (Suppl.) (Stockh.) 344:109–120.

Bergman, P., B. Sjögren, and B. Hakansson. 1962. Hypertensive form of congenital adrenocortical hyperplasia. Acta Endocrinol. 40:555–564.

Bidlingmaier, F., M. Wagner-Barnack, O. Butenandt, and D. Knorr. 1973. Plasma estrogens in childhood and puberty under physiologic and pathologic conditions. Pediatr. Res. 7:901–907.

Bradbury, J. T. 1941. Permanent after-effects following masculinization of the infantile female rat. Endocrinology 28:101–106.

Broster, L. R., C. Allen, J. Patterson, A. W. Greenwood, G. F. Marrian, and G. C. Butler. 1938. The Adrenal Cortex and Intersexuality. Chapman and Hall, Ltd., London.

Brown, W. W., F. P. Toyama, and W. Gonzales. 1970. Multiple uterine leiomyomas developed in the presence of a high androgen environment secondary to adrenogenital syndrome. Obstet. Gynecol. 35:255–259.

De Crecchio, L. 1865. Sopra un caso di apparenze virili in una donna. Morgagni 7:1951.

Gabrilove, J. L., D. C. Sharma, and R. I. Dorfman. 1965. Adrenocortical 11β-hydroxylase deficiency and virilism first manifest in the adult woman. N. Engl. J. Med. 272:1189–1194.

Gandy, H., and R. E. Peterson. 1968. Measurement of testosterone and 17-ketosteroid in plasma by the double isotope dilution derivative technique. J. Clin. Endocrinol. Metab. 28:949–977.

Gold, J. J., and A. Scommegna. 1960. The use of corticoids in obstetrics and gynecology. Clin. Obstet. Gynecol. 3:1068–1082.

Goldzieher, J. W. 1967. Oestrogens in congenital adrenal hyperplasia. Acta Endocrinol. 54:51–62.

Greenblatt, R. B., J. M. Manautev, S. L. Clark, and A. P. Rosenberg. 1958. Suppression of adrenal cortical activity in treatment of menstrual disorders. Metabolism 7:25–39.

Hall, K., and B. Hökfelt. 1966. Clinical and steroid metabolic studies in four siblings with congenital virilizing adrenal hyperplasia. Acta Endocrinol. 52:535–549.

Horton, R., E. Romanoff, and J. Walker. 1966. Androstenedione and testosterone in ovarian venous and peripheral plasma during ovariectomy for breast cancer. J. Clin. Endocrinol. Metab. 26:1267–1269.

Huffman, J. W. 1941. Effect of testosterone propionate upon reproduction in the female. Endocrinology 29:77–79.

Jones, H. W., and G. E. S. Jones. 1954. The gynecological aspects of adrenal hyperplasia and allied disorders. Am. J. Obstet. Gynecol. 68:1330–1365.

Jones, H. W., Jr., and B. S. Verkauf. 1971. Congenital adrenal hyperplasia: age at menarche and related events at puberty. Am. J. Obstet. Gynecol. 109:292–297.

Keye, W. R., Jr., and R. B. Jaffe. 1974. Modulation of pituitary gonadotropin response to gonadotropin-releasing hormone by estradiol. J. Clin. Endocrinol. Metab. 38:805–810.

Kim, M. H., A. H. Hosseinian, and C. Dupon. 1974. Plasma levels of estrogens, androgens and progesterone during normal and dexamethasone treated cycles. J. Clin. Endocrinol. Metab. 39:706–712.

Kirkland, J., R. Kirkland, L. Librik, and G. Clayton. 1974. Serum gonadotropin levels in female adolescents with congenital adrenal hyperplasia. J. Pediatr. 84:411–414.

Kirschner, M., and J. B. Jacobs. 1971. Combined ovarian and adrenal vein catheterization to determine the site(s) of androgen overproduction in hirsute women. J. Clin. Endocrinol. Metab. 33:199–209.

Korth-Schutz, S., L. S. Levine, and M. I. New. 1976. Serum androgens in normal and prepubertal and pubertal children and in children with precocious puberty. J. Clin. Endocrinol. Metab. 42:117–124.

Kovacic, N. 1959. Congenital adrenal hyperplasia and precocious gonadotropin secretion in a 6 year old girl. J. Clin. Endocrinol. Metab. 19:844–847.

Lloyd, C. W., J. Lobotsky, D. T. Baird, J. McCracken, and J. Weisz. 1971. Concentration of unconjugated estrogens, androgens and gestagens in ovarian and peripheral venous plasma of women: the normal menstrual cycle. J. Clin. Endocrinol. 32:155–166.

Mazer, M., and C. Mazer. 1939. Effect of prolonged testosterone propionate administration on the immature and adult female rat. Endocrinology 24:175–181.

Migeon, C. J. 1953. Fractionation by countercurrent distribution of urinary estrogens in normal individuals and in patients with hyperadrenocorticism. J. Clin. Endocrinol. Metab. 13:674.

Migeon, C. J., and L. I. Gardner. 1952. Urinary estrogens in hyperadrenocorticism: influence of cortisone, compound F, compound B and ACTH. J. Clin. Endocrinol. Metab. 12:1513.

Migeon, C. J., M. J. Lipsett, M. A. Kirschner, and C. W. Bardin. 1968. Physiologic basis of disorders of androgen metabolism. Combined clinical staff conference at the National Institutes of Health. Ann. Inter. Med. 68: 1327–1344.

New, M. I., and L. S. Levine. 1973. Congenital adrenal hyperplasia. In H. Harris and K. Hirschhorn (eds.), Advances in Human Genetics, pp. 251–326. Plenum Press, New York.

Peterson, R. E. 1963. Determination of urinary neutral 17-ketosteroids. In Standard Methods in Clinical Chemistry, Vol. 4, pp. 151–162. Academic Press, New York.

Pfeiffer, C. A. 1936. Sexual differences of hypophyses and their determination by gonads. Am. J. Anat. 58:195–225.

Reiter, E. O., M. M. Grumbach, S. L. Kaplan, and F. A. Conte. 1975. The response of pituitary gonadotropes to synthetic LRF in children with glucocorticoid-treated congenital adrenal hyperplasia: lack of effect of intrauterine and neonatal androgen excess. J. Clin. Endocrinol. Metab. 40:318–325.

Rivarola, M. A., J. M. Saez, H. W. Jones, A. S. Jones, and C. J. Migeon. 1967. The secretion of androgens by the normal, polycystic and neoplastic ovaries. Johns Hopkins Med. J. 121:82–90.

Rosenfield, R. L., E. N. Ehrlich, and R. E. Cleary. 1972. Adrenal and ovarian contributions to the elevated free plasma androgen levels in hirsute women. J. Clin. Endocrinol. Metab. 34:92–97.

Saxena, B. B., H. Demura, H. M. Gandy, and R. E. Peterson. 1968. Radioimmunoassay of human follicle stimulating and luteinizing hormones in plasma. J. Clin. Endocrinol. Metab. 28:519–534.

Scott, R. B., and L. R. Wharton. 1959. The effect of testosterone on experimental endometriosis in rhesus monkeys. Am. J. Obstet. Gynecol. 78:1020–1027.

Sizonenko, P. C., A. M. Schindler, I. J. Kohlberg, and L. Paunier. 1972. Gonadotropins, testosterone and oestrogen levels in relation to ovarian morphology in 11β-hydroxylase deficiency. Acta Endocrinol. 71:539–550.

Stevens, V., and J. Goldzieher. 1968. Urinary excretion of gonadotropins on congenital adrenal hyperplasia. Pediatrics 41:421–427.

Thompson, I. E., J. Arfania, and M. L. Taymor. 1973. Effects of estrogen and progesterone on pituitary response to stimulation by luteinizing hormone-releasing factor. J. Clin. Endocrinol. Metab. 37:152–155.

Vandenberg, G., G. Devane, and S. S. C. Yen. 1974. Effects of exogenous estrogen and progestin on pituitary responsiveness to synthetic luteinizing hormone-releasing factor. J. Clin. Invest. 53:1750–1754.

Wang, C. F., and S. S. C. Yen. 1975. Direct evidence of estrogen modulation of pituitary sensitivity to luteinizing hormone-releasing factor during the menstrual cycle. J. Clin. Invest. 55:201–204.

Wieland, R. G., C. De Courzcy, R. P. Levy, A. P. Zala, and H. Hirschmann. 1965. $C_{19} O_2$ steroids and some of their precursors in blood from normal human adrenals. J. Clin. Invest. 44:159–168.

Zurbrügg, R. P. 1969. Congenital adrenal hyperplasia. In L. I. Gardner (ed.), Endocrine and Genetic Diseases of Childhood, p. 424. W. P. Saunders Co., Philadelphia.

Hypothalmic Maturation in Congenital Adrenal Hyperplasia
Pulsatile Gonadotropin Output and Response to Luteinizing Hormone-Releasing Hormone Administration

Anne Colston Wentz, Silvia C. Garcia,
Georgeanna Jones Klingensmith, Claude J. Migeon, and Georgeanna Seegar Jones

The purpose of this study was to determine whether a normal sequence of gonadotropin output occurs during pubertal development in females with congenital adrenal hyperplasia. It has been previously reported that the menarche is often delayed, but studies have not determined whether this delay is related to the disease itself or to its therapy.

In normal patients, the first sign heralding the onset of puberty is the pulsatile luteinizing hormone (LH) output observed only during sleep. As puberty progresses, the pulsatile output is observed during the waking as well as the sleeping state. Administration of synthetic luteinizing hormone-releasing hormone (LRH) to the early pubertal female results in an increased follicle-stimulating hormone (FSH) output which is greater than that of LH. With continued pubertal maturation, the LRH-induced peak LH becomes progressively higher. In patients tested shortly after the first menstrual period, the LH response is within the range for normal adults, and its amplitude is dependent upon the phase of the menstrual cycle in which testing is performed.

Portions of the data presented have been published in the Journal of Clinical Endocrinology and Metabolism (42:239–246, 1976).

PROTOCOL

Ten patients with adrenal hyperplasia were studied, five of whom had not had spontaneous menses and five of whom had achieved the menarche, with the use of the following protocol. Following informed consent, an indwelling needle with a heparin lock was placed, and blood samples were withdrawn every 20 min for 5–8 hr. Following this baseline period, an intravenous bolus of 100 μg of synthetic LRH was administered. Blood samples were then withdrawn 15, 30, 45, 60, 90, 120, 150, and 180 min after the LRH infusion. All blood samples were analyzed for LH and FSH.

Serum LH and FSH were measured by double antibody radioimmunoassay (Cargille, Ross, and Yoshimi, 1969; Odell, Ross, and Rayford, 1967). The lower limits of sensitivity were 10.7–15.7 ng/ml for LH and 39.2–58.4 ng/ml for FSH. The cumulative interassay variation was 5.8% for LH and 5.3% for FSH. The normal adult female range exclusive of the midcycle peak was 30–90 ng/ml for LH and 150–350 ng/ml for FSH.

All samples from each patient were assayed together, and each value represented the mean of duplicate determinations. Variation within the assay was determined for each patient, and this value was compared to the covariance for the means of each of the duplicate determinations. Thus, a variation in sample means throughout the sampling period, suggestive of episodic gonadotropin output, could readily be distinguished from expected within assay variation.

Gonadotropin results for each patient were graphed. A secretory pulse was defined as an increase from nadir to peak greater than 20% of the nadir value. The number and frequency of pulses and the average increment and percentage of increase over baseline were computed.

CASE STUDIES

The clinical findings in five patients who had not had spontaneous menarche are shown in Table 1. All five individuals had a 21-hydroxylase deficiency. Patients A and B were considered to be in excellent therapeutic control, as defined by growth parameters, bone age, and urinary 17-ketosteroid and pregnanetriol output. Patient C, who has had no further increase in height, had been under poor therapeutic management for several years, having been maintained at too low a dose of suppressive corticosteroids. Patients D and E were in poor therapeutic control because of lack of compliance. In both, urinary 17-ketosteroids were repeatedly documented at greater than 20 mg/24 hr for many years. Patient E had severe psychiatric difficulties and massive exogenous obesity. Both patients had adult skeletal maturation, but had not yet achieved menarche.

In reviewing the results of frequent sampling and LRH stimulation, Patient A (Figure 1) had a low baseline LH and no pulsatile LH activity. However, FSH pulsatile activity appeared to be regular, and the percentage of increment was statistically significant. Following LRH administration, an increase in LH values

Table 1. Clinical findings in five premenarcheal patients and five postmenarcheal patients

Patient	Age (years)	Tanner stage	Bone age (years)	Menstrual history
Premenarcheal				
A	11.5	II–III	8.8	Premenarche
B	13	III	13	Premenarche
C	15	III–IV	13 (no further growth after age 13)	Delayed
D	15	IV	Adult	Primary amenorrhea
E	24	III–IV	Adult	Primary amenorrhea
Postmenarcheal				
F	16.5	V	Adult	Regular, menarche at 13
G	17	V	Adult	Secondary amenorrhea, menarche at 13
H	21.8	V	Adult	Secondary amenorrhea, menarche at 16
J	22	V	Adult	Secondary amenorrhea, menarche at 19½
K	27	V	Adult	Irregular, menarche at 10

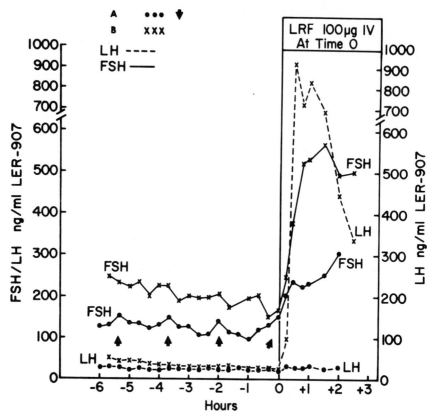

Figure 1. Pattern of gonadotropin output before and after LRF in two premenarcheal, normally developing females (patients A and B). Arrows indicate pulses. Reproduced with permission of J. Clin. Endocrinol. Metab. 42:239–246, 1976.

was not observed, whereas FSH levels were elevated. The clinical and hormonal findings suggest that this patient is prepubertal.

Patient B (Figure 1), 2 years older and in Tanner stage III, showed results expected in the individual who has just entered puberty. Baseline LH was higher, although pulsatile LH output was still not apparent. Baseline FSH values were within the adult range, and regular, significant FSH pulses had disappeared. Following LRH stimulation, both FSH and LH were increased, which is characteristic of early pubertal individuals. Thus, patients A and B, under good therapeutic control, showed results expected in normally developing individuals.

In contrast, patient C, who had not been well controlled, had no increase in height and had remained in Tanner stage III–IV for 2 years. Baseline LH and FSH values were within normal adult levels. Following LRH, she demonstrated a rise in LH and FSH which could not be distinguished from the response of the normal adult woman during the proliferative part of the cycle (Figure 2). Her

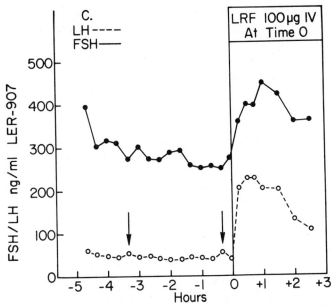

Figure 2. Pattern of gonadotropin output in a 15-year-old patient (patient C) who was poorly controlled for the past 2 years. Arrows indicate pulses.

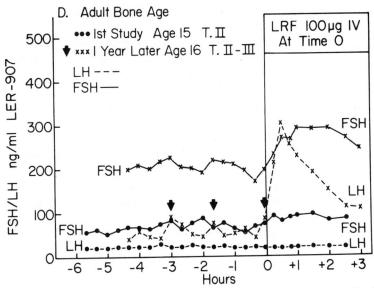

Figure 3. Pattern of gonadotropin output in patient D, studied on two occasions. The initial study was during poor therapeutic control, which had been maintained for many years. The second study was after good therapeutic control had been maintained for 3 months. Arrows indicate pulses.

clinical findings were not compatible with her hormonal response, and she is thought to have delayed menarche, possibly related to undertreatment.

Patients D and E, both with adult bone age, had primary amenorrhea. Both were under poor therapeutic control during most of their lives and were clearly out of control when studied. Patient D, when studied at age 15 (Figure 3), had the lowest values of both FSH and LH observed (mean LH was 22 ng/ml and mean FSH was 67 ng/ml) and had no response following LRH administration. These findings were compatible with her clinical picture. Patient E had low baseline values of LH (mean 30 ng/ml), with no response to LRH and normal adult levels of FSH (mean 222 ng/ml). Statistically significant FSH pulsations were observed, although the response of FSH following LRH administration was lower than that observed in patient B (peak 373 ng/ml). This pattern is clearly atypical, being neither prepubertal nor adult.

Patient D was restudied 1 year later, after therapeutic control had been maintained for 3 months. Some breast development had occurred, and 17-ketosteroid and pregnanetriol values were normal. Pulsatile LH output was observed (Figure 3), and both FSH and LH increased following LRH. Improved therapy appears to be associated with normalization of gonadotropin parameters.

Thus, in this small series of individuals who have not achieved menarche, normal developmental progression of gonadotropin output and the expected response to LRH administration were documented only in those individuals who were maintained at cortisone acetate doses appropriate for body surface. In those individuals in whom therapeutic control was poor, prepubertal or atypical response patterns were observed.

The clinical findings in five individuals who had achieved spontaneous menarche are shown in Table 1. Patient F is the only individual with an 11β-hydroxylase deficiency and she always maintained normal therapeutic and developmental parameters. Patients G and H were under poor therapeutic control for 3–4 years, and the time of onset of secondary amenorrhea correlated with the period of undertreatment. Patient J had persistent oligomenorrhea since menarche, although 17-ketosteroids were only mildly elevated during this study. More recently, proper control has been maintained and normal ovulation has been documented.

Patient F was inadvertently studied during the time of her midcycle LH surge, resulting in a high baseline LH (mean 198 ng/ml) and marked pulse amplitude (peak 2,419 ng/ml). The increase in LH and FSH following LRH administration was comparable to that observed in any adult individual tested in midcycle.

The remaining individuals all had significant episodic LH output. Pulsatile FSH output occurred sporadically and did not correlate with LH pulses. Patients H and K, with secondary amenorrhea and oligomenorrhea, showed responses within the expected range for normal reproductive age individuals. In contrast,

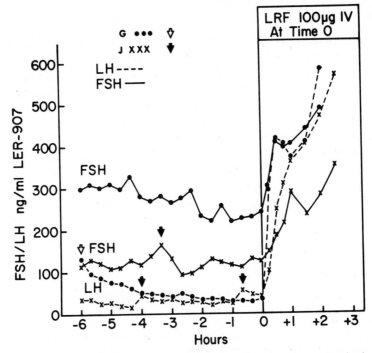

Figure 4. Response patterns before and after LRH in two postmenarcheal females (patients G and J) with secondary amenorrhea. Arrows indicate pulses. Reproduced with permission of J. Clin. Endocrinol. Metab. 42:239–246, 1976.

patients G and J, with secondary amenorrhea for 1½ and 3 years, respectively, showed atypical patterns (Figure 4). LH did not peak at 30 min as expected, but maintained increasing levels 2½ hr after LRH stimulation.

In this group of patients who had achieved spontaneous menarche, only one individual had been well controlled throughout life, and this individual was having normal menses. Two individuals had menstrual irregularities during periods of poor control, although in general their hormonal patterns were normal. The remaining two individuals, G and J, are somewhat more difficult to explain. Both had normal 17-ketosteroid values when tested. However, they had been maintained on the same dose of suppressive corticosteroids at which menarche had occurred. Thus, as surface area had increased, cortisone dosage had not been increased accordingly, possibly resulting in a subtle loss of therapeutic control. In these individuals, the pattern of gonadotropin release differed from the normal.

CONCLUSION

In this small series of patients with adrenal hyperplasia, the normal progression of gonadotropin output and the expected response to LRH administration were documented only in those individuals who were maintained at appropriate corticosteroid doses. In those in whom therapeutic control had been poor, prepubertal or atypical response patterns were observed. Whether this is due to a physiological hypothalamic immaturity or to suppression from as-yet-unidentified hormones cannot be documented. In patients in whom therapeutic control was maintained at reasonable but not optimal levels, the hormonal patterns observed were within the broad range of normal. However, the clinical responses of these patients with respect to menarche and menstrual history indicated minor dysfunction. Thus, a normal sequence of gonadotropin output may be expected to occur during pubertal development in properly treated females with adrenal hyperplasia.

REFERENCES

Cargille, C. M., G. T. Ross, and T. Yoshimi. 1969. Daily variations in plasma FSH, LH and progesterone in the normal menstrual cycle. J. Clin. Endocrinol. Metab. 29:12–19.
Odell, W. D., G. T. Ross, and P. L. Rayford. 1967. Radioimmunoassay for luteinizing hormone in human plasma or serum: physiological studies. J. Clin. Invest. 46:248–255.

Plasma Sex Steroids and Gonadotropins in Pubertal Girls with Congenital Adrenal Hyperplasia
Relationship to Menstrual Disorders

Gail E. Richards,[1] *Dennis M. Styne,*[1] *Felix A. Conte,*
Selna L. Kaplan, and Melvin M. Grumbach

The achievement of optimal management of patients with virilizing congenital adrenal hyperplasia (CAH) is a difficult task. A particularly perplexing problem is that of reproductive function, including fertility. Neither the frequency of menstrual irregularities in many patients with 21-hydroxylase deficiency, the most common variety of CAH, nor the fertility rate has been well documented. From the earliest descriptions of the treatment of this condition, it is apparent that a major factor in normal cyclic menstruation is adequate adrenal suppression. After initiation of glucocorticoid therapy, patients with a bone age of 12 years or more often undergo pubertal development (Wilkins et al., 1952), and pregnancy with normal offspring has been described in patients with virilizing CAH who have been treated (Speroff, 1965).

Of the adolescent female patients under treatment for virilizing CAH in this clinic, 25% had not had the onset of menses by 17 years of age (Table 1), in agreement with the findings of Jones and Verkauf (1971). All patients who reached menarche did so at the normal time. Those patients who did not have menses by 17 years may comprise a distinct subgroup. This chapter presents a preliminary report of an investigation of the factors which might contribute to menstrual irregularity in patients with CAH.

[1] Recipients of Research Fellowships in Pediatric Endocrinology from the National Institute of Arthritis, Metabolism, and Digestive Diseases and the National Institute of Child Health and Human Development, National Institutes of Health, United States Public Health Service.

This work was supported in part by grants from the National Institutes of Child Health and Human Development and the National Institute of Arthritis, Metabolism, and Digestive Diseases, National Institutes of Health, United States Public Health Service.

Table 1. Age of menarche in patients with congenital virilizing adrenal hyperplasia

Age (years)	No. of patients	Menstruating	Not menstruating
13	17	5	12
14	17	6	11
15	13	9	4
16	13	9	4
17	12	9	3

MATERIAL AND METHODS

Six patients were selected for a preliminary study of the hormonal milieu in young women with 21-hydroxylase deficiency. The patients were divided into three categories: prepubertal, pubertal but premenarcheal, and postmenarcheal (Table 2).

The prepubertal patient (S. B.) was a 4 years 6 months-old girl (bone age 10 years) with compensated 21-hydroxylase deficiency who had not had glucocorticoid therapy and was studied during adrenal suppression with dexamethasone. Three patients (J. I., M. V., and J. C.) were pubertal but had not had menses. They were 13 years 3 months, 13 years 7 months, and 19 years 3 months of age, with bone ages of 13 years 9 months, 15, and adult, respectively. Growth was only slightly retarded (height was 0.7–2.5 S.D. below the mean). The diagnosis of 21-hydroxylase deficiency had been made in all within the first 2 years of life. One patient had been treated sporadically until the age of 2 years 3 months. All had onset of breast development in the 10th year, and all had the salt-losing form of CAH. Two patients (A. R. and C. L.), 22 years 5 months and 16 years

Table 2. Pertinent clinical findings in six female patients with congenital virilizing adrenal hyperplasia

Patient	Prepubertal S. B.	Pubertal premenarcheal			Postmenarcheal	
		J. I.	M. V.	J. C.	C. L.	A. R.
Age (years/months)	4/6	13/2	13/7	19/3	16/11	22/2
Age at diagnosis (years/months)	4/6	2/3	0/8	2 weeks	2 weeks	6/9
Height (S.D.)	+3	−2.5	−2	−0.7	Mean	−4.6
Weight (S.D.)	+1	Mean	−1.3	−1.4	−0.4	−0.7
Bone age (years)	10	13/9	15	Fused	Fused	Fused

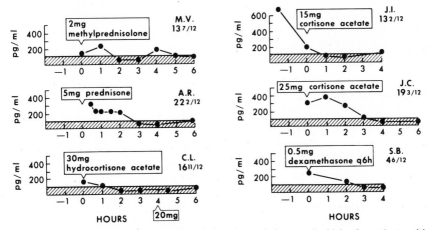

Figure 1. Plasma ACTH after the first morning dose of glucocorticoid in six patients with congenital adrenal hyperplasia. Patient C. L. received a second dose of glucocorticoid 4 hr after the beginning of the study. The *shaded area* indicates the normal range.

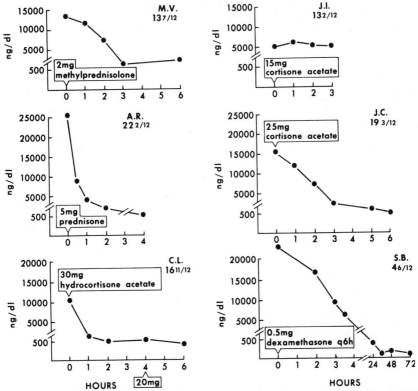

Figure 2. Plasma 17-hydroxyprogesterone after the first morning dose of glucocorticoid in six patients with congenital adrenal hyperplasia. Patient C. L. received a second dose of glucocorticoid 4 hr after the beginning of the study.

11 months old, had the onset of breast development at about 8 years and menarche in the 13th year. Menses had been irregular in both patients. Glucocorticoid and mineralocorticoid therapy was initiated in the younger patient (C. L.) at 2 weeks of age; her final height was normal. The 22-year-old patient had not been diagnosed until 6 years 9 months of age; her final height was −4.6 S.D.

At the time of study, several different glucocorticoid preparations were being used, including cortisone acetate, hydrocortisone acetate, methylprednisolone or prednisone, equivalent to 19–50 mg/m^2/day of cortisone acetate in variously divided doses. Cortisone acetate equivalents were calculated by the commonly accepted conversion factors in the ratio of 5 mg of prednisone to every 25 mg of cortisone acetate. Dosage had been stable for several years. Urinary 17-ketosteroids rarely had been above 15 mg/day, the upper limit of normal for postpubertal females in this laboratory. The mean urinary pregnanetriol concentration was 10 mg/day at the time of investigation.

Plasma adrenocorticotropic hormone (ACTH), testosterone, 17-hydroxyprogesterone, estrone, and estradiol were measured at hourly intervals after the patient's first morning dose of glucocorticoid. The response of pituitary gonadotropes to synthetic luteinizing hormone-releasing factor (LRF) was used as a means of assessing the hypothalamic-pituitary-gonadal axis function. All deter-

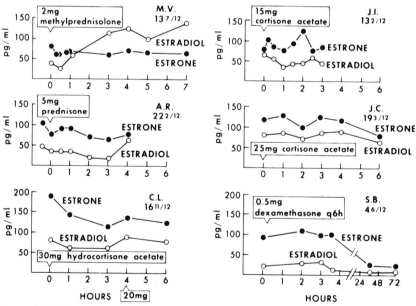

Figure 3. Plasma estrone and estradiol after the first morning dose of glucocorticoid in six patients with congenital adrenal hyperplasia. Patient C. L. received a second dose of glucocorticoid 4 hr after the beginning of the study.

minations were made by radioimmunoassay: LER-960 was the standard for the luteinizing hormone (LH) assay and LER-869 for the follicle-stimulating hormone (FSH) assay, according to previously described methods (Jenner, Grumbach, and Kaplan, 1970; Jenner et al., 1972; Kelch, Kaplan, and Grumbach, 1973; Rees and Cool, 1971; Roth, Grumbach, and Kaplan, 1973; Sizonenko et al., 1970).

In all patients, plasma ACTH was elevated above the normal range before the first morning dose of glucocorticoid (Figure 1). Normal levels should be less than 100 pg/ml. In every patient, a single dose of glucocorticoid reduced the ACTH level to within the normal range within 2–3 hr.

Levels of plasma 17-hydroxyprogesterone were markedly elevated in all patients before the morning dosage of medication (Figure 2). Although glucocorticoid reduced 17-hydroxyprogesterone significantly, none of the values fell within the normal range (<150 ng/dl) after a single dose of medication. In the previously untreated patient (S. B.), 17-hydroxyprogesterone was suppressed to normal levels 36 hr after dexamethasone (0.5 mg/6 hr).

Plasma estrone and estradiol were in the normal adult female range in the five pubertal patients (Figure 3). Because none were having regular menses, the

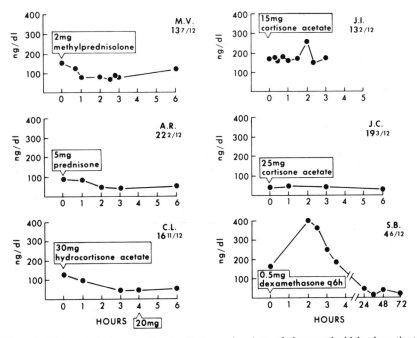

Figure 4. Plasma testosterone after the first morning dose of glucocorticoid in six patients with congenital adrenal hyperplasia. Patient C. L. received a second dose of glucocorticoid 4 hr after the beginning of the study.

Table 3. Response to LRF of a 4½-year-old untreated female patient (bone age 10 years) with a 21-hydroxylase defect

	Patient S. B.	Treated prepubertal CAH		Prepubertal controls	
LH (ng/ml) (LER-960)					
Basal	<0.5	0.83 ±	0.17	0.79 ±	0.07
Peak	0.7	1.7 ±	0.1	1.76 ±	0.14
Increment	0.7	1.1 ±	0.2	0.93 ±	0.09
Area	79.0	162 ±	39	111.1 ±	15.6
FSH (ng/ml) (LER-869)					
Basal	0.9	1.4 ±	0.32	1.43 ±	0.21
Peak	2.5	8.1 ±	1.6	5.26 ±	1.87
Increment	1.6	7.0 ±	1.5	3.92 ±	2.0
Area	302	1,043 ±	145	637 ±	295

phase of the cycle could not be determined with accuracy. There was no significant suppression of estrone or estradiol after a single dose of glucocorticoid. In patient S. B., however, estrone and estradiol were elevated to the pubertal range but declined to prepubertal levels 36 hr after dexamethasone (0.5 mg/6 hr). Patient M. V. had a rise in estradiol from midpubertal levels to high adult levels 4 hr after administration of glucocorticoid.

In all patients, plasma testosterone was clearly more than 2 S.D. above the normal adult female mean of 30 ng/dl (Figure 4). In four of five pubertal patients, the first glucocorticoid dose in the morning reduced testosterone to a near-normal female range. One patient (J. I.), who had no reduction in

Table 4. Response to LRF of three premenarcheal pubertal patients with 21-hydroxylase deficiency while on glucocorticoid therapy

	Patients			Female pubertal controls	
	J. I.	M. V.	J. C.		
LH (ng/ml) (LER-960)					
Basal	3.8	2.4	0.5	2.15 ±	0.46
Peak	7.8	16.5	3.5	6.48 ±	0.94
Increment	4.0	14.1	3.0	4.33 ±	1.12
Area	200	947	336	571.75 ±	65
FSH (ng/ml) (LER-869)					
Basal	4.1	2.7	2.7	2.01 ±	0.65
Peak	5.7	3.7	3.3	4.43 ±	1.24
Increment	1.6	1.0	0.6	2.42 ±	1.37
Area	182	105	28.75	208.98 ±	126.25

Table 5. Response to LRF in two postmenarcheal patients with 21-hydroxylase deficiency while on glucocorticoid therapy

| | Patients | | Female pubertal controls |
	A. R.	C. L.	
LH (ng/ml) (LER-960)			
Basal	0.9	0.8	2.15 ± 0.46
Peak	3.3	5.3	6.48 ± 0.94
Increment	2.4	4.5	4.33 ± 1.12
Area	269	512	571.75 ± 65
FSH (ng/ml) (LER-869)			
Basal	3.0	2.7	2.01 ± 0.65
Peak	3.3	3.0	4.43 ± 1.24
Increment	0.3	0.3	2.42 ± 1.37
Area	−22.25	20.75	208.98 ± 126.25

testosterone, had a significant decrease of ACTH into the normal range after one dose of medication.

Responses to LRF were variable. Patient S. B. had appropriate LH and FSH responses when the level of gonadotropins was plotted versus time (Table 3). Her responses were comparable to those of other treated prepubertal patients with virilizing CAH who had been reported from this laboratory (Reiter et al., 1975). Of the three patients who were pubertal but premenarcheal, two had LH and

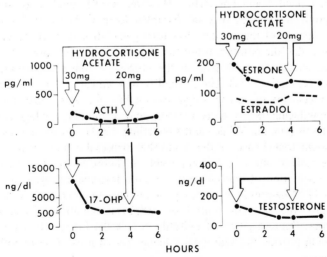

Figure 5. Plasma ACTH, estrone, estradiol, and 17-hydroxyprogesterone after the first and second morning dose of glucocorticoid in C. L., a postmenarcheal patient with congenital adrenal hyperplasia who was amenorrheic at the time of study.

FSH responses within the range of normal pubertal females (Table 4). One (M. V.) had a normal FSH response, but, although the baseline LH was normal, the response to LRF was significantly greater than the mean of our female pubertal control group. The responses of the two postmenarcheal patients were not significantly different from those of pubertal controls, but FSH responses were less than those of controls (Table 5).

The data for patient C. L. summarize the changes in levels of steroid after one dose of glucocorticoid (Figure 5). Plasma ACTH, which was abnormally elevated, returned to the normal range after medication. Plasma 17-hydroxy-progesterone, also markedly elevated, returned toward normal but did not reach the normal range after administration of glucocorticoid. Testosterone, significantly elevated, was suppressed to the normal range by a single dose. Levels of estrogen did not change significantly.

DISCUSSION

Delayed menarche and abnormal menstrual patterns in patients with 21-hydroxylase deficiency could be due to defective functioning at the level of the hypothalamus, pituitary, ovary, or uterus, or more than one of these sites. Regardless of the site(s) of dysfunction, it is hypothesized from these studies that excessive androgen production is the major factor contributing to menstrual irregularities. It has not been substantiated in humans that androgens affect the hypothalamus or higher central nervous system centers in such a way that cyclic LRF and gonadotropin release are permanently impaired, because some patients have regular menses and are fertile. However, cyclic function of the hypothalamic-pituitary complex may be disrupted temporarily by excessive androgens. The capacity of the pituitary to release gonadotropins after stimulation by LRF suggests that the pituitary is not the major site of dysfunction.

In rats, androgens participate in the process of follicular maturation and atresia (Louvet et al., 1975). The possibility of a similar effect of androgens or androgen precursors of adrenal origin cannot be eliminated. Also, the role of estrogen in inducing the ovulatory LH surge may be modified by high circulating androgen levels (von zur Mühlen and Kobberling, 1973). Finally, androgens may modify endometrial changes to the extent that menses does not occur.

On the basis of our data, it is impossible to choose among these hypotheses. Daily documentation of concentrations of gonadotropin, estrogen, and progesterone would be helpful in establishing the presence or absence of ovulation and might resolve the issue of central or peripheral causation of menstruation abnormalities. Demonstration of pulsatile or episodic LH secretion throughout the day could provide the additional evidence for an intact CNS-hypothalamic-pituitary axis.

An analogy can be drawn between the menstrual irregularities of patients with 21-hydroxylase deficiency and those with polycystic ovaries; in both conditions, testosterone levels are often elevated. Female patients with virilizing CAH before treatment sometimes have ovarian histology that is similar to that in polycystic ovaries (Sizonenko et al., 1972). Patients in this study had no ovarian or uterine abnormalities. In some patients with polycystic ovaries, suppression of the adrenal contribution to excess androgen production allows return of more normal cyclic menses (Ettinger et al., 1973). Consistent suppression of adrenal androgens might have the same effect in patients with CAH. Patient C. L. began to have vaginal bleeding when the dosage of hydrocortisone acetate (80 mg/day in three doses) was changed to 1.5 mg of dexamethasone/day in two doses. Patient J. I. has had several menstrual periods at monthly intervals since 25 mg of cortisone acetate/day in 2 divided doses was changed to 6 mg of methylpred-nisolone/day in three divided doses. M. V. has had menarche since methyl-prednisolone was increased to 6 mg in three divided doses.

The data from these patients indicate that ACTH and adrenal steroid production are usually not suppressed throughout an entire 24-hr period even when dosages of glucocorticoid are adequate to suppress urinary 17-ketosteroids into the normal range.

An optimal treatment program for congenital virilizing adrenal hyperplasia is one which suppresses androgenic effects yet allows normal growth without undue advancement of bone age. In older patients who have reached their ultimate height, it may be desirable to achieve continuous adrenal androgen suppression with glucocorticoid preparations and dosages which, while not causing a Cushingoid appearance, might be detrimental to growth in younger children. The efficacy of glucocorticoid preparations which can provide more prolonged adrenal suppression than cortisone or hydrocortisone for the treatment of menstrual irregularities in adolescent patients with CAH is currently under evaluation.

REFERENCES

Ettinger, B., E. B. Goldfield, K. C. Burell, K. von Werder, and P. H. Forsham. 1973. Plasma testosterone stimulation-suppression dynamics in hirsute women: correlation with long-term therapy. Am. J. Med. 54:195−200.
Jenner, M. R., M. M. Grumbach, and S. Kaplan. 1970. Plasma 17-OH progesterone in maternal and umbilical cord plasma in children and in congenital adrenal hyperplasia (CAH): application to neonatal diagnosis of CAH. Pediatr. Res. 4:380.
Jenner, M. R., R. P. Kelch, S. L. Kaplan, and M. M. Grumbach. 1972. Hormonal changes in puberty. IV. Plasma estradiol, LH, and FSH in prepubertal children, pubertal females and in precocious puberty, premature thelarche, hypogonadism, and in a child with a feminizing ovarian tumor. J. Clin. Endocrinol. Metab. 34:521−530.
Jones, H. W., and B. S. Verkauf. 1971. Congenital adrenal hyperplasia: age at menarche and related events at puberty. Am. J. Obstet. Gynecol. 109:292−297.

Kelch, R. P., S. L. Kaplan, and M. M. Grumbach. 1973. Suppression of urinary and plasma follicle stimulating hormone by exogenous estrogens in prepubertal and pubertal children. J. Clin. Invest. 52:1122–1128.

Louvet, J.-P., S. M. Harman, J. R. Schreiber, and G. J. Ross. 1975. Evidence for a role of androgens in follicular maturation. Endocrinology 97:366–372.

Rees, L. H., and D. M. Cool. 1971. A radioimmunoassay for rat plasma ACTH. Endocrinology 80:254–261.

Reiter, E. O., M. M. Grumbach, S. L. Kaplan, and F. A. Conte. 1975. The response of pituitary gonadotropes to synthetic LRF in children with glucocorticoid-treated congenital adrenal hyperplasia: lack of effect of intracorticoid-treated congenital adrenal hyerplasia: lack of effect of intrauterine and neonatal androgen excess. J. Clin. Endocrinol. Metab. 37:318–325.

Roth, J. C., M. M. Grumbach, and S. L. Kaplan. 1973. Effect of synthetic luteinizing hormone-releasing factor on serum testosterone and gonadotropins in prepubertal, pubertal and adult males. J. Clin. Endocrinol. Metab. 37:680–686.

Sizonenko, P. C., I. M. Burr, S. L. Kaplan, and M. M. Grumbach. 1970. Hormonal changes in puberty. II. Correlation of serum and luteinizing hormone and follicle stimulating hormone with stages of puberty and bone age in normal girls. Pediatr. Res. 4:36–45.

Sizonenko, P. C., A. M. Schindler, I. J. Kohlberg, and L. Paunier. 1972. Gonadotrophins, testosterone and oestrogen levels in relation to ovarian morphology in 11-beta-hydroxylase deficiency. Acta Endocrinol. 71:539–550.

Speroff, L. 1965. The adrenogenital syndrome and its obstetrical aspects. Obstet. Gynecol. Survey 20:185–214.

von zur Mühlen, A., and J. Kobberling. 1973. Effect of testosterone on the LH and FSH release induced by LH-releasing factor (LRF) in normal men. Horm. Metab. Res. 5:266–270.

Wilkins, L., J. F. Crigler, Jr., S. H. Silverman, L. I. Gardner, and C. J. Migeon. 1952. Further studies on the treatment of congenital adrenal hyperplasia with cortisone. II. The effects of cortisone on sexual and somatic development, with an hypothesis concerning the mechanism of feminization. J. Clin. Endocrinol. Metab. 12:277–295.

Normal Spermatogenesis in Adult Males with Congenital Adrenal Hyperplasia after Discontinuation of Therapy

Andrea Prader, Milo Zachmann, and Ruth Illig

Untreated adult males with congenital adrenal hyperplasia (CAH) generally have testicular atrophy, which is attributed to hypogonadotropic hypogonadism caused by the gonadotropin-suppressing effect of the high plasma levels of adrenal steroids.

This chapter presents four adult males with 21-hydroxylase deficiency and marked steroid changes who have normal testicular reproductive function. All four patients had received hydrocortisone treatment for some periods during childhood or adolescence or both, and all have maintained normal spermatogenesis in adult life, even after discontinuation of treatment for several years.

Table 1. Age and testicular volume

Patients	Age (years)	Testicular volume (ml)
At start of treatment		
1	9	2
2	6	3
3	7	2
4	14	14
At end of treatment		
1	18	14
2	13	10
3	16	9
4	15	14
At follow-up		
1	29	13
2	28	7
3	19	7
4	25	15

Supported by the Schweizerischer Nationalfonds zur Förderung der wissenschaftlichen Forschung (Grant No. 3.405.74).

Table 2. Urinary steroids

	17-Ketosteroids (mg/24 hr)	Testosterone[a] (μg/24 hr)	Pregnanetriol[a] (mg/24 hr)	Pregnanetriolone[a] (mg/24 hr)
Patients				
1	57.2	173	32.8	8.7
2	57.0	180	13.9	8.6
3	35.9	339	10.9	2.2
4	46.6	116	25.8	5.7
Normal	4.5–16.5	32–135	0.6 ± 0.3	0

[a]Determined by gas-liquid chromatography.

RESULTS

Table 1 shows age and testicular volume at the beginning and at the end of the treatment period and at the follow-up examination. Treatment with hydrocortisone was started between the ages of 6 and 14 years, was given for a period of 1–9 years, and was discontinued by the patients' own decisions at the age of 13–18 years. Testicular volume was normal for age before and at the end of treatment. Discontinuation of treatment had no ill effects in any of the patients. Physical examination at the age of 19–29 years revealed no anomalies, with the exception of small stature (151–166 cm) and relatively small testicular volume in patients 2 and 3. The testicular size of these two patients was at the lower limit of the normal range and below that found at the end of treatment.

Patients 1 and 2 were married and had children. Each had a sister with classic CAH who became amenorrheic as soon as treatment was discontinued.

Tables 2 and 3 summarize the results of the urinary and plasma steroid determinations. The total 17-ketosteroids, urinary testosterone, and pregnanetriol were markedly increased. The presence of large amounts of pregnanetriolone in the urine confirmed the diagnosis of 21-hydroxylase deficiency. The plasma levels of testosterone were normal, and the values of estrone and

Table 3. Plasma steroids determined by radioimmunoassay

	Testosterone (ng/100 ml)	Estrone (pg/ml)	Estradiol (pg/ml)
Patients			
1	681	426	141
2	1,020	272	55
3	327	586	454
4	930	119	64
Normal			
Males	612 ± 172	31 ± 7	21 ± 5
Females	35 (20–70)	75 (20–182)	121 (17–290)

Table 4. Plasma gonadotropins determined by radioimmunoassay[a]

| | Plasma LH (ng/ml) | | Plasma FSH (ng/ml) | |
	Basal	Peak after LHRF (25 μg/m^2 intravenously)	Basal	Peak after LHRF (25 μg/m^2 intravenously)
Patients				
1	1.1	5.4	1.9	4.6
2	0.8	2.7	0.8	1.6
3	1.1	3.5	2.8	6.1
4	0.8	3.4	2.4	3.4
Normal	1.5 ± 0.8	6.2 ± 1.3	2.0 ± 0.7	2.8 ± 1.7

[a]Standard preparations used: LH(LER-960), 1 mg = 4,620 I.U. second IRP; human pituitary FSH, 1 mg = 3,500 I.U. second IRP.

estradiol were markedly elevated. Plasma luteinizing hormone (LH) and follicle-stimulating hormone (FSH) were measured before and after stimulation with luteinizing hormone-releasing factor (LHRF) (Table 4). Basal LH levels were low normal, and the LH response to LHRF was subnormal in three patients. Basal FSH levels and the FSH response to LHRF were normal. Sperm counts of all patients were in the upper normal range (86–181 million/ml).

DISCUSSION

The results show that these four adult male patients with 21-hydroxylase deficiency are fertile in spite of grossly abnormal steroid findings and in spite of relatively small testes in two of them.

Most untreated men with CAH are clinically unremarkable, with the exception of small stature, small testes, and sterility. The hypogonadism is probably caused by the suppressing effect of the elevated adrenal steroid levels on the release of gonadotropins. Treatment with glucocorticoids which suppress the excessive adrenal steroid production allows a normal testicular development.

In a minority of untreated male patients, the testes show a normal or even increased size due to either hyperplastic adrenocortical tissue in the atrophic testes or to normal testicular maturation. Of 24 adult patients reported in the literature (Siebenmann, manuscript in preparation), 21 had testicular atrophy and only 3 had normal testicular maturation (Bahner and Schwarz, 1961; Kiessling and Schwarz, 1966; Stewart, 1960). In addition, Wilkins, Blizzard, and Migeon (1965) mention two untreated brothers with normal spermatogenesis. It seems, therefore, that spontaneous gonadal maturation in male patients with CAH is relatively rare, but still more frequent than in female patients, in whom it is unknown or extremely rare. The cause of spontaneous testicular maturation in these patients is unknown. It is unlikely to be due to a genotypic CAH variant, because the patient reported by Bahner and Schwarz (1961) had an adult sister with fully expressed CAH.

We do not know of any published report of adult males with normal spermatogenesis after discontinuation of therapy. However, unpublished data from the Johns Hopkins group give the following additional information: one of the two brothers mentioned by Wilkins, Blizzard, and Migeon (1965) was treated for 8 days at the age of 13 and is now married with two children. One other adult male patient discontinued treatment 6 years ago and now has two children, aged 4 and 2.

The following question arises: Do the four patients in this study have spontaneous testicular maturation unrelated to treatment or is their normal testicular function a consequence of the earlier steroid therapy which was discontinued several years earlier?

These four patients were not specifically selected. A total of nine adult male patients were observed. Four of them are still being treated. Five discontinued steroid treatment; four of this group are presented here. In the fifth patient a sperm count could not be performed, but all other results were similar to those of the four patients. Unfortunately, there was no opportunity to study an adult male patient who had never been treated.

It seems unlikely that all of our five patients underwent spontaneous testicular maturation. The marked urinary steroid changes and the full expression of CAH with amenorrhea in the affected sisters of patients 1 and 2 tend to exclude an unusually mild form of CAH. It is, therefore, possible that earlier treatment is responsible for testicular maturation in some patients. In the first three patients, this assumption is more likely than in the last patient. They had normal testicular growth under steroid treatment and a reduction of testicular volume after discontinuation of therapy. The fourth patient already showed pubertal testicular size at the start of treatment and no reduction after treatment, as would be expected in a patient with spontaneous testicular maturation.

If the normal spermatogenesis of most of these patients is the consequence of earlier treatment, it would follow that treatment is necessary for the induction, but not for the maintenance, of normal spermatogenesis.

The steroid and gonadotropin findings explain the normal spermatogenesis to some extent only. Normal tubular function requires the presence of FSH and testosterone. In the plasma of these patients, both are present in normal concentration for adult males. In contrast, LH appears to be slightly decreased, and the estrogens are markedly increased.

The normal plasma testosterone level in the patients studied is of interest. It may be assumed to be of predominantly adrenal origin. In children with untreated CAH, plasma testosterone is increased. It is not known whether it is also increased in adult males who have never been treated. The high urinary testosterone in the presence of normal plasma testosterone can be explained by the hepatic conversion of androstenedione and other adrenal steroids into testosterone glucuronide.

It is surprising that the increased estrogens do not suppress the gonadotropins and do not induce gynecomastia. There appears to be a resistance to estrogens at the hypothalamic and peripheral level. This may possibly be explained by a displacement of estrogens by other adrenal steroids at the receptor level.

SUMMARY

Four adult males with 21-hydroxylase deficiency who were treated late during childhood or adolescence or both and who have discontinued treatment several years ago were studied. All of them have normal spermatogenesis, normal plasma testosterone, slightly low LH and normal FSH, and very high plasma estrogens, with a resistance to estrogens at the hypothalamic and the peripheral level. It seems likely, but cannot be proven, that in some of these patients testicular maturation has not been spontaneous but has been induced by the previous treatment and that in these patients the maintenance of normal testicular function does not require continuous therapy.

REFERENCES

Bahner, F., and G. Schwarz. 1961. Congenitale Nebennierenrindenhyperplasie beim Mann mit normaler Keimdrüsenfunktion und Fertilität. Acta Endocrinol. (Kbh.) 38:236–246.

Kiessling, W., and G. Schwarz. 1966. Zur Genese des Hypogonadismus beim kongenitalen adrenogenitalen Syndrom. Arch. f. Klin. Exp. Dermatol. 227: 684–687.

Siebenmann, R. E. Die Pathologie der kongenitalen adrenogenitalen Syndrome, manuscript in preparation.

Stewart, J. S. S. 1960. A fertile male with untreated adrenal hyperplasia. Acta Endocrinol. (Kbh.) Suppl.51:661.

Wilkins, L., R. M. Blizzard, and C. J. Migeon. 1965. *In* The Diagnosis and Treatment of Endocrine Disorders in Childhood and Adolescence, Ed. 3, p. 410. Charles C Thomas, Springfield, Illinois.

Gonadotropin-Adrenal-Testicular Axis in Males with Congenital Adrenal Hyperplasia and Idiopathic Sexual Precocity

Salvatore Raiti, Noel Maclaren, and Fatui Akesode

As part of a study of gonadotropin production rates in various pubertal disorders, it was surprising to find very high follicle-stimulating hormone (FSH) production in two young boys with untreated congenital adrenal hyperplasia (CAH). Therefore, previous reports on gonadotropin excretion were reviewed and gonadotropin studies were carried out in other males with treated or untreated CAH.

Increased gonadotropin excretion has been found in patients with untreated congenital adrenal hyperplasia. Escamilla (1947) reported slight increase in follicle-stimulating hormone in about half of the 13 patients studied. Brown (1958) found that in two untreated females the urinary FSH excretion was slightly higher than in three girls and 1 boy with isosexual precocious puberty. Kovacic (1959) found increased total gonadotropins in one 6-year-old untreated girl. Stevens and Goldzieher (1968) studied eight patients, five aged 4–10 years and three aged 10–29 years. Four of the five children showed FSH excretion in the adult range. Four of five children also had increased luteinizing hormone (LH) excretion, two being only slightly increased and two being in the adult male range. Following therapy with cortisone, prednisone, or dexamethasone, the FSH excretion decreased in three patients, but showed no change in the three other patients. The LH excretion showed either no change or was increased.

Kirkland, Librik, and Clayton (1974) studied three adolescent and adult affected females receiving cortisol replacement therapy. They found normal plasma concentrations of FSH and LH, but no midcycle gonadotropin peaks. Normal plasma FSH and LH concentrations following prolonged therapy were reported by Molitor, Chertow, and Fariss (1973). On the other hand, Penny, Olambiwonnu, and Frasier (1973) reported normal or low plasma FSH and LH concentrations in a 6-year-old male before treatment. Within 8 days of therapy, there was a considerable rise in the plasma concentrations of FSH and LH,

Table 1. Clinical and laboratory studies

Patient	Chronological age (years/months)	Height age (years/months)	Skeletal age (years/months)	Urinary 17-KS (mg/24 hr)	Plasma FSH (mI.U./ml)	Plasma LH (mI.U./ml)
Congenital adrenal hyperplasia						
J. W.	3 weeks	10 weeks	12 weeks	7.6	<1	7.0
T. W.	4 weeks	Normal	Normal	1.6	<1	6.0
P. M.	1/0	1/10	2/8	3.0	4.0	7.5
J. S.[a]	3/11	3/10	4/6	2.1	4.5	2.5
M. B.	6/6	9/6	10/0	8.8	8.0	3.0
J. A.[a]	12/4	10/0	12/5	3.1	5.0	5.0
J. M.	81/0	12/6	Adult	51.2		
Idiopathic precocious puberty						
J. A.						
(a)	4/0	7/0			1.0	<3.0
(b)	4/6	7/6	10/5		<4.0	<4.0
C. D.						
(a)	3/0	7/6	10/0		3.0	16.0
(b)	4/6	9/0	14/0		2.0	8.0

[a]Previously diagnosed and treated.

followed, by rises in plasma testosterone concentration and by sexual maturation. Sohval and Soffer (1951) reported excess gonadotropins in the urine in 9 of 22 patients with CAH during the 1st week or two of therapy.

This chapter reports the studies on the FSH and LH production rate and excretion, and on plasma adrenal steroid concentrations in seven untreated or partially treated males with CAH. The findings in these patients are compared with those in two boys with idiopathic sexual precocity because their plasma testosterone and Δ^4-androstenedione concentrations are produced predominantly by the testes rather than by the adrenal glands.

CASE REPORTS (TABLE 1)

Congenital Adrenal Hyperplasia

Case 1 M. B., a non-salt-loser, was diagnosed at age 6½ years. Rapid growth and pubic hair were first noticed at 3 years of age. When first seen in this laboratory, he had about 50 pubic hairs, but no axillary or facial hair or acne. His penis was 4 cm long and 1 cm in diameter. His testes measured 3 X 2 cm bilaterally. On completion of his diagnostic and gonadotropin studies, he was given suppressive, followed by maintenance, cortisol replacement therapy. Three months later his parents refused to give him any further therapy, and he was lost to follow-up.

Case 2 P. M., who had 11-hydroxylase deficiency, has been reported by Raiti et al. (1975), but the data on his production rates of FSH and LH were not included. Therapy began soon after 1 year of age and has been continued. At age 3½ years, he was restudied while on treatment. His penis was 5 cm long and 2 cm in diameter. His testes measured 1.5 X 1.0 cm bilaterally. He had no pubic hair.

Case 3 T. W., a salt loser, aged 1 month, was studied following hospitalization for undiagnosed hyponatremic dehydration.

Case 4 J. W., a salt loser, aged 3 weeks, was also studied followed hospitalization for undiagnosed hyponatremic dehydration.

Case 5 J. S., a non-salt-loser, appeared normal at birth and was said to have normal urinary 17-ketosteroid (17-KS) excretion. When first seen at 9 months of age, he had a large penis and pigmented nipples. His diagnosis was confirmed by urinary steroid studies. At age 3 years 11 months, his cortisone therapy was reduced from 25 mg (5,5 and 15 mg) to 5 mg twice a day for 3 months. Blood and 24-hr urines were collected at monthly intervals for 3 months.

Case 6 J. A., a non-salt-loser, was diagnosed at 3 years of age. He presented with rapid growth, pubic hair, and facial acne. Therapy was begun and continued. At age 12 years 4 months, he still had about 50 pubic hairs, but no axillary or facial hair. His penis was 6 cm long. His testes measured 2 X 2 cm bilaterally. Prednisone therapy was reduced from 2.5 mg three times a day to 2.5 mg/day for 2 months; it was then stopped completely for 1 month and restarted when the study was complete. Blood and 24-hr urines were collected at monthly intervals.

Table 2. Production rates (urinary method)

1. Treat patient with KI for 1 day before test and until test is complete.
2. Prepare human FSH (hFSH) or human LH (hLH) labeled with ^{125}I at low specific activity. Sterilize.
3. After voiding, inject 2–3 μCi intravenously.
4. Collect all urine (48 hr for hLH; 72 hr for hFSH).
5. Precipitate 10 ml of urine pool at pH 5.5 with acetone. Resuspend in phosphate-buffered saline solution.
6. React aliquots of infused hormone and of urine precipitates with excess antibody. Check for nonspecific binding.
7. Calculate amount injected (immunological cpm) and amount excreted (immunological cpm).
8. Measure unlabeled FSH and LH excreted in urine.
9. Calculate specific activity (S.A.) of excreted hormone.
10. Calculate production rate = $\dfrac{\text{amount injected (cpm immunological)}}{\text{S.A.} \times \text{time (days)}}$

Case 7 J. M., a non-salt-loser, aged 81, was diagnosed following study of his excessive virilization, which at first was thought to be caused by a tumor. He had not fathered any children nor had he married.

Idiopathic Sexual Precocity

Case 8 J. A., aged 4 years, had stage 2 pubic hair when first studied. His testes measured 4 X 2 cm bilaterally. He was restudied 6 months later. His pubic hair was at stage 3, but his testicular size had not changed.

Case 9 C. D. was first diagnosed and studied at stage 3 puberty when he was 3 years old. He was restudied 1½ years later, by which time his sexual maturation was nearly complete.

METHODOLOGY

The production rates (PR) of FSH and LH were measured by the methods of Raiti et al. (1970, 1975) (Table 2). These techniques are similar to those for

Table 3. Urinary excretion of FSH or LH

1. Collect 24-hr urine.
2. Take 10-ml aliquot. Add 0.1 ml of 25% human serum albumin.
3. Bring pH to about 5.5 using dilute acetic acid.
4. Precipitate by adding 20 ml of reagent grade acetone or 40 ml of 95% alcohol.
5. Leave overnight at 4°C.
6. Centrifuge for 5 min. Discard supernatant.
7. Resuspend precipitate in 10 ml of phosphosaline buffer.
8. Bring pH to 7.0 using 1N ammonium hydroxide.
9. Measure FSH or LH by appropriate radioimmunoassay.
10. Calculate total excretion for 24-hr period.

measuring cortisol production rates except that immunological methods are used to characterize the injected and the excreted labeled hormone. The metabolic clearance rate (MCR) was measured by the methods of Kohler, Ross, and Odell (1968) and Coble et al. (1969).

The urinary excretion of FSH and LH was measured by the method of Raiti and Blizzard (1968) (Table 3). The urinary proteins were precipitated at pH 5.5 and at refrigerated temperatures with the use of alcohol (5 volumes) or acetone (2 volumes). The dried precipitate was dissolved in the buffer of the radioimmunoassay. Appropriate aliquots were then used in the FSH or LH radioimmunoassay. The plasma testosterone and Δ^4-androstenedione concentrations were measured by radioimmunoassay (deLacerda et al., 1973; Murphy, 1971).

RESULTS

Congenital Adrenal Hyperplasia

24-Hour Urinary 17-KS Excretion All undiagnosed cases showed elevated urinary 17-KS excretion for age of the patient (Table 1). The 17-KS excretion in patient J. S. after 3 months of reduced therapy was slightly increased for age. In patient J. A., the 17-KS excretion surprisingly remained within the normal range.

FSH Studies The plasma FSH concentrations in patients J. S. and J. A. were normal for age (4.2 ± 0.7 mI.U./ml) (Raiti et al., 1969), but were elevated

Table 4. FSH studies

Patients	Chronological age (years/months)	MCR (ml/min)	Excretion (I.U./day)	PR (I.U./day)
Normal male adults		14.3–18.9	8.5 ± 3.6	21.9–47.6
Congenital adrenal hyperplasia				
J. W.	3 weeks		0.31	
T. W.	4 weeks		0.21	
P. M. (a)	1/0	3.6	6.2	41.5
(b)	3/6		1.7	10.3
J. S. (a)	3/11		2.9	
(b)	4/1		4.1	
M. B.	6/6	9.2	6.7	40.2
J. A. (a)	12/4		6.4	40.2
(b)	12/7		7.6	
J. M.	81/0		13.6	
Idiopathic precocious puberty				
J. A.	4/0		2.2	17.9
C. D. (a)	3/0	6.4	3.2	21.8
(b)	4/6	6.6	2.2	21.8

in patient M. B. and probably elevated in patient P. M. at 1 year of age (Tables 1 and 4). In patients J. W. and T. W., the plasma FSH was barely detectable.

The 24-hr urinary excretions of FSH in the untreated patients M. B. and P. M. were elevated both for age and for the degree of sexual development and were within the range found in adult males (Raiti et al., 1969). When patient P. M. was restudied after 2½ years of constant suppressive therapy, his urinary FSH excretion fell to a concentration which was normal for his age. Patients J. S. and J. A. showed normal 24-hr FSH excretion during therapy and a small but significant rise after the 3 months of inadequate therapy. Patient J. M. showed FSH excretion in excess of the normal range for adult males (deLacerda et al., 1973). In the two neonates, the FSH excretion prior to therapy was low.

The PRs of FSH (Raiti et al., 1970) were measured in patients P. M. and M. B. before therapy, and both were at the upper limit of the normal range for adult males. Following 2½ years of suppressive therapy, the PR of FSH in patient P. M. fell to 25% of the initial value and to a level well below the normal adult range. Prior to therapy, the metabolic clearance rate of FSH was in the adult range for patient M. B., but was much lower in patient P. M.

LH Studies Before therapy, patient P. M. showed a plasma LH concentration which was elevated for age and more consistent with that of a male at stage 2 or 3 of sexual development (Johanson et al., 1969) (Tables 1 and 5). The plasma concentration in patient M. B. was normal for age, but low for the degree of virilization (Johanson et al., 1969). Following reduction and/or cessa-

Table 5. LH studies

Patients	Chronological age (years/months)	MCR (ml/min)	Excretion (I.U./day)	PR (I.U./day)
Normal male adults		14.3–18.9	22.3–45.1	247.7–464.5
Congenital adrenal hyperplasia				
J. W.	3 weeks		0.35	
T. W.	4 weeks		1.1	
P. M. (a)	1/0	8.8	5.9	166
(b)	3/6		4.7	139
J. S. (a)	3/11		5.1	
(b)	4/1		2.9	
M. B.	6/6	11.9	11.8	141
J. A. (a)	12/4		10.0	
(b)	12/7		7.4	
J. M.	81/0		16.4	
Idiopathic precocious puberty				
J. A. (a)	4/0		5.0	122.0
(b)	4/6		9.2	398.2
C. D. (a)	3/0	28.3	5.6	459.2
(b)	4/6	13.5	11.8	197.2

Table 6. Pituitary-testicular-adrenal axis

Patients	Plasma testosterone (μg/100 ml)	Plasma Δ^4-androstenedione (μg/100 ml)	LH PR (I.U./24 hr)	FSH PR (I.U./24 hr)
Normal male adults	575 ± 150	190.0 ± 20.0	247.7–465.5	21.9–47.6
Congenital adrenal hyperplasia				
J. W.	144.3	97.8		
T. W.	39.4	34.0		
P. M. (a)	154.0	378.0	166	41.5
J. S. (b)	133.3	69.2		
M. B.	246.0	576.0	141	40.2
J. A. (b)	58.8	31.1		
J. M.				
Idiopathic precocious puberty				
J. A. (a)	123		122.0	17.9
(b)	243		398.2	
C. D. (a)	444.5	38.2	459.2	21.8
(b)	120.0	97.7	204.9	21.8

tion of therapy, patients J. S. and J. A. had normal plasma LH concentrations for age and for the degree of virilization. In the two neonates, the plasma LH concentrations appeared to be elevated.

Before therapy, patients P. M. and M. B. showed 24-hr urinary excretions of LH which were elevated for age and were consistent with stage 2 or 3 of sexual development (Baghdassarian et al., 1970). The urinary excretion of LH in patient J. S. while on therapy was elevated for age, but was normal for age in patient J. A. The urinary LH excretion decreased significantly in both of them after 3 months of inadequate therapy. The untreated adult J. M. showed a low urinary LH excretion. The LH excretions were also low in the two untreated neonates.

The PRs and MCRs of LH in patients P. M. and M. B. were below the adult range before suppressive therapy and in P. M. after suppressive therapy.

Plasma Testosterone and Δ^4-androstenedione (Table 6) All plasma testosterone concentrations were 10–20% of those found in normal adult males, although patient M. B. had a much higher concentration. The plasma Δ^4-androstenedione concentrations were considerably elevated in patients P. M. and M. B., but were well below the normal adult range in the other patients studied.

Idiopathic Precocious Puberty

Patient J. A. progressed from stage 2 to stage 3 of puberty. Patient C. D. progressed from stage 3 to stage 5 of puberty. The four studies of these two patients can be viewed as a continuum. Their FSH excretion was low, but their production rates had reached the normal adult range by stage 3 of puberty. The MCR for FSH in C. D. was below the normal adult range. The PR for LH increased from stage 2 to stage 3 of puberty and then fell again at the end of puberty. In C. D. at midpuberty, the MCR was high, but returned to normal toward the end of puberty. The plasma testosterone concentrations were highest at midpuberty. The Δ^4-androstenedione concentrations were in the normal adult range.

DISCUSSION

Earlier gonadotropin bioassay studies showed increased excretion in patients with untreated CAH (Brown, 1958; Escamilla, 1947; Kovacic, 1959; Sohval and Soffer, 1951; Stevens and Goldzieher, 1968). Most of these assays were nonspecific, but Brown (1958) and Stevens and Goldzieher (1968) did measure both FSH and LH specifically, and both found considerable elevation of FSH excretion and slight or moderate increase in LH excretion. The plasma FSH and LH radioimmunoassay studies (Kirkland, Librik, and Clayton, 1974; Molitor, Chertow, and Fariss, 1973; Penny, Olambiwonnu, and Frasier, 1973) have shown normal concentrations prior to therapy.

These plasma FSH studies showed some increase in concentrations in the two older untreated patients, but very low concentrations in the two neonates. The plasma concentrations remained in the normal range in the two patients in whom therapy was decreased for 3 months.

The FSH urinary excretions were more striking and were in the adult range for normal males. Similar results were found by Stevens and Goldzieher (1968) by using bioassays. The FSH excretion in the 81-year-old male was higher than for adult males. Increases in urinary FSH excretion were found following 3 months of inadequate therapy in patients J. S. and J. A. There was considerable suppression in FSH excretion in patient P. M. during adequate maintenance therapy. The PRs of FSH were at the upper limit of the normal range for adult males in the two patients so studied. One of them showed a 75% suppression of FSH production during adequate maintenance therapy.

The plasma LH concentrations in the untreated or poorly treated patients were probably normal for age in three patients and probably elevated in patient P. M. and in the two neonates. Normal plasma concentrations were previously reported (Kirkland, Librik, and Clayton, 1974; Molitor, Chertow, and Fariss, 1973; Penny, Olambiwonnu, and Frasier, 1973). The urinary excretion of LH was increased in two of the untreated patients (P. M. and M. B.) and in one of the treated patients (J. S.). The 81-year-old patient showed a low excretion of LH compared to normal adult males, in spite of considerable virilization. The excretion was low in both of the neonates. It was surprising that when therapy was reduced or stopped in patients J. S. and J. A., the LH excretion decreased although the FSH excretion increased. The slight decrease in LH excretion in patient P. M. during suppressive therapy would be expected as a consequence of reduction of testosterone production. The PRs of LH in patients P. M. and M. B. were well below the normal range for adult males. The findings of this study were consistent with the bioassay results of Brown (1958) and Stevens and Goldzieher (1968).

The two patients with precocious puberty were included for contrast, because their virilization was due to androgens of testicular rather than adrenal origin. The plasma FSH concentrations were low for age and for degree of sexual development in both patients. One patient (J. A.) showed low and one (C. D.) showed elevated plasma LH concentration for age, although normal for the degree of sexual development. In contrast to the patients with CAH, the FSH excretion was normal for age in these patients with idiopathic precocious puberty. The PRs of FSH were below or at the lower limit of the normal adult male range. On the other hand, their urinary LH excretion was increased for age. Their PRs of LH reached and remained in the normal adult range as puberty advanced.

Two of the CAH patients (T. W. and J. A. (b)) showed very low plasma testosterone and Δ^4-androstenedione concentrations. Modest rises in plasma testosterone concentration were seen in patients J. W., P. M. (a), and M. B., the latter being consistent with the LH PR. Both P. M. (a) and M. B. showed very high plasma Δ^4-androstenedione concentrations and also very high FSH PRs, tempting the speculation of a cause and effect relationship. In the patients with precocious puberty, the rises in plasma testosterone were associated with increase in LH PRs. The plasma Δ^4-androstenedione concentrations were well below the normal adult range.

Thus, the virilization resulting from two separate organs was associated with different patterns of gonadotropin production and excretion. Whereas the adrenal virilization of CAH was associated with a more striking increase in FSH PR and excretion, the virilization of testicular origin was associated with more striking changes in LH PR and excretion, although the FSH changes were also significant. Such increased testicular activity may have resulted from a pituitary or hypothalamic disorder, because no cause for the precocious puberty was found.

It could be speculated that the more remarkable changes in FSH in CAH could be associated with any or all of three stimuli: the adrenal androgens, adrenal estrogens, or increased pituitary activity secondary to increased ACTH production.

Testosterone, Δ^4-Androstenedione, Pregnanetriol, and CAH

It is possible that any or all of these steroids stimulate pituitary production of FSH in the pubertal child. A direct feedback control between testosterone and LH is expected. It is feasible that Δ^4-androstenedione produced in excessive amounts (beyond the normal adult male range) might act directly as a stimulus for FSH production. Such greatly increased plasma concentrations of Δ^4-androstenedione, as well as increased testosterone PRs, have been previously reported (Camacho and Migeon, 1966; Rivarola, Saez, and Migeon, 1967), although no gonadotropin studies were included. Increased plasma 17-hydroxy-progesterone alone or in combination with these other steroids conceivably could act as the stimulus for increased FSH production, although this has not been reported.

Estrogens and CAH

Several groups have reported increased urinary estrogen excretion in untreated patients. Wilkins et al. (1951) reported significantly increased urinary estroids in patients aged 2½–18½ years. These fell considerably after cortisone therapy. Tamm, Apostolakis, and Voight (1966) found that urinary estrogen excretion increased in a 15-year-old patient after therapy was stopped. Therapy with human chorionic gonadotropin did not alter the excretion, but following ACTH therapy there was a significant rise in estriol excretion. They found similar increased estriol excretion in orchiectomized patients after ACTH, but not after human chorionic gonadotropin therapy. Goldzieher (1967) studied 11 patients aged 4–36 years, including three adult castrates. He found a marked increase in the production rates of estrone and estradiol in the older untreated patients and adults, which were not related to the changes in urinary 17-ketosteroids or pregnanetriol. Administration of human chorionic gonadotropin produced no effect, whereas ACTH therapy produced a marked increase in urinary estrogen excretion. Gabrilove, Nicolis, and Sohval (1973) reported one 16½-year-old affected and untreated male with gynecomastia. His total urinary estrogen excretion was increased.

Vorys, Ullery, and Stevens (1965) showed that small doses (0.02 and 0.05 mg/day) of ethinyl estradiol produced a 2-fold rise in urinary excretion of FSH in women, but higher doses (0.07 and 0.1 mg/day) produced no effect or slight suppression. Premarin (conjugated natural estrogens) had little or no effect on FSH, but stimulated a significant and rapid increase in LH excretion. In a 47-year-old male with a feminizing adrenal tumor, Rose et al. (1969) found increased production rates of estradiol and estriol. The urinary gonadotropin excretion (bioassay by the mouse uterine weight method) was increased, but the plasma FSH and LH concentrations (measured by radioimmunoassay) were normal.

Increased ACTH and Gonadotropins

Stevens and Goldzieher (1968) speculated that with a steroid enzyme defect there might be pituitary overactivity not only of ACTH but also of FSH and LH. Butt et al. (1963) studied eight patients with Stein-Leventhal syndrome. During and following dexamethasone therapy for 5 days, there was a significant rise of urinary FSH excretion, followed by an increased estriol excretion. They suggested that suppression of ACTH by corticoid therapy produced the compensatory rise in FSH. Sohval and Soffer (1951) drew attention to case records of adrenocortical hyperfunction with increased urinary gonadotropin excretion, and Goldzieher and Green (1962) reported strong evidence for the occasional coexistence of a hyperadrenocortical state and polycystic ovaries.

CONCLUSIONS

These studies conclude that with prolonged virilization caused by adrenal androgens (CAH), a significant elevation in FSH and a modest elevation in LH production and excretion are to be expected. These abnormal changes persist into adult life in untreated cases, as found in our 81-year-old man. It is postulated that these FSH changes are caused by increases of either Δ^4-androstenedione or even pregnanetriol or by increased adrenal estrogen production or by pituitary overactivity, not only for ACTH, but also for FSH production. On the other hand, virilization due to idiopathic precocious puberty is associated with modest rises of FSH and more marked increases in LH production and excretion as puberty advances. It is presumed that this is the normal sequence of gonadotropin changes during pubertal development. In these patients, the FSH and LH production remains in the normal adult range once puberty is complete.

ACKNOWLEDGMENTS

The authors wish to thank Mr. Glen E. Taylor for his technical help with all the FSH and LH studies and the National Institute of Arthritis, Metabolism, and Digestive Diseases, United States Public Health Service, for the immunochemical hFSH and hLH and their antisera.

REFERENCES

Baghdassarian, A., H. Guyda, A. Johanson, C. J. Migeon, and R. M. Blizzard. 1970. Urinary excretion of radioimmunoassayable luteinizing hormone (LH) in normal male children and adults, according to age and stage of sexual development. J. Clin. Endocrinol. 31:428−435.

Brown, P. S. 1958. Human urinary gonadotropins. I. In relation to puberty. J. Endocrinol. 17:329−336.

Butt, W. R., A. C. Crooke, F. J. Cunningham, and R. Palmer. 1963. The effect of dexamethasone on the excretion of estriol and follicle stimulating hormone in patients with Stein-Leventhal syndrome. J. Endocrinol. 26:303−304.

Camacho, A. M., and C. J. Migeon. 1966. Testosterone excretion and production rate in normal adults and in patients with congenital adrenal hyperplasia. J. Clin. Endocrinol. 26:893−896.

Coble, Y. D., Jr., P. O. Kohler, C. M. Cargille, and G. T. Ross. 1969. Production rates and metabolic clearance rates of human follicle stimulating hormone in premenopausal and postmenopausal women. J. Clin. Invest. 48:359−363.

deLacerda, L., A. Kowarski, A. Johanson, R. Athanasion, and C. J. Migeon. 1973. Integrated concentration and circadian variation of plasma testosterone in normal men. J. Clin. Endocrinol. 37:366−371.

Escamilla, R. F. 1947. Diagnostic significance of urinary hormonal assays: report of experience with measurements of 17-ketosteroids and follicle stimulating hormone in the urine. Ann. Intern. Med. 30:249−290.

Gabrilove, J. L., G. L. Nicolis, and A. R. Sohval. 1973. Nontumorous feminizing adrenogenital syndrome in the male subject. J. Urol. 110:710−713.

Goldzieher, J. W. 1967. Estrogens in congenital adrenal hyperplasia. Acta Endocrinol. 54:51−62.

Goldzieher, J. W., and J. A. Green. 1962. The polycystic ovary. I. Clinical and histologic features. J. Clin. Endocrinol. 22:325.

Johanson, A. J., H. Guyda, C. Light, C. J. Migeon, and R. M. Blizzard. 1969. Serum luteinizing hormone by radioimmunoassay in normal children. J. Pediatr. 74:416.

Kirkland, J., L. Librik, and C. Clayton. 1974. Serum gonadotropin levels in female adolescents with congenital adrenal hyperplasia. J. Pediatr. 84:411−444.

Kohler, P. O., G. T. Ross, and W. D. Odell. 1968. Metabolic clearance and production rates of human luteinizing hormone in pre- and postmenopausal women. J. Clin. Invest. 47:38−47.

Kovacic, N. 1959. Congenital adrenal hyperplasia and precocious gonadotropin secretion in a 6 year old girl. J. Clin. Endocrinol. 19:844−846.

Maclaren, N. K., C. J. Migeon, and S. Raiti. 1975. Gynecomastia with congenital virilizing adrenal hyperplasia (11β-hydroxylase deficiency). J. Pediatr. 86: 579—581.

Molitor, J. L., B. S. Chertow, and B. L. Fariss. 1973. Long-term follow up of a patient with congenital adrenal hyperplasia and failure of testicular development. Fertil. and Steril. 24:319—323.

Murphy, B. E. P. 1971. Sephadex column chromatography as an adjunct to competitive protein binding assays of steroids. (New Biol.) Nature 232:21—24.

Penny, R., O. N. Olambiwonnu, and S. D. Frasier. 1973. Precocious puberty following treatment in a 6 year old male with congenital adrenal hyperplasia: studies of serum luteinizing hormone (LH), serum follicle-stimulating hormone (FSH) and plasma testosterone. J. Clin. Endocrinol. 36:920—924.

Raiti, S., and R. M. Blizzard. 1968. Measurement of immunologically reactive follicle stimulating hormone in human urine by radioimmunoassay. J. Clin. Endocrinol. 28:1719—1723.

Raiti, S., R. M. Blizzard, R. Penny, and C. J. Migeon. 1970. Production rate of follicle stimulating hormone in adult males. In W. R. Butt, A. C. Crooke, and M. Ryle (eds.), Gonadotropins and Ovarian Development, pp. 185—198. E. and S. Livingstone, Edinburgh.

Raiti, S., T. P. Foley, Jr., R. Penny, and R. M. Blizzard. 1975. Measurement of the production rate of human luteinizing hormone using the urinary excretion technique. Metabolism 24:937—941.

Raiti, S., A. Johanson, C. Light, C. J. Migeon, and R. M. Blizzard. 1969. Measurement of immunologically reactive follicle stimulating hormone in serum of normal male children and adults. Metabolism 18:234—240.

Raiti, S., C. Light, and R. M. Blizzard. 1969. Urinary follicle-stimulating hormone excretion in boys and adult males as measured by radioimmunoassay. J. Clin. Endocrinol. 29:884—890.

Rivarola, M. A., J. M. Saez, and C. J. Migeon. 1967. Studies of androgens in patients with congenital adrenal hyperplasia. J. Clin. Endocrinol. 27:624—630.

Rose, L. I., G. H. Williams, K. Emerson, and D. B. Villee. 1969. Steroidal and gonadotropin evaluation of a patient with a feminizing tumor of the adrenal gland: in vivo and in vitro studies. J. Clin. Endocrinol. 29:1526—1532.

Sohval, A. R., and L. J. Soffer. 1951. The influence of cortisone and adrenocorticotropin on urinary gonadotropin excretion. J. Clin. Endocrinol. 11: 677—687.

Stevens, V. C., and J. W. Goldzieher. 1968. Urinary excretion of gonadotropins in congenital adrenal hyperplasia. Pediatrics 41:421—427.

Tamm, J., M. Apostolakis, and K. D. Voight. 1966. The effects of ACTH and HCG on the urinary excretion of testosterone in male patients with various endocrine disorders. Acta Endocrinol. 53:61—72.

Vorys, N., J. C. Ullery, and V. Stevens. 1965. The effects of sex steroids on gonadotropins. Am. J. Obstet. Gynecol. 93:641—648.

Wilkins, L., R. Lewis, R. Klein, L. I. Gardner, J. F. Crigler, Jr., E. Rosemberg, and C. J. Migeon. 1951. Treatment of congenital adrenal hyperplasia with cortisone. J. Clin. Endocrinol. 11:1.

PSYCHOLOGICAL, INTELLECTUAL, AND EDUCATIONAL ASPECTS

Dating, Romantic and Nonromantic Friendships, and Sexuality in 17 Early-treated Adrenogenital Females, Aged 16-25

John Money and Mark Schwartz

This chapter is one of a series from the Psychohormonal Research Unit of the Johns Hopkins Hospital and University concerning the behavioral sequelae of congenital adrenal hyperplasia (CAH). In previous publications (Baker and Ehrhardt, 1974; Ehrhardt and Baker, 1974; Ehrhardt, Epstein, and Money, 1968; Ehrhardt, Evers, and Money, 1968; Lewis, Ehrhardt, and Money, 1970; Money and Lewis, 1966; Money and Schwartz, 1976), interview and IQ data were reported on samples of girls with this syndrome during childhood and early adolescence. This chapter presents follow-up information on adrenogenital girls treated early in life with cortisone who are now in late adolescence and early adulthood (ages 16–25). Specifically, information on their dating, romantic and friendship interests, and sexual functioning is presented.

SAMPLE SELECTION AND DESCRIPTION

The 17 CAH patients of this study belonged to the generation of females who grew up since 1950 and who from early childhood received the benefit of cortisone therapy for the successful control of postnatal masculinization. They were chosen from a total of 47 females, between the ages of 16 and 25, under treatment in the Pediatric Endocrine Clinic. Patients were included who were regularly followed in the clinic or lived within commuting distance so as to be recalled to the Psychohormonal Unit for a follow-up interview to augment the longitudinal record already on file in the unit. There was no known bias in sampling. The only exception might be that offspring of middle class parents

This work was supported by Grant HD-00325 from the United States Public Health Service and by funds from the Grant Foundation, New York.

Table 1. Descriptive data on 17 patients with early treated adrenogenital syndrome

	M.I.	S.U.	U.P.	P.I.	M.E.	O.W.	H.I.	W.A.	S.N.
Date of birth	04/25/56	08/27/55	05/29/50	11/12/53	07/21/55	07/07/59	10/29/56	03/28/49	11/11/54
Original clitoral size	2.5 × 0.8 cm	2.0 × 0.8 cm	2.7 × 1.3 cm	ND[a]	4 cm	2 cm	3.0 × 0.2 cm	2 cm	2.5 × 1.2 cm
Age of clitorectomy	2 years	2 years	5 years	2 years	3 months	2 weeks	2 years	6 years	2 years
Age diagnosis was confirmed	7 weeks	Neonatal	7 weeks	2 years	8 days	2 years	ND	3½ months	Neonatal
Salt loser	Yes	No	Yes	No	Yes	Yes	Yes	No	Yes
First born	Yes	Yes	No	No	No	No	No	No	No
Age first seen	7 weeks	1 month	7 weeks	17 years	3 years	5 years	1½ years	6½ years	1 week
Age last seen	19 years	20 years	25 years	22 years	19 years	16 years	18 years	26 years	18 years
Present age (1975)	19 years	20 years	25 years	22 years	20 years	16 years	19 years	26 years	21 years
Bedwetting until teenage	Yes	No	No	No	No	No	Yes	No	Yes
Number of siblings	0	2	1	3	3	1	2	1	1
Menarche	16 years	None	14 years	14 years	14 years	None	13 years	11 years	14 years
Hirsutism in teenage	No	Yes	No	No	No	Yes	No	No	No

[a]ND, no data.

continued

Table 1—*Continued*

	E. N.	F. L.	W. E.	L. O.	J. O.	P. O.	W. I.	T. A.
Date of birth	02/28/58	09/23/50	04/06/54	03/23/49	03/17/57	08/20/56	03/12/58	02/18/53
Original clitoral size	2.8 × 1.2 cm	2 cm	2.5 × 1.2 cm	2 × 1.3 cm	1.5 × 1 cm	2.5 × 1.4 cm	2.5 × 1 cm	2.4 × 0.9 cm
Age of clitorectomy	2 years	4 years	5 years	2 years	2 years	2 years	2 years	5½ years
Age diagnosis was confirmed	Neonatal	5 months	Neonatal	2 months	3 days	6 weeks	1 week	5 months
Salt loser	No	No	No	Yes	Yes	Yes	Yes	No
First born	No	No	Adopted	Yes	Yes	No	Yes	Yes
Age first seen	7 months	2 months	5 years	1 month	15 days	6 weeks	6 months	5 months
Age last seen	17 years	25 years	21 years	20 years	18 years	17 years	17 years	22 years
Present age (1975)	17 years	25 years	21 years	26 years	18 years	19 years	17 years	22 years
Bedwetting until teenage	No	Yes	No	No	No	No	Yes	Yes
Number of siblings	1	1	1	3	1	1	1	2
Menarche	13 years	None	10 years	19 years	12 years	None	None	16 years
Hirsutism in teenage	No	Yes	No	No	No	No	No	No

[a]ND, no data.

wealthy enough to afford interstate travel to a distant hospital were over-represented.

In all but three cases, the patient and one parent were interviewed at least biennially, during their scheduled endocrine follow-up, throughout childhood. In the three exceptions, one child was seen more sporadically because of distance, and two were followed elsewhere when young. Recent interviews to augment the existing longitudinal information in the psychohormonal files were also obtained. Each hospital interview lasted at least 2 hr and was either completely recorded on tape or summarized on tape by the interviewer and patient at the end of the interview.

Information from the combined pediatric endocrine and psychohormonal files pertinent to the present study was independently abstracted and tabulated by two individuals.

Table 1 lists relevant descriptive data on the patients. Thirteen have been followed in the Pediatric Endocrine Clinic and its Psychohormonal Unit since infancy. Four were treated and followed hormonally elsewhere early in life, before first being seen for psychohormonal study. In 16 of the cases, the correct diagnosis was made neonatally or within the 1st year. In two cases, the diagnosis was not established until age 2. Twelve of the patients had a clitorectomy within the first 2 years of life. Clitorectomy was delayed to ages 4, 5, or 6 in the remaining five cases. The mean age of menarche was 13 years 10 months, except

Table 2. Information on high school grades, IQ, and college attendance in 17 patients with early-treated adrenogenital syndrome

High school grade average	
Grade	No. of patients
A	4
B	4
C	4
D	3
Quit school	2
Intelligence	
IQ	No. of patients
90–99	3
100–109	4
110–119	4
120–129	5
No data	1
Postsecondary education	
Institution	No. of patients
College or specialty school	9
No college	5
Plan to attend college after high school	1
Do not plan to attend after high school	2

Table 3. Interview data on aspects of dating and romance in 17 patients with early-treated adrenogenital syndrome

I. Dating	
A. Has had the experience of being escorted by a male friend alone and has attended mixed social events	8
B. Has had the experience of being escorted by a female friend alone and has attended mixed social events	0
C. Has had the experience of being escorted by both a female and male friend alone and has attended mixed social events	3
D. Has not been escorted by a male or female alone but has attended mixed social events	3
E. Has not been escorted by a male or female alone and has not attended mixed social events	3
II. Age of first interest in attending mixed social events or dating	
A. Age 13−15	2
B. Age 16−17	5
C. Age 18−19	6
D. Age >19	1
E. Age >17 and no dating yet	3
III. Frequency of dating, escorted by a male friend alone or a female friend alone	
A. 1−5 times	2
B. 6−10 times	1
C. More than 10 times	8
D. 0 times	6
IV. Dating partners	
A. Has dated one partner more than three times	
1. Heterosexual partner only	6
2. Homosexual partner only	0
3. Heterosexual and homosexual partners	2
B. Has never dated one partner more than three times	3
C. Does not date	6
V. Age of first romantic involvement	
A. Heterosexual partner	
1. Age 13−15	1
2. Age 16−17	2
3. Age 18−19	4
4. After age 19	1
5. No romantic involvement with a heterosexual partner	9
B. Homosexual partner	
1. Age 13−15	1
2. Age 16−17	0
3. Age 18−19	0
4. After age 19	2
5. No romantic involvement with a homosexual partner	14

424   Money and Schwartz

Table 4. Interview data on aspects of sexual practices, arousal, and imagery in 17 patients with early-treated adrenogenital syndrome

I. Sexual practices

   A. Heterosexual exclusively
     1. Frequent experience — 2
     2. Moderate experience — 0
     3. Infrequent experience[a] — 3
   B. Homosexual exclusively
     1. Frequent experience — 0
     2. Moderate experience — 0
     3. Infrequent experience — 1
   C. Bisexual
     1. Frequent heterosexual experience and infrequent homosexual — 0
     2. Moderate heterosexual experience and moderate homosexual — 1
     3. Infrequent homosexual experience and infrequent heterosexual[a] — 1
   D. Autosexual only
     1. Frequent — 0
     2. Moderate — 0
     3. Infrequent — 1
   E. No experience claimed — 8

II. Erotic dreams and/or fantasies

   A. Exclusively heterosexual — 6
   B. Exclusively homosexual — 1
   C. Bisexual — 4+?1
   D. Autosexual — 0
   E. No erotic dreams and/or fantasies claimed — 3
   F. No data — 2

III. Sexual arousal

   A. Most sensitive area for sexual arousal
     1. Breasts — 1
     2. Vulva — 3
     3. Breasts and vulva — 3
     4. Other areas — 0
     5. Not aroused anywhere — 2
     6. No experience claimed — 8
   B. Sexual climax (orgasm)
     1. Yes — 2
     2. No — 6
     3. No experience claimed — 9
   C. Vaginal lubrication
     1. Yes — 9
     2. No — 0
     3. No experience claimed — 0
     4. No data[b] — 8

Continued

Table 4—*Continued*

___

III. Sexual arousal—*Continued*

    D. Patient's own estimate of level of "sex drive"

        1. Above average   2

        2. Average   6

        3. Below average   1

        4. No estimate[b]   8

    E. Primary stimuli of sexual arousal

        1. Tactual   8

        2. Visual   1

        3. Narrative   1

        4. No stimuli are arousing   1

        5. No experience claimed   6

    F. Stimuli which can provide sexual arousal

        1. Visual only   1

        2. Tactual and narrative   3

        3. Tactual and visual   5

        4. Tactual, visual, and narrative   2

        5. Not able to be aroused   1

        6. No experience claimed   5

___

[a]In two patients, the vaginal opening was too small for the penis to penetrate.

[b]These questions have just recently been added to the schedule of inquiry, so completion of information on lubrication and the estimated level of "sex drive" is awaited.

for five girls who have not begun menstruating at ages 16, 17, 19, 20, and 25. Three patients became hirsute during teen age owing to partial noncompliance in taking cortisone therapy.

Table 2 presents information on high school grades, IQ, and college attendance for the 17 patients. The high school grade averages were surprisingly lower than those one might expect from the IQ distribution. Three of the five patients with below average high school grades had IQs above 110. The only variable that could be associated with poor grades was unstable family life.

FINDINGS

Dating and Romance

Inspection of Table 3 disloses that the 17 women were, as a group, delayed in reaching the dating age and in having their first romance. This delay was not related to unattractiveness of appearance, in the opinion of the authors. In fact, the 17 women, as a group, were more than usually attractive in physique and appearance. The only exception was one obese woman. Four others were overweight, but not markedly so.

The delay in dating and romance also was not related to a more generalized social inhibition or withdrawal, but was specifically related to the establishment of a pair bond characterized by intimacy, romance, and eroticism. Even those older women who had the highest dating frequency in their social history had a limited experience with respect to number of partners. Among the 17 girls, 9 reported that they had been romantically attracted to a partner in a serious way. The onset of these relationships tended to be later into teen age, and they were of a relatively short duration. It was as if they were relationships of convenience and comradeship, rather than of profound erotic attachment. In only one case was the relationship sustained. The couple is still married. One other woman married. She became romantically attracted to a man after writing to him and seeing his photographs. They eventually arranged to meet. In 1 week they were married, before he left for a 2-year army enlistment. After 1 year they lived together for 1 week, then separated in preparation for a divorce.

The one woman who considered herself a lesbian reported that she was in love with a heterosexual woman. The partner, made anxious by the erotic implication of the friendship, terminated it.

Sexual Practices, Arousal, and Imagery

Information on sexual functioning is based on the eight women who had sexual experience with a partner and one other who reported masturbation experience only. The eight ostensibly asexual women ranged in age from 16–25 (median 19½ years).

The information presented in Tables 4 and 5 discloses that the majority of the nine sexually experienced women were satisfied with their ability to become aroused, but that satisfaction with erotic sensitivity was variable. Two women had vaginal openings that were too small for penetration during intercourse. Dilation was necessary in both cases. Two other women had difficulty maintaining a genital erotic response after the preliminary arousal phase. One of these women reported that each time the partner touched her she felt as if a doctor were examining her. The other woman who had little genital erotic feeling blamed it on long-term failure to take cortisone. This patient was also slightly hirsute.

The other five women were satisfied with their erotic sensitivity, although only two claimed to have experienced orgasm. These two had frequent sexual

Table 5. Reported experience of bisexualism in fantasy and/or practice[a]

	Present age	
Reported psychosexuality	16–19 (n = 7)	20–26 (n = 10)
Bisexual fantasy only	0	2 + ?1
Bisexual fantasy and experience	0	2
Homosexual fantasy and lesbian experience	0	1
Heterosexual fantasy and experience	4	2
Sexuality denied	3	2

[a]This table summarizes Table 4, sections I and II.

experience. One was married. She reported that her breasts were more sensitive than her vulvar region. The second was a recalcitrant 17-year-old who claimed having had sexual intercourse with more than 10 partners. She was the only patient who claimed also to have multiple orgasms.

Six of the women could become aroused by visual erotica. Touch, however, was the primary mode of sexual arousal in five of these six cases. The one exception was a woman who reported no dating experience.

Only one patient reported a strong genitopelvic component to erotic stimulation. She spoke openly about sexual arousal, including the fact that she had erotic feelings in fantasy toward her older brother. The other sexually experienced woman reported a "ticklish sensation" and a "tightening" of the vaginal muscles in response to erotic stimulation. When these women became aroused they were not able to pinpoint any specific vulvar area of eroticism, including the area of the amputated clitoris.

Four of the patients were able to be bisexually aroused, and a fifth only homosexually. One other 20-year-old woman reported by letter that she was homosexual. She is not included in this sample, because she was unavailable for follow-up. Three of these women had had sexual experience with a woman partner. The remaining two could be sexually aroused by both men and women, but did not know if they would ever be able to have homosexual experiences. A sixth woman did not discuss bisexuality, but her evasive answers could be interpreted to suggest that she quite likely is bisexually aroused. The openly bisexual reports included a history of attraction to females since elementary

Table 6. Interview data on aspects of nonromantic friendships in 17 patients with early-treated adrenogenital syndrome

I. Friendships during teen age	
A. Casual and close friendships	5
B. Casual friendships only	7
C. Casual acquaintanceships	4
D. Comradeship within the family only	1
II. Invites friends to home	
A. Frequently	5
B. Occasionally	4
C. Never	8
III. Has difficulty making friends	
A. Yes	8
B. No	9

Table 7. Compliance in taking cortisone and family life stability or instability in 17 patients with early-treated adrenogenital syndrome

| | Family life | | |
	Stable	Unstable[a]	No. of patients
Compliance	6	2	8
Partial compliance	2	4	6
No compliance	0	3	3

[a]Unstable refers to parental divorce or separation, death of one parent, and/or parental psychopathology.

school. This history was not freely reported until after age 20. The possibility of still more bisexual disclosures at a later date cannot be ruled out.

Nonromantic Friendships

Table 6 shows that none of the 17 patients was strongly gregarious. They all reported that they seldom made an effort to establish a friendship, especially if distance was a barrier. Five of the patients reported that they had no close or casual friends. Four did have casual acquaintanceships in school. The fifth isolated herself from social contact outside of her family. Several of the patients judged themselves hard to get close to, and their parents concurred. Four who had no close school friends had difficulty establishing close friendships when they left home to attend college.

Compliance in Taking Cortisone

Compliance in taking medication (Table 7) constitutes a problem which has peripheral relevance to the topics of this chapter. Only eight of the patients had a long-term history of consistent compliance. If they had a stable family life, they had at least partial compliance. Patients from unstable homes commonly had a greater degree of noncompliance; these same patients also had an increased risk for gender confusion in teen age. Four of them used such terms in self-reference as "butch," "not all female," or "half man, half woman." Such ambivalence was incongruous with the medical self-knowledge each patient was given over the years, with a minimal number of technical terms. Hirsutism or erotic bisexuality, or both, may have exaggerated the problem in three of the cases.

DISCUSSION

Four characteristics common to females with the early treated adrenogenital syndrome during late adolescence and early adulthood are 1) relative diffidence in establishing friendships, 2) late onset of dating and romance, 3) possible bisexuality in imagery or experience, and 4) inhibition of erotic arousal or expression, or both. It is possible that all four of these characteristics are related, although there is no final and absolute proof to this effect.

If they are related, they may all stem from 1) a delayed effect of excess prenatal androgenization on certain brain pathways, 2) an unknown side effect of long-term cortisone therapy (more specifically, under the dosages given during the past 25 years), or 3) a secondary effect of a chronic condition requiring pharmacological treatment and a history of related genital surgery and repeated examination of the sex organs throughout childhood and adolescence.

It is not yet possible to formulate a definitive explanation. It is possible that all three explanations may be contributory. The first alternative, however, deserves special attention because of extensive experimental animal evidence, primates included, on the postnatal effects of prenatal androgen. In relation to the hypothalamus, prenatal androgen influences oxidative metabolism (Mogui-levsky, 1966), protein content (Scacchi et al., 1970), serotonin level (Ladosky and Gaziri, 1970), ribonucleic acid metabolism (Clayton, Kogara, and Kraemer, 1970), nuclear volume (Dörner and Staudt, 1968), and neural connections (Raisman, 1974). The primate evidence parallels that of the clinical study of prenatally androgenized human beings.

In adrenogenital girls exposed to excess fetal androgen, the postnatal effect on behavior is manifested initially in a strong degree of tomboyish behavior (Ehrhardt and Baker, 1974; Money and Ehrhardt, 1972; Money and Schwartz, 1976). Girls thus affected play very well with boys in their competitive games, but the boys do not establish close friendships with them, as they would if the same girls were being reared and habilitated as boys. Other girls also do not establish close friendships with girls prenatally androgenized due to CAH. The transition to teen age, accompanied by pubertal hormonal feminization, is accompanied by tomboyism, but not by enough erotic attraction toward boys to permit the tomboyish adrenogenital girl to feel a close psychological kinship with her female contemporaries.

At the same time, she does not experience an extreme repudiation of femininity, as one sees in a female-to-male transexual. Nor is she able to accept bisexuality or lesbianism and to be nonjudgmentally at ease with it—at least in most cases. Thus, she is left as something of a social isolate.

The alternative to social isolation is engrossment in career achievement, characteristic of many adrenogenital patients. It takes many years for the adrenogenital woman to feel completely at ease with her femininity in an erotic sense. Not all individuals are affected to the same degree, and those who come from stable homes adjust much better than those who do not.

The difficulty in achieving womanhood following a history of excess fetal androgenization of the sexual anatomy and of certain sex-related aspects of brain functioning stands in contrast to the ease of reaching masculinity when the same genetic and gonadal female is assigned and habilitated as a boy (Money and Daléry, in this volume).

Prenatal hormones may have facilitated bisexuality in the women of the present study. Although the sample size is presently too small for definitive conclusions, more women reported bisexual experience or erotic imagery, or both, than would be expected by chance. Sorenson (1973) interviewed a large sample of adolescents (age 13–19). Fewer than 1% reported having a recent homosexual experience. Three patients (18%) in this sample reported recent homosexual experience, and they plus two others (29%) reported bisexual or homosexual imagery.

Clitorectomy did not necessarily destroy erotic sensitivity, although it may have reduced it. Other vulvar areas are obviously sensitive enough to compensate for clitoral absence. That is not to say that the consideration of clitorectomy should be undertaken lightly. Follow-up of the women, as they gain more extensive sexual experience, will be necessary before the effect of clitoral absence can be fully ascertained.

SUMMARY

Seventeen adrenogenital women, 16 to 26 years old, belong to the first generation of adults regulated on cortisone therapy since infancy. They are the first such patients studied for adult eroticism and sexuality. The findings indicated an elevated prevalency of 1) relative difference in establishing friendships, 2) late onset of dating and romance, 3) possible bisexuality in imagery or experience, and 4) inhibition of erotic arousal or expression, or both. It is possible that all four of these characteristics are related, although there is no final and absolute proof to this effect.

REFERENCES

Baker, S. W., and A. A. Ehrhardt. 1974. Prenatal androgen, intelligence and cognitive sex difference. In C. R. Friedman, R. Richard, and R. Vande Wiele (eds.), Sex Differences in Behavior. John Wiley and Sons, Inc., New York.

Clayton, R. B., J. Kogara, and H. C. Kraemer. 1970. Sexual differentiation of the brain: effects of testosterone on brain RNA metabolism in newborn female rats. Nature 226:810–812.

Dörner, G., and J. Staudt. 1968. Structural changes in the preoptic anterior hypothalamic area of the male rat following neonatal castration and androgen substitution. Neuroendocrinology 3:136–190.

Ehrhardt, A. A., and S. W. Baker. 1974. Fetal androgens, human central nervous system differentiation, and behavioral sex differences. In C. R. Friedman, R. Richard, and R. Vande Wiele (eds.), Sex Differences In Behavior. John Wiley and Sons, Inc., New York.

Ehrhardt, A. A., R. Epstein, and J. Money. 1968. Fetal androgens and female gender identity in the early-treated adrenogenital syndrome. Johns Hopkins Med. J. 122:160–167.

Ehrhardt, A. A., K. Evers, and J. Money. 1968. Influence of androgen and some aspects of sexually dimorphic behavior in women with the late treated adrenogenital syndrome. Johns Hopkins Med. J. 123:115–122.

Ladosky, W., and L. C. J. Gaziri. 1970. Brain serotonin and sexual differentiation of the nervous system. Neuroendocrinology 6:168–174.

Lewis, V. G., A. A. Ehrhardt, and J. Money. 1970. Genital operations in girls with the adrenogenital syndrome: subsequent psychologic development. Obstet. and Gynecol. 36:11–15.

Moguilevsky, J. A. 1966. Effect of testosterone in vitro on the oxygen uptake of different hypothalamic areas. Acta Physiol. Lat. Amer. 16:353–356.

Money, J., and A. A. Ehrhardt. 1972. Man and Woman, Boy and Girl: The Differentiation and Dimorphism of Gender Identity from Conception to Maturity. The Johns Hopkins University Press, Baltimore.

Money, J., and V. G. Lewis. 1966. IQ, genetics and accelerated growth: andrenogenital syndrome. Bull. Johns Hopkins Hosp. 118:365–373.

Money, J., and M. Schwartz. 1976. Fetal androgens in the early-treated adrenogenital syndrome of 46, XX hermaphroditism: influence on assertive and aggressive types of behavior. Aggressive Behav. 2:19–30.

Raisman, G. 1974. Evidence for a sex difference in the neuropil of the rat preoptic area and its importance for the study of sexually dimorphic function. Aggression 52:42–51.

Scacchi, P., J. A. Moguilevsky, C. Libertun, and J. Christot. 1970. Sexual differences in protein content of the hypothalamus in rats. Proc. Soc. Exp. Biol. Med. 133:845–848.

Sorenson, R. 1973. Adolescent Sexuality in Contemporary America: Personal Values and Sexual Behavior, Ages 13–19. World Publishing, New York.

Hyperadrenocortical 46, XX Hermaphroditism with Penile Urethra
Psychological Studies in Seven Cases, Three Reared as Boys, Four as Girls

John Money and Jean Daléry

This chapter is one in a series of studies from the Psychohormonal Research Unit of The Johns Hopkins University and Hospital on the effects of excessive fetal androgenization on subsequent behavior and gender identity in chromosomal 46, XX females with the adrenogenital syndrome. The adrenogenital syndrome is the result of a genetically recessive inborn error of metabolism due to an enzymatic defect in the biosynthesis of cortisol. By way of consequences, there is an excessive secretion of fetal adrenal androgen, which in turn causes varied degrees of fetal masculinization of external and internal genital structures in the genetic female. The excessive amounts of adrenal androgen secretion are not limited to the fetal stages; it continues into the postnatal period unless cortisone replacement therapy is given. When the treatment is started soon after birth and is well regulated, the physical handicaps are minimized.

In the most extreme degree of masculinization, when excessive androgen is produced before the 12th week of fetal life, the urethra extends along the shaft of the hypertrophied clitorine organ, opening at the tip of the glans, so as to form a clitorine penis indistinguishable from a normal penis. The labioscrotal folds are completely fused, to the extent that they look like an empty scrotum. In this anatomic type, the patient can at birth easily be mistaken for a male with bilateral cryptorchidism. This type is often referred to as Prader's type V

This work was supported by Grant HD-00325 from the United States Public Health Service and funds from the Grant Foundation, Inc., New York, and from La Fondation de l'Industrie Pharmaceutique pour la Recherche, Paris.

(Prader, 1954). Different subtypes of this syndrome occur; masculinization may be the only manifestation or it may be associated with a tendency to salt loss or with hypertension. A direct relationship between the degree of masculinization of the genitalia and the salt-losing tendency has been reported (Qazi and Thompson, 1972; Verkauf and Jones, 1970). In addition, the salt-losing subtype

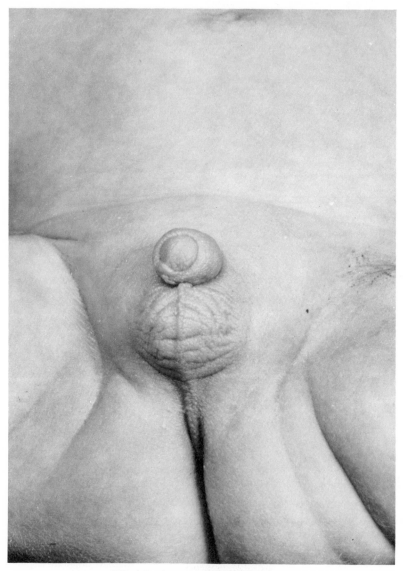

Figure 1. Aspects of genitalia at birth.

may suffer sporadic life-threatening manifestations in times of illness or injury and requires additional treatment for salt loss.

Cortisone replacement therapy, clitorectomy, and vaginal exteriorization are required when the patient is to live as a female. Cortisone and testosterone replacement therapy and removal of the internal sex organs and the gonads are required when the patient is to live as a male.

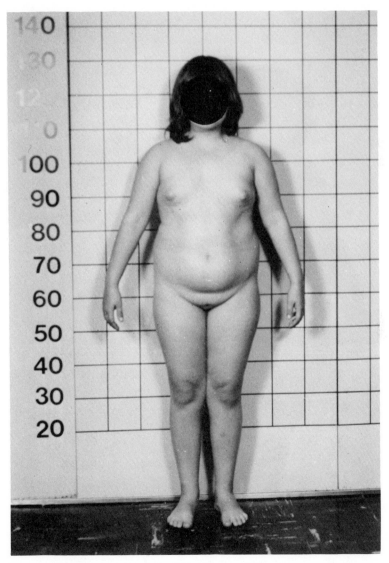

Figure 2. Girl at the age of 10.

PURPOSE OF STUDY

The purpose of these studies is to show that complete embryonic differentiation of a penis in a genetic female does not preclude assignment, rearing, and habilitation as a girl with a feminine gender identity—albeit tomboyish—but, conversely, is also consistent with assignment, rearing, and habilitation as a boy with a masculine gender identity.

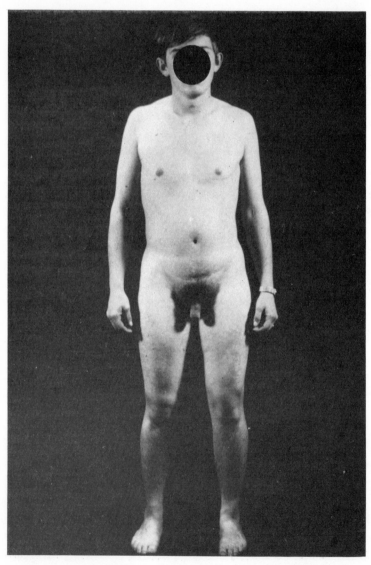

Figure 3. Boy at the age of 19.

Table 1. Descriptive data of sample ($n = 7$)

	E. U.	O. A.	O. I.	A. O.	U. T.	O. O.	I. I.
Date of birth	4.10.57	5.17.51	1.31.49	4.29.71	11.7.64	10.21.63	8.3.63
Original sex assignment	Male at birth	Male at birth	Male at birth	Female at 6 days	Male at birth; female at 19 days	Male at birth; female at 8 weeks	Male at birth; female at 1 year
Age at first psychological report	13 years	19 years 6 months	6 years 4 months	6 days	19 months	8 weeks	1 year
Age at last follow-up	18 years 2 months	24 years 3 months	26 years 6 months	4 years 1 month	10 years 5 months	11 years 7 months	12 years 1 month
Age at surgery	13 years	3 years 6 months	7 years 5 months	16 days; 2 years 6 months	1 month; 20 months	10 weeks; 2 years 9 months	1 year; 3 years
Age at beginning of cortisone therapy	3 years 6 months	11 days	4 years 7 months	6 days	19 days	21 days	2 months
Age at determination of genetic status	12 years 2 months	1 month	7 years 5 months	6 days	19 days	8 weeks	10 months
Penile size in cm (age)	5 X 2 (13 years)	6 X 2.5 (19 years 6 months)	6.5 X 2.5 (5 years 6 months)	2.5 X 3.0 (3 days)	3 X 1.5 (19 days)	3.5 X 1.4 (8 weeks)	2 X 1.2 (11 months)
Prosthetic testes	Yes	No	No	No	No	No	No
Salt-losing syndrome	No	Yes	Not proved	Yes	Yes	Yes	Yes
Family history of ambiguous genitalia	No	Yes[a]	No	Yes[b]	No	Yes[c]	No
Age at beginning of puberty	2 years 6 months	11 years 6 months	3 years 6 months	Prepubertal	10 years	11 years	11 years
Height in cm (age)	152 (18 years 2 months)	160 (24 years 3 months)	152 (26 years 6 months)	96.2 (3 years 9 months)	135.8 (10 years 5 months)	133.8 (11 years 7 months)	140 (12 years 1 month)
Weight in kg (age)	58 (16 years)	62 (24 years 3 months)	78 (26 years 6 months)	13.5 (3 years 9 months)	38.2 (10 years 5 months)	40.1 (11 years 7 months)	91 (12 years 1 month)

[a] Sibling with abnormal penis died at 3 weeks.
[b] Sibling with ambiguous genitalia died at 1 week.
[c] Two siblings with ambiguous genitalia died at 11 and 30 days.

SAMPLE SELECTION AND CHARACTERISTICS

The criteria for inclusion in this sample were 3-fold: first, the diagnosis was adrenogenital syndrome; second, the chromosomal sex was female; and, third, the patients presented at birth the extreme degree of masculinization of the external genitalia with penile urethra and fusion of the labioscrotal folds (Figures 1–3).

Ten patients met these criteria. One, born in 1955, died in an acute adrenal crisis in 1958; two others born in 1973 and 1974 were too young to be reported here. The seven remaining patients are reported herein (Table 1). Six of them were referred to the Psychohormonal Research Unit from the Pediatric Endocrine Clinic of the Johns Hopkins Hospital. The seventh one was seen by one of the authors in the Children's Hospital in Boston, courtesy of Dr. John Crigler. These patients were divided into two groups, according to their sex of rearing.

Group I included three patients who were declared males without ambiguity at birth and were raised from birth as males. The syndrome of adrenal hyperplasia was recognized before the genetic status; and surgical correction, namely, hysterectomy and ovariectomy, was performed still later. Additionally, E. U. had prosthetic testes implanted in his scrotum when he was 13. Because in two cases the adrenogenital syndrome was not recognized neonatally and cortisone replacement therapy was not started until later, both developed signs of precocious puberty. As a consequence, the excessive acceleration of the bone growth created a discrepancy between physique age and chronological age in childhood. The premature fusion of the epiphyses explains the characteristic short stature in adulthood (Table 1). Patients of this group will be referred to as boys, according to their sex of rearing.

Group II included four patients raised as females. Three of them were declared males at birth and were reannounced as females. Because of the death of an older sibling with ambiguous genitalia, a suspicion of female hermaphroditism was raised for the fourth one at birth, and no sex was declared. She was announced a girl at the age of 6 days. For all four, adrenal hyperplasia, as well as the genetic status, was recognized early in life. The first stage of surgical correction of the genitalia, namely clitorectomy and division of the scrotal fusion, was performed without delay; the second stage, namely, exteriorization of the vagina, was performed later (see Table 1). Patients of this group will be referred to as girls, according to their sex of rearing.

In summary, the seven patients reported here had a concordant prenatal history, but the postnatal history was completely discordant for patients of group I and those of group II.

PROCEDURE

The basic procedure for the present study was to compile material from the patients' files. This was completed by a contemporary interview with the patient and such members of his or her family as were available. Additionally, extended telephone interviews were given to the three men and one girl who lived too distant for a contemporary visit to the Johns Hopkins Hospital. A standard data schedule of topics was followed, but the interviews themselves were flexible. Interviews were recorded completely or summarized on tape. The information relevant to this study was abstracted from the transcripts and then tabulated.

FINDINGS

Rehearsal of Sex-coded Roles in Play Habits and Domestic Activities

For little girls, rehearsal of parental and domestic roles in play habits and child caregiving is a socially accepted and recommended stereotype in our society. A little girl traditionally rehearses her future motherhood by playing the mother with her dolls and her future as a housewife by helping her mother with the domestic activities.

The four girls did not follow exactly the stereotypic pattern. They played with dolls only rarely. They preferred traditional boys' toys, such as cars, trucks, guns, and blocks. They liked to ride their bikes or motorbikes. I. I.'s favorite hobby was building models of cars. In the game of house, A. O. and U. T. rehearsed the role of the mother. O. O. preferred the role of the father; she pretended to go to work on her motorbike and expected her friend, who played the role of the mother, to have supper ready when she came back. She also played the role of doctor; with a physician's kit, she gave shots to her sick dolls. When she was 5 years old, her mother observed her playing as if she were pregnant. The mother reported, "She put a whole bunch of clothes underneath her dress and said, 'I am pregnant; I will soon have my baby.'"

The three boys followed more closely the socially stereotyped pattern. None of them was interested in doll play. So far as a retrospective study can tell, their boyish play habits were unremarkable. When old enough, at age 12, E. U. liked to ride his motorbike with a friend in the desert near his home, to build models of funny cars, and to hunt and fish with his father. As a teen-ager, he raised steers for financial gain as part of a school farm project. O. I. liked to ride his bike and to play Tarzan and cowboys. All three were interested in playing ball games with other boys.

The seven patients had in common their lack of interest in infant caregiving. When asked by their mothers to help with the housework, the three boys did so reluctantly. They preferred to play outside with their friends. When he was 13 years old, E. U. said, "I have to empty the trash, sweep the carpet, wash the truck and the car. I don't specially appreciate it." Occasionally, O. A. and O. I. helped their mothers with the cooking. When he was 8, O. I. explained to us in a very proud way that he knew how to cook better than his father and that he had to teach him: "I can cook nearly about everything. My daddy can't even cook soup."

The girls, W. T. and O. O., complained a lot about working in the house, but they did it for the reward of being allowed to play outdoor games. A. O. did not engage in any domestic work. I. I. cleaned her room and made her bed, but she did not help her mother with the housework and did not cook.

Romantic Interests in Boyfriends and Girlfriends

As reported by his mother, E. U. had his first date when he was around 12. The couple danced together at school dances and held hands. At one time he wanted to kiss the girl, but she refused. At the age of 13, when queried about what it means to have a girlfriend, he replied, "Well, it means that you like each other; you just don't care about anybody else . . . Friendship, that's just when you see them every so often, but you never call them or anything. Whenever you're a little bit more than friendship, you like her a little bit more, and you call her, and this kind of stuff. And you spend money on her, and your wallet gets a little lighter than it usually is." At the time of the last psychological report, he had had four different girlfriends. He had dated the last one for more than 1 year and was expecting to marry her.

Before he married, O. A. had four or five different girlfriends, the first when he was around 13 years old, with whom he engaged in kissing and petting.

O. I. reported having his first girlfriend when he was around the age of 8. He engaged in petting and kissing with her when he was 9. More than 17 years later, he was able to recall her and to describe her physically. He claimed having had 19 different girlfriends before he met his future wife.

The four girls were too young to make appropriate statements on their romantic interest in boyfriends. One can infer from older patients with adrenal hyperplasia, but with a lesser degree of genital masculinization at birth, that they will be "late bloomers" with respect to romantic interest in boys and that the threshold barrier to erotic awakening will be rather high.

When she was 10 years old, U. T. doubted that she would go out with a boyfriend if she were old enough and if her parents gave permission, adding, "I have more important things I would like to do, like playing basketball." When she was 10 years old, O. O. declared that she knew that some of her friends went to boys' houses and talked about which boy they liked best, but she was not interested in doing it. I. I. did not have a boyfriend; her only interest in boys was to compete with them and to comment on their performances in ball games.

Physical Energy, Tomboyism, and Cosmetic Interests

In early childhood, the three boys showed intense athletic interests, including outdoor preference, participation in rough sports, and competitiveness with other boys. These activities were not associated with fighting and aggression, which were conspicuous by their absence. Athleticism was commensurate with physique age rather than with chronological age. In early adulthood, O. A. was the only boy who still engaged in regular sports. The two others, by reason of their short stature in adulthood, secondary to premature bone maturation before effective cortisone regulation, were somewhat restricted in their interests in competitive sports and outdoor activities.

The four girls followed the behavioral pattern of other girls with the adrenogenital syndrome often referred to as tomboyism (Ehrhardt, Epstein, and Money, 1968). Their tomboyism included high energy expenditure in rough outdoor play. They showed a preference for boys over girls in their peer contact, and they liked competitiveness with boys. U. T. explained when she was nine years old, "I'd better be good [at sports], 'cause I substitute for a boy in the football game. I was not afraid of the ball, and he was. I was the only girl . . . Two other girls are better than me in soccer, but I am the best at baseball." The mother of O. O. commented, "O. has a lot of initiative and determination." Later she added, "She is more out to have a lot of fun. I think she is a tomboy." This tomboyism was considered by the parents of the girls as a socially acceptable pattern. None of them tried to discourage it, and there was no excess of parental pressure toward more stereotypic femininity. The girls enjoyed being tomboyish in play and were not rejected by their peers. This tomboyism did not include hyperactivity or aggressiveness. It was not accompanied by an overt desire to be a boy.

In keeping with their energetic outdoor recreation, the girls preferred to wear utilitarian and functional clothes, like slacks, overalls, and shirts, rather than attractive dresses. They wore dresses on special occasions such as church attendance or visits to the hospital. The same preferences applied to accessories such as jewelry and hair styling.

The clothing habits of the boys were unremarkable for a boy.

Reaction to Physical Handicaps

The four girls and one of the boys presented a severe salt-losing tendency. Consequently, the diagnosis of hyperadrenocortical hermaphroditism was recognized, and replacement therapy was initiated early in life. Under well regulated hormonal therapy the prognosis for physical development is variable, but within the normal range.

The girls can anticipate fertility. The three men knew of their inability to induce a pregnancy. One man and his wife decided to have children and, at the time of the last psychological report, had started a pregnancy by donor insemination.

In childhood, two of the men did not benefit from early cortisone therapy, because adrenal hyperplasia was not recognized until they developed signs of precocious puberty. When the first signs of precocious development were noticed, the parents did not expect abnormal sexual behavior. Mrs. I. explained her attitude toward the precocious appearance of pubic hair: "When he got about three and a half years old, I noticed one day when I was bathing him, it seemed like he had a little straggly black hair and I kept trying to wash it off; and it would not come off . . . His father is just a bear of hair; he has got it all over his body, on his back, shoulders and everything. Well, I thought maybe the child might have inherited all that hair. I just thought maybe he was going to be like his father. I did not know nothing much about boys."

Because a faulty plan of case management was decided upon by an insufficiently informed physician, E. U. developed breasts about the age of eleven years, in anticipation of menarche. This mortified him, and he tried to hide it from his friends and from his family. At the age of 13, he commented, "It started 2 years ago . . . It was embarrassing. I kept quiet. You are just always scared that somebody will find out about it and they may start kidding you. I thought I would just have to live life like that . . . One month ago, my mother told me about plastic surgery, that it could be removed . . . I was overjoyed. I really could not wait until I could get here." His local doctor had told him he was a female and should change to live as a girl, but he refused. Mrs. U. had no doubt about her son's masculinity. When E. was 13, she said, "He has a sister, and they are just completely different. He does not think like a girl. He does not have the same interests, and right now the thing that I think made me very sure of it is that he has a girlfriend; and that to me was a relief—when he did—because that was just the clincher, that he was not a girl. So I just think he is a boy."

The three boys were told that their sex glands had to be removed, because they could not descend into the scrotum, an explanation which made the monthly testosterone injection more acceptable. The lack of testes, as well as the inability to induce a pregnancy, did not create any evident behavioral problem. O. I. and O. A. knew the possibility of having artificial testes implanted, but were not interested in it. E. U. was satisfied with his artificial testes.

Although their adult height was only 5 feet (152 cm), E. U. and O. I. did not overtly complain about it. O. I. commented, "I am short, I am fat, but I have no complex."

Sexual Practices and Fantasies

According to disclosures of the mothers and according to direct inquiry, none of the seven patients reported socially unacceptable childhood investigative sexual curiosity and play. On the other hand, there was no extreme shyness about appearing naked either in front of members of the family or during a physical examination.

The four girls were too young at the time of the last psychological report to give relevant information on sexual practices and fantasies.

The three patients reared as boys, being adult at the time of the last psychological report, provided detailed information pertaining to their sex lives (Table 2). All three began their sex lives before marriage and found sexual intercourse pleasurable. Neither of the two married men reported extramarital sex. None of the three had difficulty in getting and maintaining an erection. E. U. appeared somewhat dissatisfied with his sex life and complained, at a time

Table 2. Sexual function of the three males

	E. U.	O. A.	O. I.
Age at first masturbation	No information	13 years	9 years
Age at first vaginal intercourse	16 years	19 years	20 years
Premarital sex including vaginal intercourse	Yes	Yes	Yes
Frequency of intercourse	Once a week	Three times a week	2–3 times a week
Erotic stimuli	Visual	Touch	Visual
Erotic zones	No information	Genitalia	Genitalia
Attitude toward oral sex	No information	No experience	Pleased
Self-rating of satisfaction with sex life	Slightly dissatisfied	Very pleased	Very pleased

when receiving insufficient androgen, about his penis not getting hard enough to go deep enough. The other two, as well as their wives, were perfectly satisfied with their sexual function. All three reported orgasm by masturbation and by vaginal intercourse. They all reported that they ejaculated a small amount of a watery liquid. They could not have a repeat orgasm over a short period of time in the manner typical of a woman. O. I. claimed, besides having pleasurable vaginal intercourse two to three times a week, that he masturbated two to three times a day. None of them reported any erotic behavior or fantasies toward men.

Social Mixing with Peers and Siblings

All seven patients were able to mix with and to be accepted without difficulty by their peers either at school or in their neighborhoods or families. The four girls preferred social mixing related to competitive rough play and sports, rather than long-term relationships with a single friend.

School Achievement and Career

The three boys finished their schooling around the age of 18. None went to college. E. U. obtained average grades in high school. From the age of 18 he worked with his father, who owns a farm supply business. Because of bad grades, O. A. dropped out of 8th grade at school when he was 17, worked as a cook for 4 years, and is presently working in construction with his father. O. I. dropped out of school around the age of 17 and is presently employed in a factory doing manual work.

At the time of the last report, A. O. was too young to attend school. U. T. obtained good results in the 5th grade and expected to be either a nurse or a veterinarian. O. O. was in the 6th grade, doing very well academically and expecting to be either a doctor or an artist. I. I. had average academic achievement in the 6th grade and expected to become a car racer.

DISCUSSION

Seven constitute too few cases on which to report a basic psychological finding. But seven patients who are chromosomal and gonadal females with complete masculinization of the external genitalia are a large sample. Weldon, Blizzard, and Migeon (1966) reported an endocrine study of five adrenogenital patients with penile urethra and reviewed the relevant literature. O. I., U. T., O. O., and I. I. of this present report were included in their report also. O. I.'s medical history has been reported by Jones and Scott (1971). The cases of O. I. and O. O. have also been reported by Money (1970) and Money and Ehrhardt (1972).

The present report raises the pragmatic question of whether, in the future, a 46, XX adrenogenital baby born with a fully formed penis should be assigned and reared as a boy or a girl. For those assigned as boys, the evidence of this study, based on three patients, suggests a rather smooth development from fetal through pubertal masculinization. In fetal life, masculinization involves the external genitalia and, inferentially, pathways in the brain that subserve certain limited aspects of sexually dimorphic behavior, which can be summed up as tomboyism. For the 46, XX adrenogenital baby assigned, reared, and habilitated surgically and hormonally as a boy, tomboyism (more accurately, boyism) is smoothly incorporated postnatally into a masculine differentiation of gender identity and role. In teen age, there is no romantic and erotic impediment to maturation as a male or to the establishment of an erotic partnership with a woman; and the issue of infertility can be coped with.

For the 46, XX adrenogenital baby born with a penis and assigned, reared, and habilitated surgically and hormonally as a female, tomboyism can be incorporated postnatally into a socially acceptable tomboyish version of a feminine differentiation of gender identity and role, although there are certain constraints regarding erotic functioning. These constraints, it has been known for some time (Money and Ehrhardt, 1972), involve delayed onset of romantic and erotic pair-bonding with a male partner. Until new evidence on psychosexual functioning became available (Money and Schwartz, in this volume), it was not known that tomboyism in the 46, XX adrenogenital patient of the postcortisone era, hormonally regulated since birth and reared and habilitated as a girl, might be associated in teen age and young adulthood with an increased likelihood of bisexuality or lesbianism in imagery or practice, or both.

Bisexuality may be considered either an advantage or a disadvantage, depending on one's personal ideology regarding sexuality. In the mores of our time, bisexuality is still rather heavily stigmatized, despite a lessening of the stigma in recent years. Consequently, it is not easy for the contemporary teen-aged adrenogenital girl with a bisexual disposition and a weak degree of erotic attraction toward boys to negotiate her psychosexual development. One 18-year-old patient, in despair over, among other things, the failure of a lesbian romance, committed suicide as these studies were concluded.

The issue of sex assignment in the case of the 46, XX adrenogenital baby born with a penis is one of competing values, namely, of preserving fertility as a female versus increasing the probability of a smoother path through adolescence to psychosexual maturity and erotic function as a male. The medical profession is divided. Perhaps the masculine alternative is beset with fewer difficulties overall. Certainly in cases in which the child grows and differentiates a masculine gender identity and role before the chromosomal and gonadal status is diagnosed, a sex reassignment by edict would be a great folly. It would, in fact, be as unwise as an enforced sex reassignment for any growing boy. Gender identity cannot be changed by edict once it has become differentiated.

SUMMARY

The seven chromosomal and gonadal females reported here with the adrenogenital syndrome were born with a penis as a result of extreme fetal androgenization. Four of them were reared as girls and differentiated a female gender identity with tomboyism. The other three were reared as boys, differentiated a male gender identity, and performed sexually as men with women partners. Sex reassignment for them, as for any similar patient who had differentiated a boy's gender identity, was unthinkable. On sex assignment of the neonate with the same syndrome, medical opinion is divided. Fertility as a female must be weighed against greater ease of psychosexual development and erotic pair-bonding as a male. The authors suggest the latter is beset with fewer difficulties.

REFERENCES

Ehrhardt, A. A., R. Epstein, and J. Money. 1968. Fetal androgens and female gender identity in the early-treated adrenogenital syndrome. Johns Hopkins Med. J. 122:160–167.

Jones, H. W., Jr., and W. W. Scott. 1971. Genital Anomalies and Related Endocrine Disorders, Ed. 2. The Williams and Wilkins Company, Baltimore.

Money, J. 1970. Matched pairs of hermaphrodites: behavioral biology of sexual differentiation from chromosomes to gender identity. Engineering Sci. (California Institute of Technology) 33:34–39.

Money, J., and A. A. Ehrhardt. 1972. Man and Woman, Boy and Girl: The Differentiation and Dimorphism of Gender Identity from Conception to Maturity. The Johns Hopkins University Press, Baltimore.

Prader, A. 1954. Der Genital befund beim Pseudohermaphroditismus feminimus des kongenitalen adrenogenitalen Syndroms. Helv. Paediatr. Acta 9:231–248.

Qazi, Q. H., and M. W. Thompson. 1972. Genital changes in congenital virilizing adrenal hyperplasia. J. Pediatr. 80:653–654.

Verkauf, B. S., and H. W. Jones. 1970. Masculinization of the female genitalia in congenital adrenal hyperplasia: relationship to the salt losing variety of the disease. South. Med. J. 63:634–638.

Weldon, V. V., R. M. Blizzard, and C. J. Migeon. 1966. Newborn girls misdiagnosed as bilaterally cryptorchid males. N. Engl. J. Med. 274:829–833.

Males and Females with Congenital Adrenal Hyperplasia
A Family Study of Intelligence and Gender-related Behavior

Anke A. Ehrhardt and Susan W. Baker

Patients with congenital adrenal hyperplasia (CAH) have not only been the subject of many endocrinological studies, but they have also been of great interest to behavioral scientists. This chapter attempts to synthesize what is presently known about cognitive functioning and gender-related behavior in females and males with CAH.

In the 1950's, Money and his collaborators studied the effects of abnormal prenatal and postnatal sexual maturation on gender identity formation and other aspects of psychosexual differentiation (Money, 1955; Money, Hampson, and Hampson, 1955; Money, Hampson, and Hampson, 1957). Their detailed investigation and long-term follow-up of those late treated patients contributed to our knowledge of the effects of abnormal physical development on gender-related behavior. The most important outcome of these earlier clinical studies was the formulation of a theory on gender identity differentiation stressing, in particular, the importance of postnatal environmental influences such as those involved in the rearing of a child.

More recently, in the 1960's and 1970's, stimulated by animal experimental evidence on the effects of fetal sex hormones on parts of the central nervous system, research interest shifted to early treated children who grew up without the additional complication of abnormal postnatal physical sexual development (Money and Ehrhardt, 1972). Presently, evidence is available from a number of studies on cognitive development and gender-related behavior of CAH children compared to various control groups.

447

INTELLIGENCE AND COGNITIVE DEVELOPMENT

Full IQ: Review

It has been documented and is generally accepted that men and women do not differ in overall intelligence. One can expect that any group of males and females in the normal population, chosen on a random basis without socioeconomic or any other bias, will have a normal distribution of IQ scores and a mean IQ of 100 on the basis of standard intelligence tests.

Therefore, it was somewhat surprising when Money and Lewis (1966) found an elevated mean IQ of 109.9 and a significant increase in high IQs of above 110 (namely, 60% instead of 25%) in a clinical sample of 70 patients with CAH. This finding cannot be explained by a theory that all patients with endocrinopathies coming to a place like The Johns Hopkins Hospital tend to have higher IQs because of a socioeconomic bias. By testing representative clinical samples of patients with various endocrine conditions, Money and his collaborators established the fact that the tendency toward higher IQ in a group of patients with the same hormonal abnormality is the exception rather than the rule. Most groups of patients with endocrinopathies show a normal distribution in IQ (Money et al., 1967). As documented by Money and Lewis (1966), the unusual result in their study of intelligence in patients with CAH also cannot be attributed to any specific descriptive variable of their sample; for instance, it cannot be related to the sex of the patient (both subgroups of males and females showed the same tendency toward higher IQ), to social background (patients living in Baltimore were not significantly different from patients who came from a great distance), to age at initiation of therapy (no difference could be shown between late versus early treated groups), or to any other characteristic of the various subsamples. Thus, the question was raised as to whether the elevation of IQ was related to some aspect of the syndrome itself, either to the increased adrenal androgen production before or after birth, or both, or to the genetic transmission of the syndrome.

The hypothesis that exposure to abnormal levels of fetal androgens may be related to elevation in IQ was strengthened by a study on 10 girls with progestin-induced hermaphroditism (Ehrhardt and Money, 1967). In this instance, the fetus was exposed to high levels of androgenic substances due to maternal intake of steroids to prevent miscarriage. The drugs sometimes had an unexpected virilizing effect on a genetically female fetus. The hormonal abnormality was limited to the prenatal phase. No hormonal abnormality was observed in the affected children after birth.

Test results of the sample of females with the progestin-induced condition included a mean full IQ of 125, no one in the sample having an IQ below 100 and 6 girls having IQs above 130. The authors noted a relationship between IQ and educational level of the parents and a social bias toward the upper end. However, the degree of elevation of IQ was still somewhat unusual.

A completely independent study was carried out in England at about the same time and should be mentioned in this context. Dalton (1968) reported an educational follow-up study of children (both male and female) who had been exposed to progesterone administered to their mothers for relief of toxemic symptoms. The dosages varied from 50–300 mg/day by intramuscular injections. In no case was evidence of genital masculinization observed. For the educational follow-up, the author selected two control groups to be matched with the progesterone children. One group consisted of next born children listed in the labor ward register whose mothers had a normal pregnancy and delivery. The second control group included children delivered to women who had toxemia during pregnancy without hormonal treatment. The children were 9–10 years of age at the time of the follow-up. Educational ratings were solicited from teachers of the children in the various groups on a blind basis. The results showed that progesterone children received significantly more "above average" grades than did those of either control group in all academic subjects. There was also a positive correlation between high dosage and early treatment and above average school achievement. Dalton concluded that prenatal treatment with progesterone was likely to be related to enhanced school performance.

Although the last study did not involve children with CAH, Dalton's results are important for this consideration of abnormal hormonal exposure and intelligence. They support the evidence that prenatal exposure to abnormal levels of sex hormones may be in some way related to enhanced intellectual development. If so, this relationship may not be limited to androgenic substances. Dalton's work is also noteworthy because her findings come from another center in a different country.

One other recent study which was reported by Perlman (1973) should be mentioned. Perlman confirmed the elevation of full IQ (mean 112.0; S.D. 14.91) in a sample of 17 females and males with CAH. Her patient sample was not significantly different in IQ from a matched control group. Both patient and control samples were not representative, however, for all social classes, but were biased toward the upper end.

Thus, in the early 1970's, considerable evidence was accumulated to suggest that abnormal levels of androgens (and possibly other hormones) in children with CAH may be related to a positive effect on the fetal brain mediating enhanced intellectual development after birth.

Full IQ: Buffalo Family Study

In 1971, a study at the Buffalo Children's Hospital was designed to serve several purposes. The first purpose was to assess the intelligence of a representative sample of patients with CAH in another hospital population and to determine whether the finding of an elevated mean full IQ could be confirmed. The second goal was to compare CAH patients with a relevant control group which would share as much as possible the same socioeconomic and parental background. A family study including patients, parents, and siblings seemed the best approach to reach this goal. If the prenatal exposure to excess androgens was a critical factor for the elevation in IQ of the CAH patients, the sibling group without CAH and the parent sample should have a normal distribution of full IQs with a mean not significantly different from 100. Furthermore, the distribution of IQ scores and the mean full IQs should differ for the siblings and parents compared to the patients. The third purpose of the family study was to assess differential abilities.

The sample for this family study consisted of 27 patients with CAH with a sex ratio of 17 females to 10 males. This is clearly a representative sample of the clinical population seen in the Pediatric Endocrine Clinic, considering that at the time of this study only 31 patients with CAH had been seen since the clinic's inception 10 years before. The age range was 4 yr 3 mo to 19 yr 9 mo for females and 4 yr 8 mo to 26 yr 3 mo for males, with most of the patients and siblings in middle childhood and early adolescence. Because several families had more than one child with CAH, these studies actually dealt with a total of 21 families. Although not all siblings and parents were available for the study, a representative sample of unaffected family members was evaluated. The total sibling sample consisted of 11 females and 16 males. Eighteen mothers and 16 fathers participated in the study. The families came from social classes II to V, according to the Hollingshead index (Hollingshead, 1957), with a greater number from lower than from middle and higher classes. The sample was clearly not biased toward the upper end.

All patients were under long-term treatment with replacement of cortisone. The females had also undergone surgical correction of the external genitalia, usually in infancy or early childhood.

To assess general intelligence level, a widely used standard intelligence measure—one of the three Wechsler Intelligence Scales, chosen according to the age of the subject—was administered to patients, siblings, and parents. On all three tests the subject obtained a full IQ (mean 100; S.D. 15), our measure of general intelligence.

The mean full IQ of the complete sample of patients ($n = 27$) was 112.74 (S.D. 16.52) and was significantly different from the norm (z test; $p \leqslant 0.01$; one-tailed). The elevation of IQ was mainly due to an unusually high number of IQs above 110 (59% instead of the expected 25%). There were also too few children with IQs below 100, according to the expected norm. One mentally retarded boy was included in the sample; his mother was also retarded.

The finding of IQ elevation in the patient sample is remarkably similar to previous findings (Figure 1). Money and Lewis (1966) and Perlman (1973) found similarly elevated mean IQs with very similar frequency distributions.

Next the findings on the patient sample were compared with the results on the siblings and parents. Both mean full IQs in the sibling sample (110.59; S.D. 17.46) and in the parent sample (107.06; S.D. 14.75) were significantly elevated

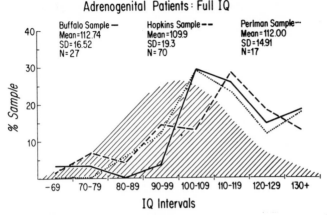

Adrenogenital Patients: Full IQ

Figure 1. Mean full IQs and frequency distributions of three independent samples of CAH patients tested at different hospitals compared with the normal distribution. Reprinted with permission from John Wiley and Sons, Inc., Sex Differences in Behavior, (1974).

from the norm (z test; $p \leqslant 0.01$; two-tailed), but not significantly different from each other (Figure 2). The three distributions were not as similar as the three different hospital distributions (Figure 1), but they were not significantly different from each other.

This finding of elevation in IQ in patients with CAH, with no significant difference between them and their siblings without CAH (Baker and Ehrhardt, 1974), has recently been confirmed by McGuire and Omenn (1975). The result also agrees with the observation by Money and Lewis (1966) on a small number of siblings.

Thus, at this point the fact seems fairly well established that patients with CAH have a tendency toward enhanced intelligence development as measured by full IQ scores on standard tests. They are not different, however, in this respect from their parents and siblings without the disease.

The finding is puzzling and difficult to explain. These data were analyzed from many different angles to assess any possible relationship with specific variables of any subsample (Baker and Ehrhardt, 1974). Obviously, the finding cannot be attributed specifically to the prenatal or postnatal hormonal abnormalities, or both, involved in congenital adrenal hyperplasia, because patients did not differ in IQ from unaffected siblings and parents. It also cannot be explained by a social class bias, because the socioeconomic background of the sample was clearly representative. If anything, the sample may have been a little biased toward the lower end. This finding cannot be supported by a theory that all patients who come to specialty clinics tend to have higher IQs, because studies on other endocrine samples did not confirm this assumption (Meyer-Bahlburg, 1975; Meyer-Bahlburg et al., 1974; Money et al., 1967). Following the same line

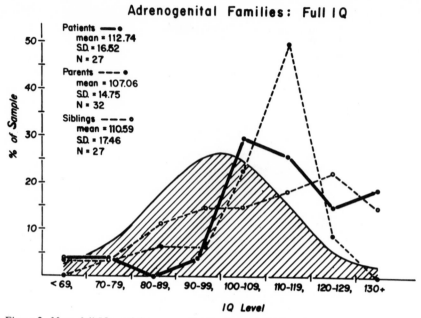

Figure 2. Mean full IQs and frequency distributions of CAH patients, parents, and siblings in the Buffalo sample. The *shaded area* represents the expected normal distribution. Reprinted with permission from John Wiley and Sons, Inc., Sex Differences in Behavior (1974).

of reasoning, it is also unlikely that IQ elevation in studies with CAH patients should be solely due to outdated norms of the Wechsler scales.

As an alternative hypothesis to explain the elevation of IQ in families who have children with CAH, it is necessary to consider the genetic aspect of the condition. Because the transmission is autosomal recessive, both parents have to be carriers to produce a child with CAH. The majority of the unaffected siblings should also be carriers. Statistically, it is expected that, of four children born to two heterozygote carriers, one will have CAH, two will be heterozygote carriers, and one will be unaffected genetically. It is conceivable that the recessive genetic trait may be linked somehow to another trait favoring postnatal intellectual development. This theory would be compatible with the finding of an elevated mean IQ in all three samples of patients, siblings, and parents. We are at the brink of being able to reliably determine heterozygote carriers. Once this is easily possible, the sibling sample can be divided into carriers and noncarriers. The critical test will be whether these two subsamples differ in intelligence.

As an alternative to genetic causation, there is the possibility of an as-yet-unknown selection process of families who bring their children with CAH to pediatric endocrine clinics. If this kind of process exists, it seems to be unrelated to social class, because our socioeconomic data did not suggest a bias toward the upper end.

Full IQ: Salt Losers Versus Non-salt-losers

In several studies, the analysis of data on full IQ has included the evaluation of a possible relationship to special features of congenital adrenal hyperplasia. No significant differences have been reported between patients with the different types of the disease.

Nevertheless, the results of full IQ in salt-losing patients versus non-salt-losing patients deserves some comment. Information on this matter has accumulated from three studies (Table 1). Money and Lewis (1966) had 15 patients (14 females and 1 male) with salt loss in their sample of 70. The mean IQ for the group of 15 was 105.1 (S.D. 12.6) versus a mean IQ of 110.6 (S.D. 18.4) for the group of 55 non-salt-losers. The difference was not statistically significant. McGuire and Omenn (1975) reported a mean full IQ of 100.44 for their subsample of 9 salt losers (5 females and 4 males) and a mean full IQ of 109.64 for the 22 non-salt-losers. This difference was also not statistically significant.

The Buffalo study consisted of 15 salt losers (9 females and 6 males) from 13 families and 12 non-salt-losers (8 females and 4 males) from 8 families. The mean full IQ for the salt losers was 110.20 (S.D. 14.39) and 115.92 (S.D. 19.02) for the non-salt-losers. If the retarded boy (with the retarded mother) is excluded from the sample of non-salt-losers, the mean full IQ was 120.55 (S.D. 10.72). The difference is not statistically significant.

The mean full IQ for the 20 siblings of the salt losers was 108.4 (S.D. 15.69), and, for the 7 siblings of the non-salt-losers, the mean full IQ was 116.86 (S.D. 21.91). Without the brother of the retarded boy, the mean full IQ was 115.00 (S.D. 23.39). Of the 13 families with salt-losing CAH children, IQ data were available on one or both parents in 11 of the families. The total number of parents was 20. If both parents' scores were available, the mean score of the mother's and father's IQ was used. For the sample of parents of salt losers, the mean full IQ was 108.05 (S.D. 12.52). Seven families were represented for the

Table 1. Mean full IQ in salt losers versus non-salt-losers in three studies on patients with CAH

Authors	Salt losers		Non-salt-losers	
	n	Full IQ	n	Full IQ
Money and Lewis (1966)	15	105.1	55	110.6
McGuire and Omenn (1975)	9	100.44	22	109.64
Ehrhardt and Baker (1974)	15	110.20	12	115.92
			(11)	(120.55)

non-salt-losers with a total of 12 parents. The mean full IQ was 103.07 (S.D. 15.89).

In all three independent studies, there appears to be a tendency for salt losers to perform somewhat below the non-salt-losers. In this family study, this was not related to social class or to parental IQ. The difference in the same direction between the two sibling subsamples cannot be explained.

Although not of statistical significance, the agreement among the three studies makes it less likely that this result is due to pure chance. Therefore, the difference in mean full IQs may be indicative of a slight disadvantage for the salt losers compared to the non-salt-losers. This could be related to the added complications of their disease, with phases of dehydration and weakness and frequent hospitalizations in some cases.

Because the results are merely tentative, one cannot draw any conclusions at this point. However, these observations may serve as a hypothesis to be tested in future research.

Differential Abilities: Buffalo Family Study

Another purpose of our family study was the assessment of differential abilities. Although there are many stereotypes about sex differences in intellectual and cognitive abilities in the normal population, upon careful review of the literature one finds very few consistent results (Maccoby and Jacklin, 1974). Until about age 10, differences in performance between the sexes are usually developmentally unstable. They vary with the age of the girls and boys involved in the particular study reported. Generally, it is believed—and it is shown in several but not all studies—that girls do better in a variety of verbal skills than boys. The reports on the superiority of boys in spatial tests are quite consistent after the age of 10–11 years, although the differences between the sexes are often small. Some studies have reported than men do better than women on tests of quantitative abilities but in this area the findings are also conflicting.

In spite of the inconclusive picture for normal samples of females and males, it seemed worthwhile to assess differential abilities in children with CAH and in their families. If fetal hormones are involved in normal sex differences for cognitive abilities, it can be postulated that CAH females who were exposed to abnormally high levels of fetal androgens might have a different pattern than their female siblings and might be more similar to their male siblings. It could also be speculated that males with CAH, possibly exposed to even higher prenatal androgen levels than normal males, might demonstrate a pronounced male pattern of differential cognitive abilities.

In this context, findings of this study on comparison of verbal and performance IQs and of the various subtest scores on the Wechsler scales are reported. In addition to the Wechsler scales, results have been obtained on the Primary Mental Abilities (PMA) tests (Thurstone, 1963), which measure specific abilities based on a factor analysis model.

The Wechsler Scales are divided into two sections of subtests referred to as the verbal part and the performance part. Six verbal subtests are pooled to give a verbal IQ (mean 100; S.D. 15), and five subtests, including various visual-motor tasks, are pooled to give a performance IQ (mean 100; S.D. 15).

Data for all six groups (male and female patients, brothers and sisters, mothers and fathers) were analyzed and no significant difference was found in verbal IQs between any of the groups. The analysis of performance IQs also did not result in any significant finding supporting our hypotheses (Baker and Ehrhardt, 1974).

The results on the various subtest scores were compared by use of the clusters of subtests found by Cohen (1957, 1959) on the basis of a factor analysis. Cohen differentiates between a verbal comprehension factor and a perceptual factor. A third factor (freedom from distractibility) is not consistent over all ages and, therefore, was not included in our data analysis. Our data for differences between and within groups on verbal comprehension and perceptual factors were analyzed, and no significant differences were found between patients with CAH and other groups. Several trends were in the expected direction, but did not reach statistical significance (Baker and Ehrhardt, 1974).

Our findings of no significant differences between verbal and performance IQs for the patient samples agree with previous findings by Lewis, Money, and Epstein (1968). In addition, these studies established that the patients were not significantly different from their siblings and parents in performance on the Wechsler subtests, as shown by the comparison of verbal and performance IQs and the Cohen factors.

For the Primary Mental Abilities tests, norms are given in deviation quotients with a population mean of 100 and a standard deviation of 16. Three of the tests (verbal, number, and spatial) are administered consistently from kindergarten throughout high school. Data analysis in this study was based on these three tests for the patients and siblings only, because the validity of the norms is more questionable for the age groups of the parents.

As seen in Figure 3, the most striking finding is the decline on the number deviation quotient for both males and females with CAH. Within-group comparisons resulted in a significant difference for both groups between their scores on the verbal and spatial tests and their scores on the number test. Neither sibling group showed a similar decline. Between-group comparisons on the number tests showed that all patients scored significantly lower than all siblings ($p \leqslant 0.05$; two-tailed). By contrast, the results on the verbal and spatial tests were unremarkable and not significantly different between the various groups.

Thus, the only significant finding on differential abilities on the Primary Mental Abilities tests was a relative inferiority on the number test for patients with CAH versus their own performance on verbal and spatial tests and versus the scores on the number test of their siblings. This was true for both males and females with CAH. This finding was unexpected and inconsistent with any

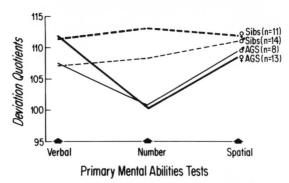

Figure 3. Mean Primary Mental Abilities (PMA) deviation quotients on three tests for four groups of the Buffalo adrenogenital (AGS) sample (20 families). The retarded family was excluded. Reprinted with permission from John Wiley and Sons, Inc., Sex Differences in Behavior (1974).

hypothesis on sex differences. It remains puzzling, especially since Perlman (1971) also found that her sample of patients with CAH scored significantly lower on an arithmetic computation test than did her control group.

It is difficult to venture a guess as to why patients with CAH may be less elevated in number abilities than in other areas and why they may be different in this respect from their siblings without CAH. Future research has to clarify whether the finding is reliable and syndrome-specific or perhaps prevalent in various pediatric clinical samples.

In general, these studies did not clarify the confusing picture of sex differences in cognitive abilities in the normal population. For the clinician, the most important finding is that patients with CAH generally do not show a specific pattern of strengths and weaknesses in cognitive abilities, with the possible exception of a relative inferiority in number abilities.

GENDER-RELATED BEHAVIOR

Female Behavior: Buffalo Family Study

Animal investigators have suggested that prenatal androgens may influence parts of the central nervous system and, thus, certain aspects of sexually dimorphic behavior. Females with CAH are known to have a history of abnormally high levels of androgens before birth and, if not treated optimally with cortisone, after birth as well. The study of their behavior is, therefore, of special interest to determine whether any behavior modifications are related to the exposure to androgen.

In Buffalo, the long-term childhood behavior of the sample of female patients with CAH ($n = 17$) was compared with that of the sample of female siblings without CAH ($n = 11$). Our methods included detailed interviews with the mothers and the children. The collected data were analyzed on rating scales, and differences between patients and siblings were statistically tested with the appropriate tests (Ehrhardt and Baker, 1974).

The most pertinent results from this investigation into the possible effects of prenatal androgens on behavior in genetic females with CAH cluster around two characteristics. First, girls with CAH expended a high level of physical energy. The behavior was long-term and specific, in the sense that the girls engaged in a high degree of rough outdoor play rather than in an elevation of general activity. The patients were significantly different in this respect from their female siblings.

Second, girls with CAH showed a conspicuously low interest in dolls, in taking care of infants, and in rehearsing other aspects of the maternal role. Their play rehearsal was more concerned with job and career roles.

The behavior pattern exhibited by females with CAH is typically called tomboyism and, therefore, it is not surprising that they were more frequently identified by themselves and others as long-term tomboys than were their female siblings.

The findings of the Buffalo family study on sibling comparisons (Ehrhardt and Baker, 1974) are in agreement with earlier studies on gender-related behavior of females with CAH and matched control groups (Ehrhardt, Epstein, and Money, 1968; Money and Ehrhardt, 1972). In all studies, females with CAH tended to have a characteristic pattern of gender-related behavior in childhood, with a high level of physical energy expenditure and preference for outdoor sport activities on the one hand and a low interest in caregiving behavior, as exhibited in doll play, attending to small infants, and role rehearsal for becoming a mother on the other hand.

To see the differences between females with CAH and females with a presumably normal prenatal hormonal history in proper perspective, it must be stressed that the typical behavior pattern exhibited by the patients did not indicate psychopathology or abnormality in any respect. Rather, it must be seen as a specific type of behavior within the normal spectrum of acceptable female behavior. Furthermore, patients with CAH did not have any gender identity conflict. They were identified as girls and liked to be girls, although they often preferred tomboyish activities to the more stereotypically feminine activities.

Of theoretical importance is the question of whether typical behavior characteristics of females with CAH can be attributed to their prenatal hormonal exposure to high levels of androgens or to any other feature of their medical syndrome. One factor may be their postnatal levels of androgens. Control with cortisone is sometimes difficult, and levels of androgens are still elevated in some patients even when treatment was initiated early, as in our clinical groups.

However, a very similar behavior pattern of high energy expenditure and low interest in parental caregiving was found in a group of girls with progestin-induced hermaphroditism (Ehrhardt and Money, 1967). In their cases, the exposure to prenatal androgenic substances was clearly limited to the time before birth, because the patients were found to be hormonally normal in their postnatal development. The agreement of findings in both patient groups makes it less likely that the postnatal hormonal abnormalities in patients with CAH are solely responsible for their behavior.

Another question which must be raised is whether the genital abnormality at birth contributes to the behavior modification in any way. Most of the females in both studies at The Johns Hopkins Hospital and at the Buffalo Children's Hospital were corrected surgically early in life and usually did not remember the operation. Nevertheless, the possibility that the knowledge of bearing a daughter with masculinized sex organs at birth might have changed the parents' attitude toward the child and contributed to the behavioral development in some respect was investigated. Parental worries and attitudes were assessed in great detail, but it was not possible to determine any common factor in the parents' behavior toward the child which might explain the typical behavior pattern found in girls with CAH.

It is impossible to completely exclude the possibility that environmental influences have contributed to the typical behavior pattern of girls with CAH. However, it seems unlikely that any of these factors is the sole explanation. Rather, the possibility that prenatal androgens may play a crucial role in the development of behavior typically consisting of a high level expenditure of physical energy and a lowered interest in parental caregiving behavior must be considered.

If prenatal hormones do have an influence on female and male behavior, their effects seem to be rather mild. The behavior changes are subtle rather than dramatic and do not include a reversal of gender identity or gender role.

Male Behavior: Buffalo Family Study

Males with CAH are usually not visibly affected by their prenatal androgen excess. If treated early and optimally with cortisone, they also do not have precocious puberty in childhood. The most interesting question in this context is whether the androgen excess before birth has any effect on the central nervous system and, thus, on postnatal behavior.

In the Buffalo family study, 9 boys with 11 "unaffected" brothers, ages 4–26 years, were compared. The patients were not significantly different in most behavior aspects assessed. They, for instance, were not more aggressive in terms of initiating fights with their peers or within the family. They were as stereotypically masculine as the sibling group in choice of playmates (boys preferred over girls), toys (cars and trucks and no dolls), and their fantasies of taking the father role in adulthood. Both patient and sibling groups showed total absence of effeminacy and a clear preference for the male gender role.

The only behavior area in which the sample of boys with CAH differed was in the area of sports and rough outdoor activities. They were more often described as having a higher energy expenditure level and were more often good athletes.

The prenatal excess of androgens may have contributed to the higher level of strength and energy in boys with CAH. Six of the nine patients had been started on cortisone treatment within the 1st month of life; three were discovered and treated later, when they showed early signs of precocious puberty. With these three boys, the high energy level may also have been due to high postnatal levels of androgens before treatment. If so, it persisted even after cortisone treatment had begun to suppress their high androgen levels.

The findings in the male sample suggest that boys with CAH are generally not different from boys without CAH in their pattern of masculine gender-related behavior (Ehrhardt and Baker, 1974). The results agree with an earlier study on late treated males with CAH (Money and Alexander, 1969).

Prenatal and postnatal androgen excess does not appear to significantly alter behavior in males, except possibly to increase energy expenditure.

CONCLUSION

General intelligence (full IQ) tends to be elevated in male and female patients with CAH. They are not different in this respect, however, from their siblings without CAH and their parents.

Patients with CAH do not have a particular pattern of cognitive strengths and weaknesses, except possibly for number abilities which are relatively inferior when compared to overall level of mental functioning.

Gender-related behavior in females with CAH tends to include an increased physical energy level and a low interest in parental caregiving. These behavior modifications are compatible with a normal female gender identity and must be viewed as variations of an acceptable pattern of feminine behavior in our culture.

Genetic males with CAH typically are not different in their gender-related behavior pattern from males without CAH, except for an increased energy expenditure level in some cases.

REFERENCES

Baker, S. W., and A. A. Ehrhardt. 1974. Prenatal androgen, intelligence and cognitive sex differences. *In* R. C. Friedman, R. M. Richart, and R. L. Vande Wiele (eds.), Sex Differences in Behavior, pp. 53–76. John Wiley and Sons, Inc., New York.

Cohen, J. 1957. A factor-analytically based rationale for the Wechsler Adult Intelligence Scale. J. Consult. Psychol. 21:451–457.

Cohen, J. 1959. The factorial structure of the WISC at ages 7–6, 10–6, 13–6. J. Consult. Psychol. 23:285–299.

Dalton, K. 1968. Ante-natal progesterone and intelligence. Br. J. Psychiatry 114:1377–1382.

Ehrhardt, A. A., and S. W. Baker. 1974. Fetal androgens, human central nervous system differentiation, and behavior sex differences. In R. C. Friedman, R. M. Richart, and R. L. Vande Wiele (eds.), Sex Differences in Behavior, pp. 33–51. John Wiley and Sons., Inc., New York.

Ehrhardt, A. A., R. Epstein, and J. Money. 1968. Fetal androgens and female gender identity in the early-treated adrenogenital syndrome. Johns Hopkins Med. J. 122:160–167.

Ehrhardt, A. A., and J. Money. 1967. Progestin-induced hermaphroditism: IQ and psychosexual identity in a study of ten girls. J. Sex Res. 3:83–100.

Hollingshead, A. B. 1957. Two factor index of social position. Yale University, New Haven, privately printed.

Lewis, V. G., J. Money, and R. Epstein. 1968. Concordance of verbal and nonverbal ability in the adrenogenital syndrome. Johns Hopkins Med. J. 122:192–195.

Maccoby, E. E., and C. N. Jacklin. 1974. The Psychology of Sex Differences. Stanford University Press, Stanford, California.

McGuire, L. S., and G. S. Omenn. 1975. Congenital adrenal hyperplasia. I. Family Studies of IQ. Behav. Genet. 5:165–173.

Meyer-Bahlburg, H. F. L. 1975. Human growth hormone deficiency in childhood and adolescence: effects on intelligence, temperament, social relations and sexuality. Presented at the Sixth International Congress of the International Society of Psychoneuroendocrinology, August 22–26, Aspen, Colorado.

Meyer-Bahlburg, H. F. L., E. McCauley, C. Schenck, T. Aceto, Jr., and L. Pinch. 1974. Cryptorchidism, development of gender identity and sex behavior. In R. C. Friedman, R. M. Richart, and R. L. Vande Wiele (eds.), Sex Differences in Behavior, pp. 281–299. John Wiley and Sons, Inc., New York.

Money, J. 1955. Hermaphroditism, gender and precocity in hyperadrenocorticism: psychologic findings. Bull. Johns Hopkins Hosp. 96:253–264.

Money, J., and D. Alexander. 1969. Psychosexual development and absence of homosexuality in males with precocious puberty. J. Nerv. Ment. Dis. 148: 111–123.

Money, J., and A. A. Ehrhardt. 1972. Man and Woman, Boy and Girl: The Differentiation and Dimorphism of Gender Identity from Conception to Maturity. The Johns Hopkins University Press, Baltimore.

Money, J., J. G. Hampson, and J. L. Hampson. 1955. Hermaphroditism: recommendations concerning assignment of sex, change of sex, and psychologic management. Bull. Johns Hopkins Hosp. 97:284–300.

Money, J., J. G. Hampson, and J. L. Hampson. 1957. Imprinting and the establishment of gender role. A.M.A. Arch. Neurol. Psychiatry 77:333–336.

Money, J., and V. Lewis. 1966. IQ, genetics and accelerated growth: adrenogenital syndrome. Bull. Johns Hopkins Hosp. 118:365–373.

Money, J., V. Lewis, A. A. Ehrhardt, and P. W. Drash. 1967. IQ impairment and elevation in endocrine and related cytogenetic disorders. In J. Zubin (ed.), Psychopathology of Mental Development, pp. 22–27. Grune and Stratton, New York.

Perlman, S. M. 1971. Cognitive function in children with hormone abnormalities. Unpublished Ph.D. thesis, Northwestern University, Chicago.
Perlman, S. M. 1973. Cognitive abilities of children with hormone abnormalities: screening by psychoeducational tests. J. Learning Disabil. 6:26–34.
Thurstone, T. G. 1963. Primary Mental Abilities. Science Research Associates, Chicago.

Adrenogenital Syndrome
The Need for Early Surgical Feminization in Girls

Viola G. Lewis and John Money

Early surgical feminization within the bounds of surgical safety is an essential part of the successful case management of an ambiguously sexed baby born with the adrenogenital syndrome. It is the best course to follow, because it is in the best interest of the patient and parents. It is also in the best interest of the professionals involved, in terms of the effort and time which ultimately have to be expended. Although pediatric endocrinologists are aware of the need for early surgical feminization in cases of adrenogenital females with ambiguous genitalia, it is necessary for the word to be spread to others who may be responsible for the patients from the moment of delivery onward. This includes obstetricians, midwives, nurses, and specialist consultants who may be called in later. What they say in making the first announcement of the baby's sex follows—one may even say haunts—the parents and baby throughout life. What should be the perfect first step in case management all too often turns into a delivery room fiasco. This is important in these days of increasing numbers of natural and Lamaze births, during which the mother is awake and the father may be present.

The first announcement of sex, along with any other information and advice given to the parents, makes a profound difference in their feelings about the child, how they will raise the child, and the information which they will in turn impart to the child, overtly or covertly. It is this initial information which sometimes sticks, regardless of anything else the parents are told over the years. Later information is assimilated in the context of the first information received.

The ideal approach is to educate every person concerned in obstetrical delivery in the techniques of dealing with parents when the baby is born with a birth defect, including birth defects of the sex organs. In the latter case, it is best to tell the parents that the baby was born with its sex organs unfinished. They have waited 9 months to learn the sex of the baby, and in this case they will unfortunately have to wait 2–3 more days.

When the size of the phallus makes it manifestly impossible to correct as a

This work was supported by Grant HD-00325 from the United States Public Health Service and by funds from The Grant Foundation, Inc., New York, New York.

penis, it is not necessary to wait for the chromatin and chromosome studies to declare the child as female. The explanation can be given that the baby was born with the genitalia unfinished and the opening covered over. In the adrenogenital syndrome, the problem arises when the phallus is large enough to be a penis and the sex assignment could be male. The well-trained obstetrician may be able to anticipate the problem if he knows that another baby in the family died under circumstances suggesting salt loss—with or without genital malformation. This information must have been obtained while the obstetrician was taking the prenatal history.

When information must be retracted or modified, parents may nod their heads and make the appropriate sounds of understanding, but one must always be sure that what they hear at this stage is what actually was said. It is best to have the parents summarize and tape record the information you hope they have absorbed in order to be sure that they have understood and have the information correctly coded in their memories. By and large, professionals today do not do a good job at explanations.

Last year, we saw for the first time a 16-year-old girl whose case demonstrated the pervasive influence of inadequate information. At another hospital, the patient was assigned male at birth. According to the mother, the assignment was made against the advice of another physician who knew that the buccal smear was chromatin positive. The diagnosis of the adrenogenital syndrome was made during the 2nd week of life, when the infant was admitted for a salt-losing crisis. A laparotomy at age 6 months revealed normal female internal reproductive organs, and the child was reassigned at that time. A clitorectomy was performed between 22 and 29 months of age. The child was referred to The Johns Hopkins Hospital at the age of 6 years for evaluation and urogenital tract repair, and again at the age of 14 years 9 months because of excessive virilization. In the absence of adequate psychological guidance, the mother, according to her own statement, always questioned the girl's gender. She could scarcely believe the information, new to her, that her 16-year-old daughter could become pregnant. She had always attempted to reinforce her daughter's femininity by constant instructions to be more lady-like. She bought her dresses and discouraged her tomboyish interest in sports. The girl disclosed that, on a recent visit with her divorced father, he had informed her that she had been born with a penis.

In her interviews, the girl herself made it apparent that she had a highly negative self-image, thinking of herself as dumb, stupid, and unattractive. Her situation was not improved by her hirsute appearance, a product of several years of irregular compliance with the recommended dosage schedule of cortisone. She was teased at school about being half man and half woman. She questioned whether she should have been a boy. At the same time, she expressed positive anticipation of marriage and motherhood.

Many of this patient's problems could have been prevented, had all of the delivery personnel known how to talk to parents in the delivery room. Students in medical school should be trained to deal with these emergencies. Unfortunately, this type of training is not yet available in most places. Nothing is more supportive to parents with a defective child than proper information right from the start.

Parents need to be reassured that their child will be able to live normally, including sexually. Explanations accompanied by pictures and diagrams are best understood because most people are visile rather than audile types. Explanations need to be at a level of conceptual understanding with which parents can cope; glands and hormones should be explained. Hormone replacement can be explained in terms of pure food like a vitamin, rather than as a drug or medication. For children, the hormone causing virilization can be characterized as "funky." For the parents to be able to teach others and, in the process, to quell any rumors about the baby's sex, it is important for them to have simple concepts— such as, the baby has "unfinished sex organs" and a vaginal opening that is "covered over." Candidness, with appropriate terms and conceptual explanations, is the best way to stop rumor mongers. Valid explanations are not only reassuring to parents, but also can be used for children at home, relatives, and close friends who will need to know (Money, 1969). They also provide the terminology with which parents can explain the condition to the child herself, at the appropriate time. A girl needs to know why she is subjected to repeated genital examinations. In some cases, she will also need an untraumatic explanation concerning the circumstances of neonatal sex reannouncement. The facts given at an early age, in simple language, prevent traumatic disclosure later by a well meaning or perhaps not so well meaning person.

The psychology of family interaction is of utmost importance to the child's psychological development. Parents who have given birth to an abnormal child may have problems in their marital and sex life. The anxieties and conflicts regarding their child add fuel to the fire, so that problems worsen. The more unstable the parents are in their relationship, the more difficult it is for professionals to deal with their misunderstandings and anxieties concerning their child's sex. Thus, being born with an abnormality into a family already beset with problems greatly increases the difficulties for the growing child.

After correct explanations, institution of early treatment, including surgical feminization, is primary in correcting the child's appearance. This is reassuring to the parents, who can then allow relatives and baby sitters to change diapers without worry. Timing of the first surgical procedure is important, especially to unstable families with a generally diminished ability to cope. In a greatly disturbed relationship, however, the benefits of early surgery may be negated. Without early surgical repair of the child, the most stable families need much advice and counseling. Even so, the evidence of their senses can override any counseling one might provide. Late surgery can prove disastrous for both parents and child.

For the girl herself, as she gets older, there is a need for long-term advice and counseling. Information about the adrenogenital syndrome, given together with sex education, aids the patient in developing a positive self-image. Although the cosmetic appearance of the genitalia is most important in childhood, during adolescence the functional utility of the vagina is of greater importance, even before the girl has decided to start her sex life.

A survey, first completed in 1970 (Jones et al., 1970; Lewis, Ehrhardt, and Money, 1970) and reinforced by the findings of Money and Schwartz (in this volume), confirms that early, correct handling helps to solve problems of parents and child. In the process of easing the burden for the patient and her parents, the professionals also benefit, because less of their time and effort is expended. The 1970 survey also demonstrated that girls from unstable families were more likely to be disturbed. Of the 29 patients reported in the 1970 study, 8 were considered disturbed and, of these, 7 were from unstable homes.

In overall case management, ideal results are obtained from a combination of 1) early, good, basic information, 2) early surgery, 3) a stable family unit, and 4) psychological support and counseling throughout therapy.

SUMMARY

Early surgical feminization is strongly advisable. It resolves parental ambiguity concerning daily routine in sex of rearing and removes restrictions on their social life associated, for example, with the baby's nudity during diapering by relatives and strangers. For the patient as she gets older, the feminine appearance of the genitalia reinforces a positive feminine self-image. For the professionals involved with the family, early surgical feminization greatly reduces follow-up time and effort. There is no point-for-point correlation between age at surgery and subsequent psychological health (Jones et al., 1970; Lewis, Ehrhardt, and Money, 1970; Money and Schwartz, in this volume), because the latter is multivariately determined. Family psychological health is one important variable. Delayed surgery is practically guaranteed to produce havoc in unstable families and to increase stress in stable families.

REFERENCES

Jones, H. W., Jr., B. S. Verkauf, V. G. Lewis, and J. Money. 1970. The relevance of surgical, psychologic, and endocrinologic factors to the long-term end result of patients with congenital adrenal hyperplasia: a study of eighty-nine patients. Int. J. Gynaecol. Obstet. 8:398–401.
Lewis, V. G., A. A. Ehrhardt, and J. Money. 1970. Genital operations in girls with the adrenogenital syndrome: subsequent psychologic development. Obstet. Gynecol. 36:11–15.
Money, J. 1969. Sex Errors of the Body: Dilemmas, Education and Counseling. The Johns Hopkins Press, Baltimore.

Education of the Patient and Parent in Congenital Adrenal Hyperplasia

Arlan L. Rosenbloom

Although there are no new or startling observations to report, it appears worthwhile to reflect on the goals and strategy for education of patients and their families. It is hoped that these reflections will serve to emphasize the need for clear cut objectives and to stimulate improved educational techniques.

Those who work with patients having diabetes and patients having adrenal hyperplasia are impressed by the similarities between the issues posed by these two conditions. Both require an understanding of the physiology of the condition and a great deal of patient and parent responsibility for management; they offer considerable opportunity for manipulation, a tendency to relax when things are going well, and a disturbing array of potentially destructive concepts. In both conditions, education has a central role and the need to co-opt the parents and the older patient as members of the treatment team is essential (Etzwiler, 1972). Although such a statement is readily greeted with much nodding approbation, the fact is that few doctors devote as much care to individualized planning and evaluation of the education program as is dedicated to metabolic diagnosis and therapy.

An educational prescription requires the establishment of reasonable and attainable goals and the planning of an approach based upon a number of individual variables, which are as follows:

1. Patient's age. Obviously the infant is not going to be the subject of an educational effort, but it is frequently forgotten that the adolescent who has been treated from infancy has changing educational requirements which might best be considered his or her business only. It is not uncommon in working with patients with diabetes to change noncompliance to a stable collaboration between patient and doctor by bypassing the parents and working directly with the child. For some youngsters, this may begin as young as 10 or 11 years, depending on many other family factors.

2. Sex of patient.

3. Age at diagnosis.

4. Intellectual level of the family. There are many patients for whom the basic

rudiments of physiology are incomprehensible and for whom concrete cause and effect must be authoritatively presented.

5. Preformed attitudes and community mythology. Factors in this area range from beliefs in causation by "bad" sexual thoughts to relatively sophisticated misconceptions of the genetics of the condition. Experience directs us to early and anticipatory dealing with these misconceptions. On several occasions, this author has been told by a mother that her daughter does not know that she had genital surgery as an infant. Many doctors have been suspicious of the male patient who is apparently adequately treated and yet continues to virilize; the most blatant example seen by this author was a physician father too proud of his herculean offspring to interrupt the process.

The time to begin an education program is from the moment of reasonable assurance that congenital adrenal hyperplasia is the problem. If the patient or parent or both are to belong to the treatment team, involvement with the diagnostic and initial therapeutic process must be immediate, with an opportunity for teaching physiology and expressing reassurance at each step. Subsequently, as has been learned with diabetes, no contact should be without an educational review. This may range from a complete review to specific aspects that need reinforcing or that have been brought up by parent questions.

The goals of the education program need to be clearly understood by those guiding it, as well as by the recipients. A method needs to be built into the management program to continuously evaluate the attainment of these goals. The goals might be stated as follows:

1. Understanding how the diagnosis was made so that there will never be a doubt that the child has the condition.
2. Understanding the effects on sexual development.
3. Understanding the necessity of treatment.
4. Understanding the specific treatment goals.
5. Knowing the effects of and signs of overtreatment.
6. Knowing the effects of and signs of undertreatment.
7. Knowing the situations which require increasing the maintenance dose and how much to increase it.
8. Skill in injection technique and knowledge of when injection of hydrocortisone is needed.
9. Understanding the meaning of tests that are performed during follow-up (e.g., sodium, potassium, roentgenogram for osseous maturation, urinary steroids).
10. Recognizing the medication and the reasons why it cannot be substituted or altered in dosage without consultation.
11. Knowing whom to call and when with problems or questions.
12. Understanding the genetic implications as they affect siblings, offspring of the patients, and other relatives.

Any educational task is made easier if its component objectives are dealt with one by one and the number and kinds of skills and knowledge to be acquired are known to all participants. The best way to accomplish this is by the production of an individualized contract which is developed between the principal teacher and the student(s). The contract may require additions or deletions as the program progresses, but it is a useful opening device at each contact. In effect, it is nothing more than a check list of goals just outlined, but it can be considerably more detailed. Such a reference point is reassuring to both patient and medical participants in the teaching exercise. Most important, it signifies a mutual commitment to the task.

An instruction manual can be a useful reinforcement of teaching, with simple illustrations and information for self-review. A manual developed for this purpose has been included at the end of this chapter. (See "Note" on page 475.)

There is no substitute for frequent contact and review, especially when application of learned behavior is expected. Thus, both the frequency of clinic visits and the continuous availability of medical personnel by telephone are important.

The lesson that emerges from experience with diabetes mellitus (Miller and Goldstein, 1972) and the work of the Quebec Network of Genetic Medicine (Clow, Reade, and Scriver, 1971) is that these complicated diagnostic, educational, and treatment problems require the expertise of a systems specialist and the skills of allied personnel who are capable of investing the large amounts of time needed in education and follow-up (Jamplis, 1975). The sensitivity to potential and manifest psychological problems, to subtle signs of overtreatment, and to informational needs is difficult to accomplish outside an adequately staffed program dealing with large numbers of youngsters with congenital adrenal hyperplasia.

A few anecdotes will emphasize the need for meeting the various educational goals in a specialized setting:

Jan was hospitalized monthly for acute episodes of adrenal insufficiency from the time of diagnosis in infancy until seen at 4 years of age. Her parents had never been taught by the medical personnel treating her to increase the oral dosage with illness or to administer hydrocortisone solution in emergencies. During the 4 years since this training was given she has had no hospitalization.

Kelly was also found to have salt-losing congenital adrenal hyperplasia in infancy. By 9 months of age she was quite Cushingoid, receiving 30 mg of hydrocortisone/day while under the care of an excellent pediatrician. Reduction in dose to a physiological replacement level caused intracranial hypertension which necessitated return to a pharmacological dose and slow reduction over several months. Normal growth and clearing of the Cushingoid appearance were achieved on a dose of 2.5 mg three times a day.

Elizabeth was first seen at 2 $\frac{1}{2}$ years of age for genital virilization. Hydrocortisone (10 mg/day) resulted in a fall of the urinary 17-ketosteroids to less than 1 mg/24 hr, but soon after beginning treatment she appeared in the clinic with obvious signs of overtreatment. Suspicion of error by the pharmacy was confirmed to be substitution of prednisone for hydrocortisone. Return to hydrocortisone, 10 mg/day in three divided doses, resulted in clearing of her Cushing's syndrome. A brief period of catch-up growth was followed by gain in height age consistent with chronological age.

John was diagnosed with salt-losing congenital adrenal hyperplasia in the intensive care nursery of a university medical center where he was kept until 3 months of age. He was discharged on 12 mg of hydrocortisone/day, which was reduced to 10 mg/day at 4 months of age because of Cushingoid facies. He was seen by a visiting specialist at 13 months of age because of progressive deviation from the third percentile and a bone age of 3 months. He was thought to have facial features of Cushing's syndrome; the roentgenograms demonstrated multiple growth lines and osteoporosis. On questioning the pharmacist, it was found that the hydrocortisone suspension had been mislabeled, and the mother noted that the apparent density of the suspension varied from time to time and with standing. The mother had never been instructed in how to dispense the medication and was having difficulty, because she did not have a calibrated syringe to do so. It was estimated that the child was getting 12.5 mg of hydrocortisone/day, which was reduced to 7.5 mg and resulted in clearing of the Cushing's syndrome and resumption of normal growth.

Tony was noted to have a large phallus when seen for bowlegs in the orthopedic clinic at 3 years of age; subsequently, the diagnosis of congenital adrenal hyperplasia was confirmed by appropriate studies in a university department of pediatrics. Although he had breast development from 6 years of age, it was not until age 10 that a buccal smear was performed and a more profound understanding of his condition developed by a newly established genetic endocrine group. With removal of his normal internal genitalia, placement of plastic testicular prostheses, and testosterone therapy, he has done well.

Emphasized by these examples are the twin issues of appropriateness of the therapeutic program and the education of the parent or patient. Sound judgment from the principal treatment agent—either parent or patient—cannot be demanded when he or she is not appropriately trained, and medical personnel must wince when compliance is achieved with a treatment program that results in secondary morbidity. Standards for education and treatment programs are clearly imperative for this condition.

REFERENCES

Clow, C., T. Reade, and C. R. Scriver. 1971. Management of hereditary metabolic disease. The role of allied health personnel. N. Engl. J. Med. 284: 1292–1298.

Etzwiler, D. D. 1972. Current status of patient education. J.A.M.A. 220:583.

Jamplis, R. W. 1975. The practicing physician and patient education. Hosp. Practice 10:93–99.

Miller, L. V., and J. Goldstein. 1972. More efficient care of diabetic patients in a county hospital setting. N. Engl. J. Med. 286:1388–1391.

MANUAL ON CONGENITAL ADRENAL HYPERPLASIA

The *adrenal glands* (Figure 1) are small organs situated on top of the kidney in each flank. They manufacture hormones (chemical "directors") and discharge them into the blood. The *medulla* or inner core of the gland makes adrenalin. The *cortex* or outer portion makes cholesterol into hydrocortisone, male hormones (androgens), and salt-retaining hormone.

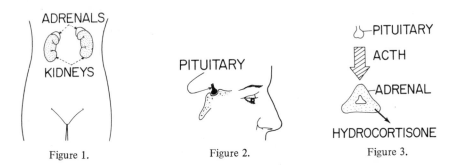

Figure 1.   Figure 2.   Figure 3.

Hydrocortisone is a hormone manufactured by the adrenal cortex. It is needed by the body to maintain an energy supply, to control the body's reaction to stress, and is necessary for life.

Androgens are male sex hormones manufactured in the testicles and in the adrenal cortex. During adolescence, they cause acne (pimples) and adult hair growth in girls. Boys make more powerful androgens in their testicles than those that come from the adrenal gland.

Salt-retaining hormone is also made in the adrenal cortex. This substance acts on the kidney to help it return salt (sodium) from the urine into the blood and to get rid of potassium. This function is essential to life.

The *pituitary gland* (Figure 2) is a pea-sized organ located on the underside of the brain about 2 inches behind the bridge of the nose. It is called the "master gland" because it makes hormones that control the thyroid, adrenal, sex, and mammary glands.

ACTH is the abbreviation of *a*drenocorticotropic *h*ormone, a protein substance made by the pituitary gland and carried by the blood to the adrenal gland, where it stimulates the making of hydrocortisone (Figure 3).

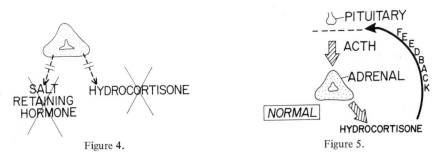

Figure 4.   Figure 5.

Congenital adrenal hyperplasia is an inherited malfunction in one of the steps required to make hydrocortisone and salt-retaining hormone (Figure 4).

Enzymes are protein substances that control the activity of chemical processes. Enzymes are the catalysts of reactions in living things. Several enzymes are involved in the making of hydrocortisone and salt-retaining hormone.

Hydrocortisone manufactured in the adrenal cortex is controlled by ACTH from the pituitary gland. When there is enough hydrocortisone in the blood to satisfy body needs, the pituitary gland decreases its production of ACTH (Figure 5).

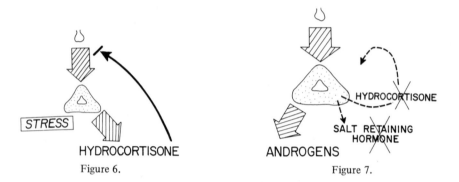

HYDROCORTISONE

Figure 6.

ANDROGENS

Figure 7.

Under stress conditions (accident, infection, surgery), the pituitary gland makes more ACTH and the adrenal gland responds by making much more hydrocortisone (Figure 6).

In *congenital adrenal hyperplasia,* the adrenal gland cannot make enough hydrocortisone. The pituitary is then not inhibited. It makes more ACTH to stimulate the adrenal gland to enlarge and work harder (hyperplasia) to make enough hydrocortisone for the body. Large quantities of the raw materials for hydrocortisone manufacture pile up. These substances are diverted into other products, mainly androgens (male hormones) (Figure 7). The most severely affected children with congenital adrenal hyperplasia are also unable to make salt-retaining hormone.

What Are the Effects of Congenital Adrenal Hyperplasia on Health?

When the block in ability to make hydrocortisone is severe, the body cannot respond adequately to stress. Children affected may die with a simple respiratory or intestinal infection or after surgery. Severely affected children who cannot make adequate amounts of salt-retaining hormone have a tendency to lose salt through their kidneys. These children fail to gain weight as infants and may lose so much salt that they develop shock and die.

Many children are able to make enough hydrocortisone to get along by enlarging their adrenal glands under the influence of large amounts of ACTH. Naturally, because of the block in the chemical assembly line, they pile up large amounts of chemicals that the gland makes into androgens. These androgens are potent stimulators of bone growth, so that children with this condition grow faster than normal. Because the bone ends close rapidly, as early as 8 years of age, untreated children end up shorter than average.

The large amount of ACTH produced is accompanied by another pituitary substance that stimulates pigment cells in the skin. This causes a tan color often seen in affected children even in infancy.

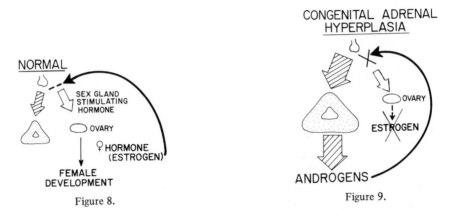

Figure 8.   Figure 9.

How Does Congenital Adrenal Hyperplasia Affect Sexual Development?

Until the 3rd month of development in the mother's womb, boys and girls have identical sex organs. Then, under the influence of male hormones made by the testicles, the boy forms a scrotum and penis. Girls who make male hormones in their adrenal glands because of congenital adrenal hyperplasia may develop similar to boys. However, their internal sex organs (uterus, tubes, and ovaries) will be completely normal. Boys born with this condition look normal as infants, but girls have a large clitoris and partial-to-complete closing of the labia (the lips at the opening of the vagina).

The boys' genitals may become adult in appearance in the first few years of life. The girls' clitoris will keep enlarging. Sexual hair will develop very early. If there is no treatment, girls will not develop fully at adolescence. This happens because the male sex hormones block the production in the pituitary gland of substances that ordinarily stimulate the ovaries to make female sex hormones (estrogen) (Figures 8 and 9).

Emergencies

Although these children are completely normal when under treatment, they are always in danger of serious collapse or death in times of stress when more hydrocortisone is needed. A few days of a dose of 3 times the regular dose is advisable whenever a person with this condition is sick enough to look and feel ill. If the child is pale and cool or if he has vomited, it is necessary to immediately give 0.5 cc of Solu-Cortef by injection. This form is rapid acting. This must also be done whenever the child is unconscious for any reason.

This Injection Must be Given Before You Call the Doctor or While Someone Else Calls Him. It Will Never Harm the Child if Given Unnecessarily.

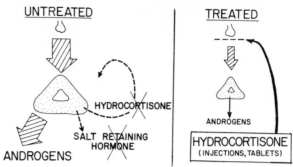

Figure 10.

Surgery

Girls with enlargement of the clitoris and closure of the labia may require plastic surgery for normal appearance, intercourse, and delivery of children. The extent of surgery and when it is done depend on the extent of the problem and the child's age when the decisions are made. Normal function can be expected because the internal female organs are not affected.

Treatment

The basic difficulty causing the problems in congenital adrenal hyperplasia is the inability to make enough hydrocortisone. Treatment involves supplying the body with this hormone in amounts that the adrenal gland would normally make. This stops the pituitary gland production of ACTH. The excessive accumulation of precursors of hydrocortisone in the adrenal gland and their conversion to androgens are then prevented (Figure 10).

Soon after treatment begins, the tan color of the skin fades, rapid growth stops, and the male sex characteristics decrease. In older girls, breast development occurs and menstruation begins, because stimulation of the ovaries is now possible.

During infancy and early childhood, the hydrocortisone may be given as a twice weekly injection. When the child is older, oral medication can be used. Some children who have an associated inability to conserve salt may need extra salt in the diet along with salt-retaining hormone treatment. Tablets of salt-retaining hormone can be placed under the skin near the shoulder blades and will last for as long as a year. The hormone can also be given as a monthly injection or as a daily tablet.

Heredity

The chemical step that is defective in congenital adrenal hyperplasia is controlled by an enzyme. Lack of this enzyme causes the inability to make hydrocortisone. The production of the enzyme is controlled by a pair of genes. Genes are areas with specific functions on chromosomes. Chromosomes are paired strands of chemicals within cells that control the inheritance of an individual. One set of chromosomes (half of the pair) comes from the mother and the other set from the father.

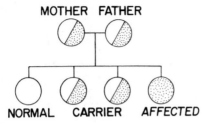

Figure 11.

Congenital adrenal hyperplasia results when two defective genes for the enzyme—one from each parent—are inherited by a child. The parents who carry the defective gene are normal, because the normal gene of the pair is dominant and the defective gene recessive. About 1 person in 50 carries this recessive gene. When that person marries another carrier, they have a 25% chance of having a child who inherits both of the abnormal genes and, therefore, has the condition. There is a 50% chance of each child being a carrier and a 25% chance of the child neither having the condition nor being a carrier (Figure 11).

Because this is a recessive trait, a person with it can have affected children only if he or she marries a carrier, a 1 in 50 chance, and then each of their children would have a 1 in 2 chance of inheriting the carrier parent's defective gene and having the condition. Brothers and sisters of children with the condition have a 2 out of 3 chance of being carriers; thus, their risk is $2/3 \times 1/50 \times 1/4$ or 1 in 300 of having an affected child. The brothers and sisters of carriers, that is, the aunts and uncles of patients, have a 1 in 2 chance of themselves being carriers. They too have a 1 in 50 chance of marrying carriers and then a 1 in 4 chance of having an affected child. Thus, the risk in first cousins of affected children is $1/2 \times 1/50 \times 1/4$ or 1 in 400. These risks go up markedly when cousins marry.

Note added in proof: The physician using this teaching manual may wish to supplement it with a listing of the various forms of glucocorticoid and mineralocorticoid therapy, their brand names, the form in which the drug comes, the dosage range, the duration of action and the indications.

DETECTION OF
HETEROZYGOUS STATE
AND PRENATAL DIAGNOSIS

Urinary Excretion of Pregnanetriolone in Parents of Children with 21-Hydroxylase Deficiency Before and After Stimulation with Adrenocorticotropic Hormone

Janos Homoki, Atilla T. A. Fazekas, and Walter M. Teller

In normal, healthy children as well as adults, pregnanetriolone (5β-pregnane-$3\alpha,17\alpha,20\alpha$-triol-11-one) (PTL) is excreted in the urine only in microgram or even nanogram amounts. The quantities reported in the earlier literature vary from 0 to 2.5 μg/24 hr, depending on the method employed (Faglia et al., 1966; Finkelstein, 1962; Kinoshita et al., 1966; Lohmeyer, 1970; Raman et al., 1965; Shearman and Cox, 1965; Zamora, Plattner, and Curtius, 1969). By gas-liquid chromatography on packed columns, Knorr (unpublished observations) found PTL values in healthy adults between <20 and 118 μg/24 hr.

Large quantities of PTL are excreted in the urine by patients with congenital adrenal hyperplasia (CAH) due to 21-hydroxylase deficiency (Bongiovanni et al., 1959; Faglia et al., 1966; Finkelstein, von Euw, and Reichstein, 1953; Fukushima and Gallagher, 1957). In addition, increased amounts of PTL are excreted in the urine of some patients with Cushing's syndrome caused by bilateral adrenal hyperplasia (Faglia et al., 1966; Finkelstein, 1962) and in patients with the Stein-Leventhal syndrome (Cox and Shearman, 1961; Travaglini and Faglia, 1971). Following the injection of adrenocorticotropic hormone (ACTH) (2 mg of Cortrophin-S Depot, Organon), normal adults excreted PTL from 116–336 μg/24 hr (D. Knorr, personal communication).

The frequency of heterozygous carriers of CAH has been reported to vary from 1:125 (Childs, Grumbach, and Van Wyk, 1956) to 1:35 (Prader, 1958). It,

This research was supported by Grant SFB-87, Project C_3, from the Deutsche Forschungsgemeinschaft.

479

therefore, was of considerable interest to determine the heterozygous state of CAH. Qazi, Hill, and Thompson (1971) detected an increased excretion of 11-oxygenated 17-ketosteroids, especially of 11β-hydroxyandrosterone, in fathers but not in mothers of children with CAH. Knorr and Butenandt (1968) found plasma concentrations of 17-hydroxyprogesterone in obligatory hetero-zygotes (parents of children with CAH) to be in the upper range of normal. After stimulation with ACTH, heterozygous carriers showed a higher increase of 17-hydroxyprogesterone concentration in serum, compared to normal controls, yet the differences were not discerning enough to advocate this determination as a test of CAH heterozygosity (Lee and Gareis, 1975). In addition, the basal urinary excretion of PTL was not discriminative (D. Knorr, unpublished observa-tions).

Following the administration of ACTH, Childs, Grumbach, and Van Wyk (1956) reported no statistically significant difference in the urinary excretion of 17-ketosteroids, pregnanediol, and pregnanetriol in heterozygous carriers of CAH and normal subjects. Knorr (unpublished observations), however, found a significant increase ($p < 0.05$) in the urinary excretion of PTL upon ACTH stimulation in parents of children with CAH of the 21-hydroxylase type. Normal persons failed to show this increase. Similar results were reported by Gleispach et al. (1974), Gleispach (1975, unpublished observations). They investigated 15 sets of parents of patients with CAH. Two mothers and one father had a resting excretion of PTL in the range of several thousand μg/24 hr; they must be considered homozygous. The remaining twenty-seven parents excreted from $<$ 5–470 μg of PTL/24 hr following the injection of 30 I.U. of ACTH/m^2 of body surface.

The validity of determinations of urinary PTL in obligatory heterozygotes of CAH of the 21-hydroxylase type before and after ACTH was re-evaluated. A highly sensitive and specific gas-liquid chromatographic procedure on capillary columns was employed.

MATERIALS AND METHOD

Subjects

Four sets of parents of patients with CAH were studied. Three couples each had one child with the simple type of 21-hydroxylase deficiency, while one couple had two children with the salt-losing form of 21-hydroxylase deficiency. Four sets of parents, each having several normal, healthy children, served as controls. In each proband, the urinary excretion of PTL was determined in the 24-hr urine specimen before and on the day of the intramuscular injection of 40 I.U. of ACTH (Synacthen, Ciba).

Method

One-twentieth volume of the 24-hr urine specimen was adjusted to pH 5.2. Hydrolysis was carried out for 48 hr with 20 mg of Helicase at 37°C. Choles-

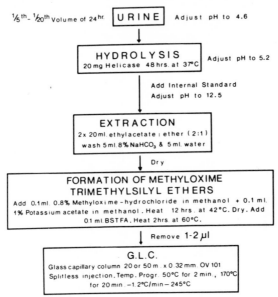

Figure 1. Flow sheet of the procedure for fractionation of urinary steroids.

terylbutyrate was used as internal standard (I.S.). Steroid extraction was carried out twice with ethylacetate-ether (2:1). The extract was then washed twice with sodium bicarbonate and distilled water. After evaporation to dryness, steroid derivatives were prepared by adding a mixture of methyloxime-HCl in pyridine and subsequently N-O-bis-trimethylsilyltrifluoroacetamide. The steroid derivatives ($1-2$ μl) were chromatographed on glass capillary columns together with n-alkans ($C_{24}-C_{34}$). The columns (50 cm $\times$ 0.32 mm internal diameter) were coated with methylsilicone. The injection was carried out without splitting (Grob and Grob, 1969). The temperature program was as follows: $50°C$ in 2 min, $170°$ isotherm for 20 min, and finally a $1.2°C$/min increase until $245°C$ was reached. The carrier gas was hydrogen. A flame ionization detector was employed. The areas under the peaks were calculated by an electronic digital integrator. The identification of a single steroid MO-TMS derivative was carried out by the methylene unit criterion (Novotny and Zlatkis, 1970). The final calculation of steroid concentration was as follows:

$$\mu \text{g of steroid/24 hr} = f \times \frac{\text{Surface area I.S.}}{\text{Surface area of steroid}} \times C \times V$$

where f = surface area of steroid standard/surface area of I.S. standard; C = concentration of steroid standard; and V = dilution factor.

In Figure 1 the entire procedure is summarized. Figure 2, A and B, shows typical chromatograms of 24-hr urines of a healthy and a heterozygous parent

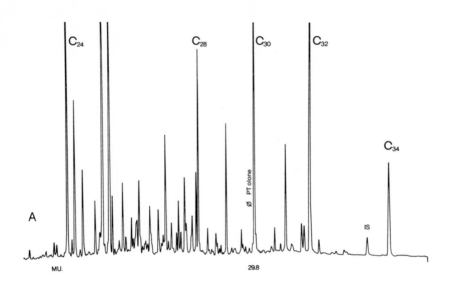

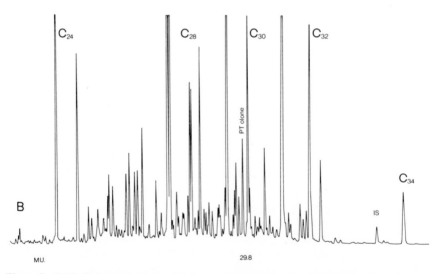

Figure 2. Original chromatograms of urinary steroids following fractionation by gas-liquid chromatography on capillary columns. *A*, normal patient after administration of 40 I.U. of ACTH; *B*, heterozygous carrier (parent) of congenital adrenal hyperplasia after administration of 40 I.U. of ACTH. Note the peak of pregnanetriolone (*PTolone*), which is absent in *A* and quite noticeable in *B*.

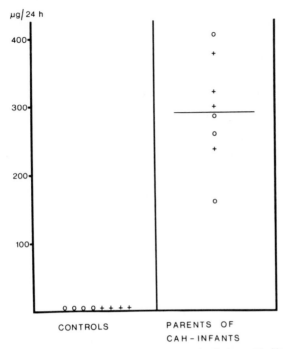

Figure 3. Urinary excretion of pregnanetriolone after stimulation with 40 I.U. of ACTH in healthy parents and parents of children with 21-hydroxylase deficiency (o, mothers; +, fathers).

after ACTH administration. The sensitivity of the method is at the level of 5 μg of steroid/24-hr urine. The recovery following hydrolysis was more than 90%. The reproducibility was checked by the coefficient of variation (18%).

RESULTS AND DISCUSSION

The parents of CAH patients excreted normal amounts of 11-oxygenated 17-ketosteroids, pregnanes, and hydroxylated corticosteroids. PTL was detectable neither in the urines of heterozygotes nor in the normal controls. Only one heterozygous father excreted 4 μg of PTL/24 hr. Following the injection of 40 I.U. of ACTH intramuscularly, control parents still showed no excretion of PTL which could be detected by our method. When challenged with ACTH, parents of children with CAH, however, excreted PTL at the mean concentration of 289 μg/24 hr (Figure 3).

These results may be interpreted as evidence that heterozygous carriers of CAH have a partial deficiency of 21-hydroxylase. Under normal conditions this defect remains unnoticeable, yet following maximal stimulation of the adrenal cortex, PTL, an abnormal metabolite of 21-deoxycortisol, can be detected in the urine. In agreement with previous authors, this study was unable to reveal an increased excretion of 11-oxygenated 17-ketosteroids and a decrease of cortisol metabolites following stimulation with ACTH in heterozygous carriers. Contrary to Knorr (personal communication) and Gleispach et al. (1974), this investigation failed to detect PTL in the urine of normal subjects before and after ACTH. On the average, our values of PTL in 24-hr urine specimens of heterozygous carriers following ACTH administration were lower than those reported by Knorr (personal communication) and Gleispach et al. (1974). These differences are most likely explained by the different methodologies employed. It is the opinion of these authors that gas-liquid chromatography on capillary columns affords maximal separation of urinary steroids and thus high specificity.

CONCLUSION

According to the results obtained in this study, this method may reliably be employed for the detection of heterozygous carriers of CAH of the 21-hydroxylase type.

SUMMARY

The urinary excretion of steroids was studied in eight parents of children with congenital adrenal hyperplasia due to 21-hydroxylase deficiency of the simple virilizing and the salt-losing type. Eight parents of normal children served as controls. Twenty-four-hr urine specimens before and after the injection of 40 I.U. of ACTH were fractionated by means of gas-liquid chromatography on capillary columns.

Before stimulation, no excretion of pregnanetriolone was detected in heterozygous and in normal parents. Following administration of ACTH, only heterozygotes showed an excretion of pregnanetriolone in the urine. This averaged 289 μg/24 hr. Employing gas-liquid chromatography on capillary columns, heterozygous carriers of congenital adrenal hyperplasia due to 21-hydroxylase deficiency may reliably be detected by their increased urinary excretion of pregnanetriolone following ACTH administration.

REFERENCES

Bongiovanni, A. M., W. R. Eberlein, J. D. Smith, and A. J. MacPadden. 1959. The urinary excretion of three C-21 methyl corticosteroids in the adrenogenital syndrome. J. Clin. Endocrinol. Metab. 19:1608–1618.

Childs, B., M. M. Grumbach, and J. J. Van Wyk. 1956. Virilizing adrenal hyperplasia: a genetic and hormonal study. J. Clin. Invest. 35:212–222.

Cox, R. I., and R. P. Shearman. 1961. Abnormal excretion of pregnanetriolone and Δ^5-pregnentriol in the Stein-Leventhal syndrome. J. Clin. Endocrinol. Metab. 21:586–590.

Faglia, G., D. Gelli, A. Liuzzi, G. Norbiato, and B. Pacini. 1966. Significato fisiopathologico e diagnostico del pregnantriolone urinario nella sindrome di Cushing. Folia Endocrinol. (Roma) 19:410–419.

Finkelstein, M. 1962. Pregnanetriolone, an abnormal urinary steroid. In R. I. Dorfman (ed.), Methods in Hormone Research, Vol. 1, p. 169. Academic Press, New York.

Finkelstein, M., J. von Euw, and T. Reichstein. 1953. Isolierung von 3α,17α,20α-trioxypregnanon (11) aus pathologischem menschlichem Harn. Helv. Chim. Acta 36:1266–1277.

Fukushima, D. K., and T. F. Gallagher. 1957. Steroid isolation studies in congenital adrenal hyperplasia. J. Biol. Chem. 229:85–92.

Gleispach, H., H. Berger, J. Glatzl, and H. Rössler. 1974. Pregnantriolonausscheidung nach ACTH-Stimulierung als Test auf vermutliche heterozygote Erbmerkmalsträger eines 21-Hydroxylasemangels. Paediatr. Paedol. 9:204–208.

Grob, K., and G. Grob. 1969. Splitless injection on capillary columns. I. The basic technique: steroid analysis as an example. J. Chromatogr. Sci. 7: 584–586.

Kinoshita, K., K. Isurugi, Y. Kumamoto, and H. Takayasu. 1966. Gas chromatographic estimation of urinary pregnanetriol, pregnanetriolone and pregnantetrol in congenital adrenal hyperplasia. J. Clin. Endocrinol. Metab. 26: 1219–1226.

Knorr, D., and O. Butenandt. 1968. Gas liquid chromatographic investigations in homozygote and heterozygote persons with congenital adrenal hyperplasia, p. 48. Presented at Seventh Annual Meeting of the European Society for Paediatric Endocrinology, Vienna.

Lee, P. A., and F. J. Gareis. 1975. Evidence for partial 21-hydroxylase deficiency among heterozygote carriers of congenital adrenal hyperplasia. J. Clin. Endocrinol. Metab. 41:415–418.

Lohmeyer, H. 1970. Pregnantriolon und adrenogenitales Syndrom. Bibl. Gynaecol. 53:48–58.

Novotny, M., and A. Zlatkis. 1970. High resolution chromatographic separation of steroids with open tubular glass columns. J. Chromatogr. Sci. 8:346–350.

Prader, A. 1958. Die Häufigkeit des congenitalen adrenogenitalen Syndroms. Helv. Paediatr. Acta 13:426–431.

Qazi, Q. H., J. G. Hill, and M. W. Thompson. 1971. Steroid studies in parents of patients with congenital virilizing adrenal hyperplasia. J. Clin. Endocrinol. Metab. 33:23–26.

Raman, P. B., R. Avzamov, N. L. McNiven, and R. I. Dorfman. 1965. A method for the determination of pregnanediol, pregnanetriol and pregnanetriolone by gas chromatography. Steroids 6:177–193.

Shearman, R. P., and R. I. Cox. 1965. Clinical and chemical correlations in the Stein-Leventhal syndrome. Am. J. Obstet. Gynecol. 92:747–754.

Travaglini, P., and G. Faglia. 1971. Pregnanetriolone excretion in Stein-Leventhal syndrome. Acta Endocrinol. (Kbh.) 68:826–832.

Zamora, E., D. Plattner, and H. Ch. Curtius. 1969. Determination of urinary pregnanediol, pregnanetriol and pregnanetriolone in normal children and adults by gas chromatography. Acta Endocrinol. (Kbh.) 62:315–318.

Congenital Adrenal Hyperplasia Caused by 21-Hydroxylase Deficiency

Plasma 17α-Hydroxyprogesterone in Patients' Relatives

Henriette Roux, Bernadette Loras, and Maguelone G. Forest

In an attempt to detect the heterozygote trait for congenital adrenal hyperplasia (CAH) due to 21-hydroxylase deficiency, this study measured plasma 17α-hydroxyprogesterone (17-OHP) because, in the biosynthetic pathway, this steroid is situated immediately before the demonstrated enzymatic defect. The results concerning plasma 17-OHP levels obtained in parents and siblings of CAH patients are presented. They are compared with those of normal subjects.

SUBJECTS AND METHODS

Subjects

Two groups were studied. A control group of 27 normal hospitalized subjects consisted of 3 men (24–40 years old), 12 women (15–53 years old), and 12 prepubertal children (2½ months–10 years old). A second group of kindred of CAH-affected subjects consisted of 6 fathers (28–49 years old), 8 mothers (27–39 years old), and 11 prepubertal siblings (3 months–10 years old). All CAH patients whose families were studied had the salt-losing form of the disease.

Methods

Adrenal stimulation was obtained by administration of either long acting adrenocorticotropic hormone ($ACTH_{1-24}$) given I.M. (1 mg/m^2/day, the maximal dose being 1.5 mg/day) or metyrapone (2–4.5 g, according to body weight), given in six divided doses every 4 hr. Blood samples were obtained at 8–9 a.m., before stimulation, and at 11 a.m., 3 hr after the last ACTH injection, or at 8 a.m., 4 hr after the last metyrapone dose. Plasma 17-OHP was measured by radioimmuno-

Table 1. Plasma 17α-hydroxyprogesterone and cortisol values in normal subjects before and after ACTH or metyrapone

	Subjects	n	17-OHP (ng/100 ml)	n	Cortisol (μg/100 ml)
Children	Basal	12	95 ± 61	11	23 ± 6.9
	ACTH	9	539 ± 250	8	71 ± 16
	Metyrapone	3	624 ± 307		
Men	Basal	3	151 ± 60	3	18.3 ± 8.0
	ACTH	1	920	1	77
	Metyrapone	2	420 and 1910		
Women	Basal follicular phase	9	43 ± 19		
	Basal luteal phase	2	157 and 166	9	18.1 ± 7.1
	ACTH	1	613	1	57
	Metyrapone				
	Follicular phase	7	560 ± 210		
	Luteal phase	1	1,644		
	Ovulation	1	1,676		

assay (M. G. Forest, 1976). Plasma cortisol was measured by a competitive protein binding technique (Loras, Roux, and Philippe, 1970).

RESULTS

Results obtained for the control group are listed in Table 1. In the adult subjects, the ACTH stimulation test (Figure 1) did not reveal any difference between the control group and the heterozygote group, either for 17-OHP values or for cortisol values.

When metyrapone was used (Figure 2), an abnormal response was possibly shown by one mother of a patient with CAH. She was tested during the follicular phase of her cycle. Looking at the group of normal women, it is interesting to note incidentally that the adrenal response to stimulation was usually higher during the luteal phase than during the follicular phase.

In children, the ACTH test (Figure 3) revealed two obviously abnormal cases. A 5-year-old girl had a high basal 17-OHP level and a response 12–15 times as high as normal. This girl is likely to be affected by either a deeply penetrant heterozygotism or by a minor form of the disease. Her genitalia were normal, but she presented some kind of adrenal decompensation during an acute febrile disease. Another type of abnormal response was found in a 3-month-old girl with normal genitalia and in good health. After ACTH stimulation both 17-OHP and cortisol increased considerably. No explanation for this case is known at the present time.

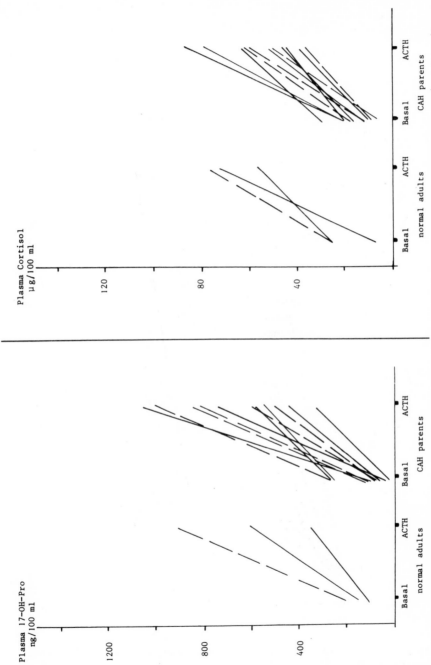

Figure 1. Plasma 17α-OHP (17-OH-Pro) and cortisol values before and after ACTH administration in normal adults and parents of CAH patients.

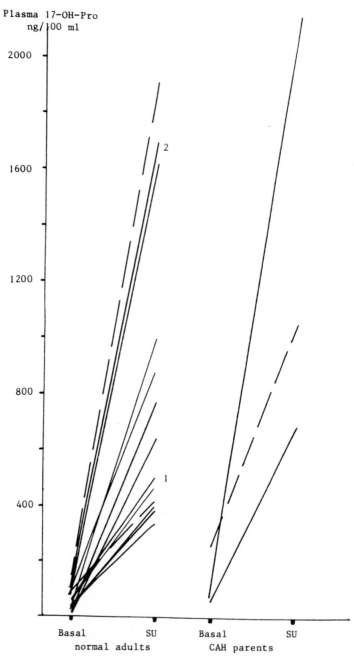

Figure 2. Plasma 17α-OHP (17-OH-Pro) values before and after metyrapone (SU) in normal adults and parents of CAH patients. Two tests were obtained from the same woman; *1* denotes a test during the follicular phase and *2* at ovulation.

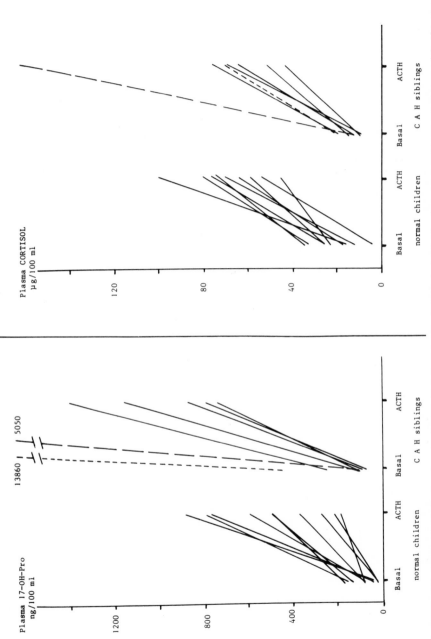

Figure 3. Plasma 17α-OHP (17-OH-Pro) and cortisol values before and after ACTH administration in normal children and siblings of CAH patients.

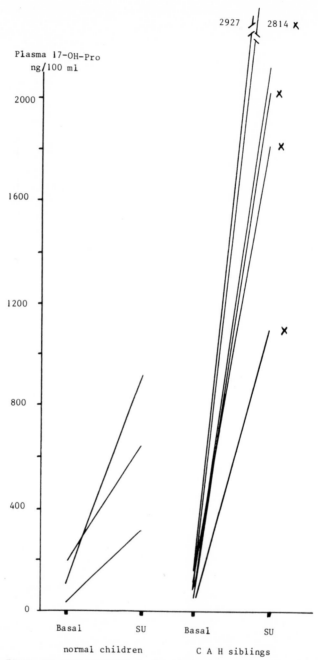

Figure 4. Plasma 17α-OHP (17-OH-Pro) values before and after metyrapone (SU) administration in normal children and siblings of CAH patients. X, the siblings of one CAH patient.

While on metyrapone stimulation (Figure 4), four to five CAH siblings had a higher than normal increase of plasma 17-OHP.

DISCUSSION

In this study, heterozygosity for CAH was not detected with our two tests of "long-term" adrenal stimulation. First, parents of CAH exhibited the same group response in 17-OHP as did normal adults, and, second, two populations among CAH siblings could not be detected. Recently, Lee and Gareis (1975) found a difference between normal adults and CAH parents by using an "acute" adrenal stimulation test.

Although this study did not separate two populations among CAH siblings, it remains that some of them had one abnormal test. Because the tests were well standardized (similar ages, doses, time of the day), it is improbable that the exaggerated responses were related to extra genetic factors. Considering a genetic cause, it can only be hypothesized that, in the CAH sibling groups, data reflect either homozygosity with a latent or minor form of the disease or a transient adrenal hypersensitivity to ACTH seen in heterozygote children.

ACKNOWLEDGMENTS

We wish to thank Drs. M. Jeune and M. David for their clinical collaboration.

REFERENCES

Forest, M. G. 1976. Use of highly specific antibodies against 17α-OH progesterone in a simplified non-chromatographic RIA and in the simultaneous determination of 4 sex hormones in human plasma. Hormone Res. (In press.)

Lee, P. A., and F. J. Gareis. 1975. Evidence for partial 21-hydroxylase deficiency among heterozygote carriers of congenital adrenal hyperplasia. J. Clin. Endocrinol. Metab. 41:415–418.

Loras, B., H. Roux, and M. P. Philippe. 1970. Dosage du cortisol plasmatique et urinaire par liaison compétitive aux protéines. Ann. Endocrinol. 31:383–388.

Test for Heterozygosity of Congenital Adrenal Hyperplasia

Dietrich Knorr, Frank Bidlingmaier, Otfrid Butenandt,
Klaus von Schnakenburg, and Wolfgang Wagner

Congenital adrenal hyperplasia (CAH) caused by 21-hydroxylase deficiency has been found to have an incidence of about 1:7,000, according to data from this laboratory (Mauthe, 1975), as well as to those reported by Prader (1958), and Prader, Anders, and Habich (1962). From this ratio, the incidence of heterozygote individuals in the normal population has been calculated as about 1:40.

Because many of the 100 children with CAH currently being followed in this clinic will become fertile, a reliable test for detecting the heterozygous carriers of this disorder is urgently needed. There is no difference in the urinary excretion of either 17-ketosteroids or total 17-hydroxycorticoids between CAH heterozygotes and normal individuals. Childs, Grumbach, and Van Wyck (1956), Fikentscher (1974) (in this laboratory), Gleispach et al. (1971), and Qazi, Hill, and Thompson (1971) studied the increase in urinary pregnanetriol and pregnanetriolone levels after ACTH stimulation. The excretion of these steroids after adrenocorticotropic hormone (ACTH) stimulation was somewhat higher in heterozygotes than in controls, but there was a wide overlap. Bergada, Rivarola, and Cullen (1965) investigated the steroid pattern after metopirone testing.

In plasma, the accumulated steroid in 21-hydroxylase deficiency is 17α-hydroxyprogesterone (Atherden, Edmunds, and Grant, 1974; Knorr, 1968; v. Schnakenburg, Bidlingmaier, and Knorr, 1974; Strott, Joshimi, and Lipsett, 1969). Therefore, the increase in the 17-hydroxyprogesterone plasma concentration in CAH heterozygotes was studied 1 hr after intravenous stimulation with 0.25 mg of a synthetic $ACTH_{1-24}$ preparation (Synacthen, Ciba). The ratio of the increase in plasma 17-hydroxyprogesterone over the increase in plasma cortisol levels (Knorr et al., 1975) was also calculated.

This work was supported by Grant SFB 51/C 10 from the Deutsche Forschungsgemeinschaft.

METHODS

The normal control group (n = 69) consisted of samples taken from the authors, healthy colleagues, and volunteering technicians. Heterozygous plasma samples (n = 38) were obtained from parents of CAH patients.

Plasma 17-hydroxyprogesterone levels were measured by a specific radio-immunoassay after Sephadex LH-20 column chromatography. Plasma cortisol concentration was determined by radioimmunoassay after a liquid-liquid partition in a water-carbon tetrachloride system.

Statistical evaluation of the results was performed separately for female and male individuals.

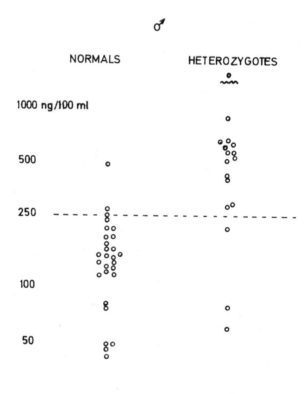

Figure 1. Individual values of increase in 17-hydroxyprogesterone plasma levels 1 hr after administration of 0.25 mg of synthetic ACTH (Synacthen, Ciba) in normal and CAH heterozygous males.

RESULTS

The mean increase in plasma 17α-hydroxyprogesterone concentration within 1 hr after ACTH stimulation in males and females was as follows. In 29 control males, a mean value of 149 ng/100 ml was found, whereas in 17 male hetero-zygotes it was 455 ng/100 ml. This difference is statistically significant at the 97.5% confidence level. In females, the mean increase of the plasma 17-hydroxy-progesterone levels were 144 ng/100 ml and 368 ng/100 ml in 40 controls and 21 CAH heterozygotes, respectively. This difference is statistically significant at the 99.9% confidence level.

If a borderline were graphically drawn between the two overlapping groups at an increase in the 17-hydroxyprogesterone plasma level of 250 ng/100 ml, 14 out of 17 male heterozygotes would be detected. Two out of 29 controls would

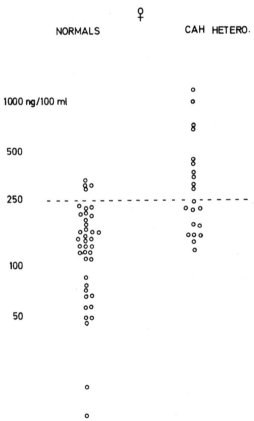

Figure 2. Increase in plasma 17-hydroxyprogesterone 1 hr after ACTH administration in normal and CAH heterozygous females (individual values).

then be considered as false positive results (Figure 1). On the other hand, only 10 out of 21 female heterozygotes would be detected, and 4 out of 40 female controls would then be falsely positive (Figure 2).

In a second step, an attempt was made to eliminate differences in the individual responsiveness of the adrenal gland by introducing the following ratio: increase of plasma 17-hydroxyprogesterone divided by increase of plasma cortisol. In normal males, the mean ratio was 8.7, whereas in heterozygote males, it was 45.0. These two mean values were found to be statistically different at the 95% confidence level. In normal females, a mean value of 6.3 was found for this ratio; in heterozygote females, on the other hand, there was an average of 16.9. The difference between these two mean values is significant at the 99.9% level.

Looking at the individual values (Figure 3) and assuming a ratio of 13 as a The frequency of spontaneous mutation causing CAH is still unknown. To be

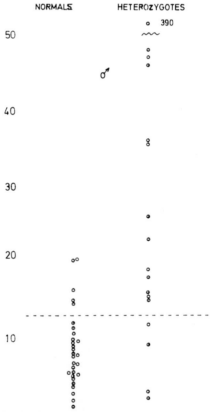

Figure 3. Ratio of the increase of 17-hydroxyprogesterone (ng/100 ml) divided by the increase of cortisol (μg/100 ml) after intravenous ACTH stimulation in normal and CAH heterozygous males.

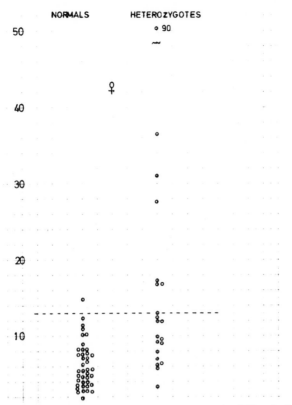

Figure 4. Ratio of the increase of 17-hydroxyprogesterone (ng/100 ml) divided by the increase of cortisol (μg/100 ml) after stimulation with ACTH in normal and heterozygous females.

borderline between normal and heterozygote individuals, 13 out of 17 heterozygote males would be detected. Using this analysis, there would be five false positive results among the 29 normal males. In the female group (Figure 4), unfortunately, the differences in this ratio were less pronounced. Only 7 out of 21 heterozygote females could be detected by using the same borderline ratio of 13. On the other hand, the ratio of only 1 out of 40 normal females exceeded this limit. The possible effects of oral contraceptives and the phase of the menstrual cycle were not considered in this study.

DISCUSSION

The method presented here detected 35–50% of all mothers and 75% of all fathers of patients with congenital adrenal hyperplasia as heterozygous carriers. completely certain, only parents having two or more children with CAH should be included in studies dealing with the detection of heterozygotes.

Furthermore, recent studies indicate that in CAH the peak 17-hydroxypro-gesterone plasma level appears somewhat earlier than 1 hr after ACTH injection (Lee and Gareis, 1975). If this finding can be confirmed, 17-hydroxyproges-terone levels should be studied during, not after, the 1st hr after ACTH administration. Studies to elucidate this time-dependence of 17-hydroxyproges-terone secretion after ACTH stimulation are currently in progress in this labora-tory.

REFERENCES

Atherden, S. M., A. T. Edmunds, and D. B. Grant. 1974. Plasma 17-hydroxypro-gesterone in newborn infants with congenital adrenal hyperplasia and in infants with normal adrenal function. Arch. Dis. Child. 49:192–194.

Bergada, C., M. A. Rivarola, and M. Cullen. 1965. Response to metopirone in parents of patients with congenital adrenal hyperplasia. Excerpta Med. Acta 99:130.

Childs, B., M. M. Grumbach, and J. J. Van Wyk., 1956. Virilizing adrenal hyperplasia. J. Clin. Invest. 35:213.

Fikentscher, E. 1974. Über die Ausscheidung von Pregnantriol und Pregnantrio-lon im Harn unter ACTH Stimulation beim congenitalen adrenogenitalen Syndrom. Inaugural dissertation, München, Germany.

Gleispach, H., H. Berger, J. Glatzl, H. Rössler, and E. Tschager. 1971. Pregnan-triolon-Ausscheidung nach ACTH Stimulierung bei mutmaßlich heterocygoten Merkmalsträgern eines 21-Hydroxylase Defektes. Paediatr. Paedol. 6:287–296.

Knorr, D. 1968. Über die gaschromatographische Bestimmung von freiem 17α-Hydroxyprogesteron im Plasma. 14. Symposion der Deutschen Gesellschaft für Endokrinologie. Springer-Verlag, New York.

Knorr, D., F. Bidlingmaier, O. Butenandt, K. v. Schnakenburg, and W. Wagner. 1975. A test for heterozygocity in congenital adrenal hyperplasia. Pediatr. Res. 9:681.

Lee, P. A., and F. J. Gareis. 1975. Evidence for partial 21-hydroxylase deficien-cy among heterozygote carriers of congenital adrenal hyperplasia. J. Clin. Endocrinol. Metab. 41:415–418.

Mauthe, I. 1975. Über die Häufigkeit des congenitalen adrenogenitalen Syn-droms in München. Inaugural dissertation, München, Germany.

Prader, A. 1958. Die Häufigkeit des congenitalen adrenogenitalen Syndroms. Helv. Paediatr. Acta 13:426–431.

Prader, A., G. J. P. A. Anders, and H. Habich. 1962. Zur Genetik des kongeni-talen adrenogenitalen Syndroms (virilisierende Nebennierenhyperplasie). Helv. Paediatr. Acta 17:271–284.

Qazi, Q. H., J. G. Hill, and M. Thompson. 1971. Steroid studies in parents of patients with congenital virilizing adrenal hyperplasia. J. Clin. Endocrinol. 33:23–26.

v. Schnakenburg, K., F. Bidlingmaier, and D. Knorr. 1974. Quick diagnosis of congenital adrenal hyperplasia (CAH) due to 21-hydroxylase deficiency by radioimmunoassay for 17-α-hydroxyprogesterone. Acta Paediatr. Scand. 63:322.

Strott, C. A., T. Joshimi, and M. Lipsett. 1969. Plasma progesterone and 17-hydroxyprogesterone in normal men and children with congenital adrenal hyperplasia. J. Clin. Invest. 48:930–939.

Detection of Heterozygote Carrier for Congenital Virilizing Adrenal Hyperplasia

James P. Gutai, A. Avinoam Kowarski, and Claude J. Migeon[1]

Population studies by Childs, Grumbach, and Van Wyk (1956) and Prader, Anders, and Habich (1962) have indicated that the mode of inheritance of congenital virilizing adrenal hyperplasia is autosomal recessive. There have been a number of unsuccessful attempts to detect the heterozygote carrier for this disorder. Childs, Grumbach, and Van Wyk (1956) used exogenous adrenocorticotropic hormone (ACTH) with no conclusive results. Cleveland, Nikezic, and Migeon (1962) attempted to unmask abnormalities in the parents of children with congenital virilizing adrenal hyperplasia (CVAH) by administering metyrapone to block 11-hydroxylation and to increase endogenous ACTH. They were unable to detect any difference between the urinary excretion of cortisol precursors of parents and those of normal controls. Qazi, Hill, and Thompson (1971) reported that fathers of children with CVAH excreted significantly greater amounts of 11-oxygenated 17-ketosteroids than male controls, but that individual heterozygotes could not be identified. Bergada, Rivarola, and Cullen (1965) reported that 5 of 15 parents of children with CVAH had an increased pregnanetriol excretion when treated with metyrapone.

The availability of rapid, specific radioimmunoassays has made possible the determination of hormone levels in blood, rather than their urinary metabolites. Lee and Gareis (1975) have measured 17-hydroxyprogesterone (17-OHP) concentrations in response to ACTH and found that they were significantly greater in parents 30 and 60 min after ACTH, but that all of them could not be detected as different from control subjects. The present chapter reports on the levels of

This work was supported by Research Grant AM-00180-24 from the United States Public Health Service. The patients were studied at the Clinical Research Center of the Department of Pediatrics, The Johns Hopkins University School of Medicine, supported by Grant 5-MOl-RR-0052 from the General Clinical Research Centers Program of the Division of Research Resources, National Institutes of Health, United States Public Health Service.

The following trivial names are used: progesterone, 4-pregnene-3,20-dione; 17α-hydroxyprogesterone, 4-pregnene-17α-ol-20-one; cortisol, 4-pregnene-11β,17α,21-triol-3,20-dione.

[1] Recipient of Traineeship Grant 5-K06-AM-21855-11 from the United States Public Health Service.

502   Gutai, Kowarski, and Migeon

plasma progesterone, 17α-hydroxyprogesterone, and cortisol in response to exogenous synthetic ACTH in control male and female subjects and in parents of children with CVAH.

MATERIALS AND METHODS

Subjects

Fourteen control subjects, nine males and five females, ranging in age from 21–32 years, were on no medication at the time of the study and had never received any steroid medication (including oral contraceptives). Five sets of parents of children with CVAH due to 21-hydroxylase deficiency, 24–42 years of age, were on no medications at the time of the study. Four of the five families had children with the salt-losing form, whereas one set of parents had a child with the simple virilizing form.

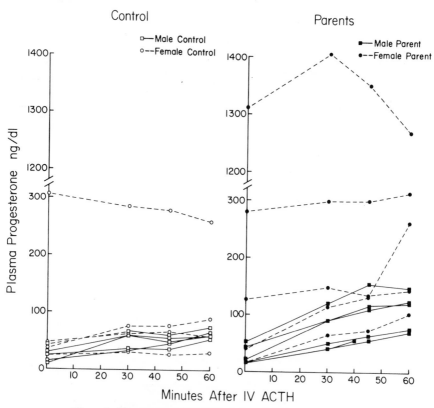

Figure 1. Plasma progesterone response to intravenous ACTH.

In each case, written informed consent was obtained prior to the start of the study. A needle was inserted into an antecubital vein and kept patent with a slow infusion of normal saline solution. Blood samples were obtained 15 min prior to and just immediately before the intravenous injection of 1.0 mg of synthetic $ACTH_{1-24}$ (Cortrosyn). Samples were also obtained 30, 45, and 60 min following ACTH administration. The blood was collected into heparinized tubes on ice, and the plasma was immediately separated and kept frozen in $-20°C$ until the time of assay.

Plasma cortisol was determined by radioassay as previously reported (Beitins et al., 1970). Plasma progesterone and 17-OHP were simultaneously determined with the use of Sephadex LH-20 chromatography and radioimmunoassay with specific antisera. The mean ± S.D. 17-OHP of 16 adult males was 94 ± 23 ng/dl and of 9 follicular phase females was 58 ± 21 ng/dl. A male plasma pool with a mean concentration of 89 ng/dl had an intra-assay coefficient of variation of 9% and an interassay coefficient of variation of 12%. The mean progesterone values of 16 adult males were 26 ± 4 ng/dl and of 9 follicular phase females were 31 ± 6 ng/dl. A male plasma pool had an intra-assay coefficient of variation of 10.6% and an interassay coefficient of variation of 12%.

Table 1. Mean plasma levels of steroids in response to ACTH

Time (min)	Progesterone (ng/dl)		17-OHP (ng/dl)		Cortisol (µg/dl)	
	Control	Parents	Control	Parents	Control	Parents
0						
Mean	59	67	114	114	10.7	9.9
± S.D.	± 93	± 88	± 76	± 93	± 6.1	± 3.2
Significance	ns[a]		ns		ns	
30						
Mean	78	112	184	330	21.9	22.7
± S.D.	± 79	± 77	± 90	± 119	± 7.9	± 5.0
Significance	ns		$p < 0.01$		ns	
45						
Mean	77	125	193	378	30.5	25.4
± S.D.	± 77	± 73	± 109	± 169	± 11.8	
Significance	ns		$p < 0.05$		ns	
60						
Mean	83	151	218	406	30.2	28.5
± S.D.	± 68	± 84	± 130	± 156	± 11.2	± 7.5
Significance	ns		$p < 0.05$		ns	

[a]ns, not significant.

RESULTS

For all three steroids, the values 15 min and just prior to ACTH administration were not significantly different when using a paired t test. Because of it, their mean was used as single pretest level.

The plasma progesterone response is shown in Figure 1, and the statistical analysis of the absolute measurements is presented in Table 1. One female parent who had markedly elevated levels of progesterone (prior to and after ACTH) was not included in the statistical analysis. The mean (± S.D.) baseline progesterone value of the control group was 59 ± 93 ng/dl, whereas the parents had a mean progesterone level of 67 ± 88 ng/dl. The parents had higher mean progesterone values at each point in time, but the difference was not statistically significant. The rate of increase was calculated as the difference between baseline value and that after ACTH divided by time. As shown in Table 2, the rate of increase of plasma progesterone from 0–30 min was significantly higher in the parents than in the controls ($p < 0.01$). The rate of increase from 0–45 min and from 0–60 min also showed a significant difference between controls and parents. It should be noted that the greatest increment of plasma progesterone was from 0–30 min.

The plasma 17-OHP response to ACTH is shown in Figure 2, and Table 1 presents the statistical analysis of the individual measurements. The response of one female parent was markedly elevated. This was the mother who also had abnormally elevated progesterone, and her value was not evaluated statistically.

Table 2. Rate of increase of plasma steroids in response to ACTH

Time (min)	Progesterone (ng/dl/min)		17-OHP (ng/dl/min)		Cortisol (µg/dl/min)	
	Control	Parents	Control	Parents	Control	Parents
0–30						
Mean	0.65	1.60	2.74	7.32	373	432
± S.D.	0.45	0.65	2.3	3.4	150	190
Significance	$p < 0.01$		$p < 0.01$		ns[a]	
0–45						
Mean	0.50	1.37	1.7	6.0	425	351
± S.D.	0.26	0.67	2.0	3.1	210	190
Significance	$p < 0.01$		$p < 0.01$		ns	
0–60						
Mean	0.53	1.46	1.8	4.9	314	307
± S.D.	0.29	0.98	1.9	2.5	122	147
Significance	$p < 0.05$		$p < 0.01$		ns	

[a]ns, not significant.

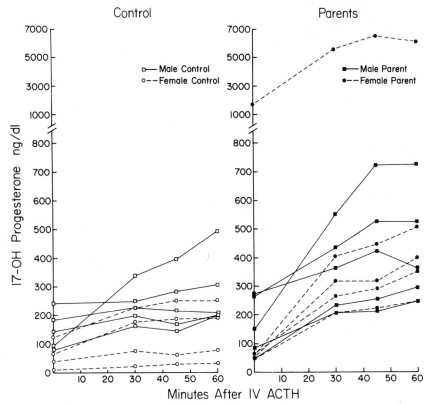

Figure 2. Plasma 17α-hydroxyprogesterone response to intravenous ACTH.

The mean baseline 17-OHP values in the controls and in the parents were identical. At 30 min the controls had a mean 17-OHP level of 184 ± 90 ng/dl, whereas that of the parents was 330 ± 119 ng/dl ($p < 0.01$). The mean plasma levels of 17-OHP at 45 and 60 min were also significantly different ($p < 0.05$). The rate of increase of 17-OHP was calculated for each group and is shown in Table 2. As with progesterone, there was a very significant difference in the rate of increase at all times between the controls and the parents. The greatest rate of increase (of 17-OHP) was from 0–30 min for both controls (2.74 ng/dl) and parents (7.32 ng/dl/min).

The cortisol response to ACTH is presented in Figure 3, and the statistical analysis of the absolute values is shown in Table 1. The mean baseline cortisol values in the controls and in the parents were not significantly different. At all times, there was no significant difference in the cortisol response to ACTH between controls and parents. There was also no significant difference in the rate of increase between the two groups.

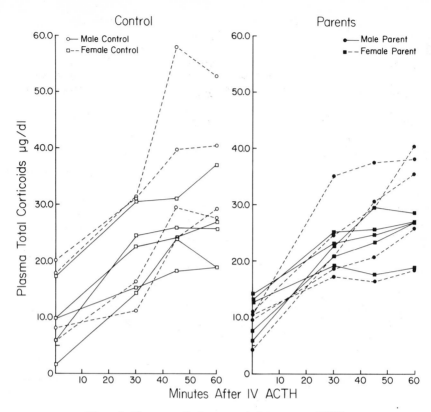

Figure 3. Plasma cortisol response to intravenous ACTH.

The sum of the rates of increase of both progesterone and 17-OHP is presented in Figure 4. One male control subject had a combined rate of increase of progesterone and 17-OHP that was above 3 S.D. from the mean, and he was excluded from the calculation of the final mean of the control group (2.4 ng/dl/min). The female parent with the combined rate of increase of progesterone and 17-OHP of 125 was excluded from the calculation of the mean combined rate of increase for the group of parents. By using a rate of 5 ng/dl/min as the upper limit of normal, nine of the ten parents had elevated values. The means of the two groups were significantly different ($p < 0.01$). One male control subject with a combined rate of increase of 9.0 ng/dl/min could not be differentiated from the group of parents.

DISCUSSION

Previous steroid studies (Bergada, Rivarola, and Cullen, 1965; Childs, Grumbach, and Van Wyk, 1956; Hall et al., 1970; Prader, Anders, and Habich, 1962; Qazi,

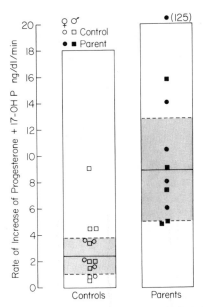

Figure 4. Sum of the rates of increase of progesterone and 17α-hydroxyprogesterone 0–30 min after intravenous ACTH. The *heavy horizontal line* is the mean, and the *shaded area* is ± 1 S.D.

Hill, and Thompson, 1971) have shown either no difference or inconsistent differences between groups of controls and groups of parents of children with CVAH, confident identification of a particular parent as a heterozygote being impossible. Recently, Knorr et al. (1975) reported the response of plasma 17-OHP and cortisol to ACTH in control subjects and parents. A significantly different ratio of 17-OHP to cortisol was obtained for the two groups, and 22 out of 30 parents could be characterized as heterozygotes. In the data presented by Lee and Gareis (1975), one of seven parents had concentrations of 17-OHP that were clearly within the control range. In the present study, a significantly different combined rate of increase of progesterone and 17-OHP in 9 out of 10 parents has been detected.

Population studies by Childs, Grumbach, and Van Wyk (1956) suggested an incidence of heterozygote of 1:128. This was probably an underestimate, because it is reasonable to believe that the sample did not include all children born in the state of Maryland who subsequently developed CVAH (Rosenbloom and Smith, 1966). Prader, Anders, and Habich (1962) examined the incidence of CVAH with 21-hydroxylase deficiency in Switzerland and predicted an incidence of the heterozygote in the general population of 1:28. It is possible that our male control subject with elevated combined increase rate of progesterone and 17-OHP was heterozygote.

The wide variation in the expression of the 21-hydroxylase gene is demonstrated by the female parent who had the highest combined increase rate of progesterone and 17-OHP (125 ng/dl/min) while her husband had one of the lowest (4.8 ng/dl/min). Yet the mother was not hirsute, had regular menses, and had no difficulty with conception. This couple had four offspring, two of them being affected males. Based upon the present test, this father would be considered a false negative.

The accurate detection of the heterozygote is of more than theoretic interest because of the implications in genetic counseling. As many homozygous patients reach reproductive age, they are concerned about the risk of this disease in their offspring. If the other parent is a normal homozygote, none of their children would be affected, but all would be heterozygote carriers. On the other hand, if the other parent is a heterozygote carrier, each child would have 1 in 2 chances of being an affected homozygote. This study is currently being enlarged to include the siblings in all families with affected children.

REFERENCES

Beitins, I. Z., M. H. Shaw, A. Kowarski, and C. J. Migeon. 1970. Comparison of competitive protein-binding radioassay of cortisol to double isotope dilution and Porter-Silber methods. Steroids 15:765–775.

Bergada, C. M., M. A. Rivarola, and M. Cullen. 1965. Response to metopirone in parents of patients with congenital adrenal hyperplasia. Excerpta Med. Int. Ser. 99:E 130.

Childs, B., M. M. Grumbach, and J. J. Van Wyk. 1956. Virilizing adrenal hyperplasia: a genetic and hormonal study. J. Clin. Invest. 35:213–222.

Cleveland, W. W., M. Nikezic, and C. J. Migeon. 1962. Response to an 11β-hydroxylase inhibitor (SU-4885) in males with adrenal hyperplasia and their parents. J. Clin. Endocrinol. Metab. 22:281–286.

Hall, R., P. A. Smith, R. A. Harkness, and G. A. Smart. 1970. A study of the parents of patients with congenital adrenal hyperplasia: detection of the heterozygote. Proc. R. Soc. Med. 63:1040–1042.

Knorr, D., F. Bidlingmaier, O. Butenandt, K. v. Schnakenburg, and W. Wagner. 1975. A test for heterozygocity in congenital adrenal hyperplasia. Pediatr. Res. 9:681.

Lee, P. A., and F. J. Gareis. 1975. Evidence for partial 21-hydroxylase deficiency among heterozygote carriers of congenital adrenal hyperplasia. J. Clin. Endocrinol. Metab. 41:415–418.

Prader, A., G. J. Anders, and H. Habich. 1962. Zur Genetik des Kongenitalen Adrenogenitalen Syndrome. Helv. Paediatr. Acta 17:271–284.

Qazi, Q. H., J. G. Hill, and M. W. Thompson. 1971. Steroid studies in parents of patients with congenital virilizing adrenal hyperplasia. J. Clin. Endocrinol. Metab. 33:23–26.

Rosenbloom, A. L., and D. W. Smith. 1966. Congenital adrenal hyperplasia. Lancet 1:666.

Heterozygous Carriers of 21-Hydroxylase Deficiency Adrenal Hyperplasia

Frank J. Gareis and Peter A. Lee

The serum 17-hydroxyprogesterone (17-OHP) response to adrenocorticotropic hormone (ACTH) stimulation has been studied among parents of children with the 21-hydroxylase form of adrenal hyperplasia with the use of two protocols (Lee and Gareis, 1975). One protocol consisted of the infusion of 50 U. of α-1−24 ACTH over 4 hr, with blood samples obtained at baseline and 2, 4, and 6 hr after beginning the infusion. Four women and three men were evaluated. The menstruating women were tested between days 7 and 10 of their menstrual cycles; two women were postmenopausal. Seven adult male controls were evaluated. Mean cortisol levels at each collection period for each of two groups did not differ. However, 17-OHP values after 2 hr of infusion were significantly higher among the parents than in the control group ($p < 0.02$). When the actual serum values at 2 hr were compared, however, there was some overlap between levels from parents and controls (Table 1). When the changes in levels between baseline and 2 hr were compared there was overlap of only one parent, a mother, into the control range (Table 1).

The second protocol involved the intravenous injection of 25 U. of α-1−24 ACTH over 2−3 min, with blood samples obtained at baseline, 30, and 60 min. Five parents, two men and three women, including the same mother whose 17-OHP values overlapped in the 4-hr infusion, were studied. The five controls were also two men and three women. The mean values of 17-OHP at 30 and 60 min differed at the 0.05 level. When actual levels at 30 min were compared (Table 1), only the previously mentioned mother was within the control range. However, if one disregards her value, there is a narrow division line between the parents and controls. When the differences between baseline and 30-min values are considered (Table 1), there is no overlap. Therefore, while the percentage of increase from baseline for the two groups overlapped considerably, if the actual change in level during the first 30 min after ACTH administration is listed, using the second protocol (rapid ACTH infusion), there is no overlap in this group of patients.

Hence, it could be suggested that, if the heterozygote is stimulated suddenly with ACTH and the response is measured promptly, he can be differentiated

Table 1. Serum 17-hydroxyprogesterone

Actual value (pg/ml)		Change from baseline (pg/ml)	
Parent	Control	Parent	Control
After 2 hr of 4-hr $ACTH_{1-24}$ infusion (50 U.)			
11,770	4,510	10,000	1,990
7,000[a]	3,900	4,830[a]	1,950
6,280[a]	3,190	4,500[a]	1,470
5,660	3,110	4,020[a]	1,140
4,810[a]	2,150	3,250	900
3,250	1,750	3,000	830
3,190[a]	1,750	1,150[a]	530
Thirty min after intravenous injection of 25 U. of $ACTH_{1-24}$			
5,385	2,150[a]	3,430	1,310[a]
3,300[a]	1,500[a]	2,820[a]	920[a]
2,870	1,340	2,150	700[a]
2,370[a]	1,290	1,590[a]	370
1,735[a]	900[a]	1,400[a]	300

[a]Females.

from controls. After prolonged stimulation the difference may not be as obvious.

REFERENCES

Lee, P. A., and F. J. Gareis. 1975. Evidence for partial 21-hydroxylase deficiency among heterozygote carriers of congenital adrenal hyperplasia. J. Clin. Endocrinol. Metab. 41:415–418.

Present Status of Prenatal Diagnosis of Congenital Adrenal Hyperplasia

Maria I. New

The numbers of disorders which can be diagnosed prenatally have increased at a rapid rate in the past 20 years (Burton, Gerbie, and Nadler, 1974; Milunsky et al., 1970). However, congenital adrenal hyperplasia (CAH) is not among those disorders in which the intrauterine diagnosis can be made unequivocally early enough in gestation to permit elective abortion.

Although amniocentesis and analysis of amniotic fluid were an established practice for monitoring pregnancy complicated by Rh incompability, it was not until 1955 (Fuchs and Riis, 1956; Makowski, Prem, and Kaiser, 1956; Serr, Sachs, and Danon, 1955; Shettles, 1956) that amniocentesis was used to determine fetal sex and not until 1960 (Riis and Fuchs, 1960) that prenatal fetal sex determination was used to recommend selective therapeutic abortions in cases of sex-linked hereditary disease.

REVIEW OF PREVIOUS INVESTIGATIONS

Jeffcoate et al. (1965) proposed amniotic fluid analysis as a means to detect congenital adrenal hyperplasia prenatally. The premise was based on the fact that fetal urine contributed to the amniotic fluid from the 20th week of gestation onward and that the fetal adrenal gland functioned by the 12th–14th week. Thus, metabolites of fetal steroid secretion were sought in the amniotic fluid near term when the fetus was at risk for congenital adrenal hyperplasia. Jeffcoate et al. (1965) studied the amniotic fluid of two fetuses at risk for CAH by determination of 17-ketosteroid and pregnanetriol. They reported elevated concentrations of both steroid metabolites in the pregnancy which resulted in a

This investigation was supported by Grant HD 72 from the National Institutes of Health, United States Public Health Service; Pediatric Clinical Research Center Grant RR 47 from the National Institutes of Health, United States Public Health Service, Division of Research Facilities and Resources; Grant CRBS-278 from the National Foundation-March of Dimes; and by Career Scientist Award I-749 and Research Contract U-2204 from the Health Research Council of the City of New York.

Table 1. Hormone levels in liquor amniotic fluid. Only fetuses 1 and 2 were at risk for congenital adrenal hyperplasia.

Case no.	Duration of pregnancy (weeks)	State of child	Sex	Weight	17-ketosteroids (μg per litre)	Pregnanetriol ($\mu g.$ per litre)
1	40	Adrenogenital syndrome	F	8 lb. (3630 g.)	104	106
2	39	Normal	F	8 lb. 7 oz. (3830 g.)	25	23
3	40	Normal	F	7 lb. 1 oz. (3210 g.)	50	24
4	39½	Normal	M	7 lb. 8 oz. (3410 g.)	25	32
5	40	Normal	F	7 lb. 7 oz. (3380 g.)	52	46
6	39	Anencephalic	F	4 lb. 13 oz. (2180 g.)	16	11

Reprinted with permission of Lancet 2:553–555 (1965).

virilized female with CAH and normal concentrations in the pregnancy resulting in a normal full term female (Table 1). Jeffcoate suggested that prenatal diagnosis of CAH might be made by demonstrating elevated concentrations of 17-ketosteroid and pregnanetriol. These findings, albeit in late pregnancy, would permit preparation for the management of the infant with CAH before delivery.

Since Jeffcoate's initial report, a total of 14 additional fetuses at risk for CAH have been studied (Breborowicz and Biniszkiewicz, 1967; Cathro, Bertrand, and Coyle, 1969; Frasier et al., 1975; Frasier, Weiss, and Horton, 1974; Merkatz et al., 1969; New and Levine, 1973; Nichols, 1969, 1970; Nichols and Gibson, 1969) (Table 2). The reports of success or failure in making the diagnosis prenatally have varied. Amniotic fluid alone has been analyzed in five cases, maternal urine alone in five cases, and a combination of both amniotic fluid and maternal urine in the remainder.

Nichols (1969, 1970) and Nichols and Gibson (1969) determined the pregnanetriol concentration of amniotic fluid in five fetuses at risk; they found high pregnanetriol levels in two cases in which the fetus proved to have CAH and normal pregnanetriol levels when the fetus was normal (Tables 3 and 4). Thus, Nichols confirmed the report of Jeffcoate et al. (1965) that amniotic fluid pregnanetriol concentration could be used for prenatal diagnosis of CAH. In studies of fetuses affected with CAH (Jeffcoate et al., 1965; Nichols, 1969, 1970; Nichols and Gibson, 1969), the pregnanetriol was measured in amniotic fluid at term or at delivery.

Merkatz et al. (1969) studied two fetuses at risk for CAH from the 20th week of gestation to delivery. The amniotic fluid concentrations of 17-ketosteroid and pregnanetriol were determined in 26 women with normal pregnan-

Table 2. Summary of attempted prenatal diagnosis of CAH

Fetus at risk	Authors	Biological fluid	Diagnosis	Sex	Steroid determination	Laboratory results
1	Jeffcoate et al. (1965)	Amniotic fluid	CAH	F	17-KS[a]	Increased
					Pregnanetriol	Increased
2	Jeffcoate et al. (1965)	Amniotic fluid	Normal	F	17-KS	Normal
					Pregnanetriol	Normal
3	Breborowicz and Biniszkiewicz (1967)	Maternal urine	CAH	M	Estriol	Increased
					17-KS	Normal
4	Cathro, Bertrand, and Coyle (1969)	Maternal urine	CAH	F	Estriol	Increased
	Oakey (1969)	Maternal urine	Normal	F	Estriol	Increased
	Oakey (1969)	Maternal urine	Normal	F	Estriol	Increased
5	Nichols (1969)	Maternal urine	Normal	?	Estriol	Normal
6	Nichols (1969)	Maternal urine	Normal	?	Estriol	Normal
7	Nichols (1969)	Maternal urine	Normal	?	Estriol	Normal
8	Nichols (1969)	Amniotic fluid	CAH	F	Pregnanetriol	Increased
9	Nichols (1969)	Maternal urine	CAH	F	Estriol	Normal
		Amniotic fluid			Pregnanetriol	Increased
10	Nichols (1969)	Maternal urine	Normal	?	Estriol	Normal
		Amniotic fluid			Pregnanetriol	0
11	Nichols (1969)	Maternal urine	Normal	?	Estriol	Normal
		Amniotic fluid			Pregnanetriol	0
12	Nichols (1970)	Maternal urine	CAH	M	Estriol	Normal
		Amniotic fluid			Pregnanetriol	Increased
13	Merkatz et al. (1969)	Amniotic fluid	CAH	M	17-KS	Normal
					Pregnanetriol	Normal
14	Merkatz et al. (1969)	Amniotic fluid	CAH	F	17-KS	Normal
					Pregnanetriol	Normal
15	New (1972)	Amniotic fluid	CAH	M	17-KS	Normal
					Pregnanetriol	Normal
16	Frasier, Weiss, and Horton (1974)	Amniotic fluid	CAH	M	Testosterone	Normal
	Frasier et al. (1975)	Amniotic fluid	CAH	M	17-OHP	Increased

[a]17-KS, 17-ketosteroids.

Table 3. Comparison of maternal urinary estriol and amniotic fluid pregnanetriol in ten fetuses at risk for adrenogenital syndrome

Source	Case	Urinary oestriol (mg. per 24 hr.)	Amniotic-fluid pregnanetriol (μg. per 1.)	Condition of newborn
Jeffcoate et al., 1965	1	Not reported	106	Adrenogenital syndrome
	2	Not reported	23	Normal
Cathro et al., 1969	3	26.5 at 26 weeks 32.4 at 29 weeks 58.8 at 34 weeks	Not reported	Adrenogenital syndrome
Nichols, 1969	4	6.5 at 28 weeks 7.1 at 32 weeks 7.5 at 36 weeks	No analysis	Normal
	5	5.8 at 30 weeks 8.1 at 34 weeks	No analysis	Normal
	6	7.3 at 31 weeks 9.0 at 35 weeks	No analysis	Normal
	7	No analysis	91	Adrenogenital syndrome
Nichols and Gibson, 1969	8	12.0 at 30 weeks 5.6 at 34 weeks	114	Adrenogenital syndrome
	9	8.0 at 32 weeks 12.2 at 36 weeks	Nil detected	Normal
	10	7.1 at 34 weeks 11.5 at 36 weeks	Nil detected	Normal

Reprinted with permission of Lancet 2:1068–1069 (1969).

cies and in two women who gave birth to infants with CAH. The fetuses with CAH could not be distinguished from the normal fetuses during early or midpregnancy, but values for both 17-ketosteroids and pregnanetriol were suggestively elevated in amniotic fluid obtained at term from the affected fetuses (Figures 1 and 2). A third fetus with CAH studied from the 32nd–40th week of gestation by the same laboratory was not detected by the determination of 17-ketosteroid and pregnanetriol in amniotic fluid even at term (New and Levine, 1973) (Figures 3 and 4). These results, therefore, are contrary to those of Jeffcoate et al. (1965), Nichols (1969, 1970), and Nichols and Gibson (1969).

Table 4. Early prenatal diagnosis of congenital adrenal hyperplasia and an attempt to treat the fetus with hydrocortisone injected intra-amniotically[a]

Days of gestation	273	278*	280*	283*	285*	287+
Pregnanetriol (μg/l)	206	227	140	90	22	20

* 25 mg hydrocortisone injected after withdrawal of amniotic fluid
+ Normal delivery

[a]The suppression of elevated pregnanetriol levels was considered an additional diagnostic feature of prenatal diagnosis of congenital adrenal hyperplasia.
Reprinted with permission of Lancet 1:83 (1970).

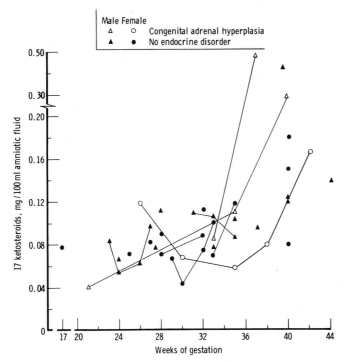

Figure 1. 17-Ketosteroid concentration in amniotic fluid throughout gestation was the same in male and female fetuses. Only at term was there a suggestive elevation of 17-ketosteroid concentration in the affected fetuses. Reprinted with permission of J. Pediatr. 75:977–982 (1969).

Maternal urine was also studied as a possible means of prenatal diagnosis of CAH. The estriol level in amniotic fluid and maternal urine is thought to reflect fetal adrenal function. Breborowicz and Biniszkiewicz (1967) and Cathro, Bertrand, and Coyle (1969) measured the estriol concentration of maternal urine in two cases in which the fetus proved to have CAH at birth. Estriol levels were markedly elevated from the 20th week until delivery (Figures 5 and 7) although 17-ketosteroid levels were not (Figure 6). These results, however, were not confirmed by the studies of Nichols (1970) and Nichols and Gibson (1969) (Table 3). Oakey (1969) also reported elevated estriol levels in maternal urine when the fetus was normal. Thus, it appears that the estriol concentration in maternal urine is not a reliable way to make the prenatal diagnosis of CAH.

Perhaps estriol should be measured in amniotic fluid rather than maternal urine. In normal pregnancy, estriol is the most abundant steroid present in amniotic fluid (Schindler and Siiteri, 1968) (Table 5). The urinary excretion of 16-hydroxylated steroids is known to be high in premature infants and

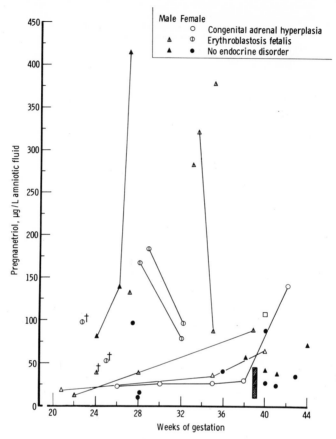

Figure 2. Pregnanetriol concentration in amniotic fluid was the same in male and female fetuses. Only at term was there a suggestive elevation of pregnanetriol concentration in the affected fetuses. The *cross-hatched bar* represents the normal range reported by Jeffcoate et al. (1965). Reprinted with permission of J. Pediatr. 75:977–982 (1969).

neonates with CAH (Reynolds, 1963). This suggests that 16-hydroxylated steroids and estriol may be present in very high concentrations in amniotic fluid when the fetus is affected with CAH. Although it has been suggested (New, 1972), the analysis of amniotic fluid for 16-hydroxylated steroids and estriol as a means of detecting CAH prenatally has not been reported.

Recently, Frasier, Weiss, and Horton (1974) and Frasier et al. (1975) have attempted the prenatal diagnosis of CAH by the measurement of specific adrenal

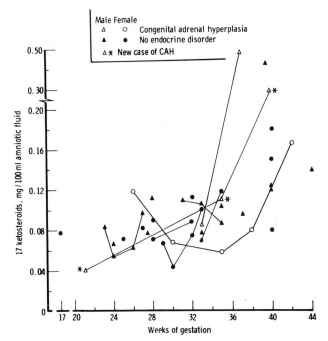

Figure 3. Variation in amniotic fluid concentration of 17-ketosteroids during gestation shown in Figure 1, with the study of an additional fetus who proved to have congenital adrenal hyperplasia. Reprinted with permission of Plenum Press, New York, Advances in Human Genetics, pp. 251–326 (1973).

steroids rather than steroid metabolites in amniotic fluid. One pregnancy which resulted in a male with CAH was studied by serial amniocentesis from the 20th week to term. Testosterone and 17-hydroxyprogesterone were measured (Figures 8 and 9). The testosterone concentration of amniotic fluid obtained from the pregnancy with the affected fetus was within the range found in control pregnancies. Although testosterone did not prove useful in prenatal diagnosis, the determination of 17-hydroxyprogesterone (17-OHP) in amniotic fluid "showed considerable promise as an in utero predictor of congenital adrenal hyperplasia" (Frasier et al., 1975). The evidence for the utility of 17-OHP in prenatal diagnosis of CAH is preliminary and additional pregnancies must be studied to confirm the findings of Frasier et al. (1975). 17-OHP is significantly elevated in cord blood of infants with CAH. Its appearance in amniotic fluid may be expected. Further studies are awaited.

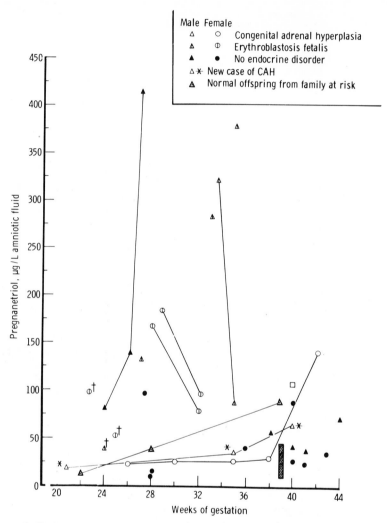

Figure 4. Variation in amniotic fluid concentration of pregnanetriol during gestation shown in Figure 2, with the study of an additional fetus who proved to have congenital adrenal hyperplasia. Reprinted with permission of Plenum Press, New York, Advances in Human Genetics, pp. 251–326 (1973).

POSSIBLE FUTURE TECHNIQUES

To date, only amniotic fluid and maternal urine have been used as biological sources of steroids for prenatal diagnosis of CAH. Other feasible methods present themselves as possible means of prenatal diagnosis; they are enumerated in Table 6.

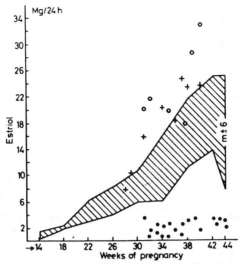

Figure 5. Urinary estriol excretion in pregnancies complicated by hypoplasia of fetal adrenals (●), hyperplasia of the fetal adrenals (○), and hyperplasia of the maternal adrenals (+). The *striped area* denotes the mean ± S.D. of the estriol levels in normal pregnancies. Reprinted with permission of Excerpta Medica Foundation, Amsterdam, Intrauterine Dangers to the Fetus (1967).

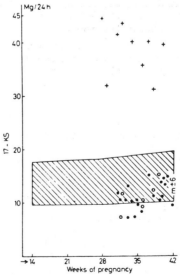

Figure 6. Urinary 17-ketosteroid excretion in pregnancies complicated by hypoplasia of the fetal adrenals (●), by hyperplasia of the fetal adrenals (○), and by hyperplasia of the maternal adrenals (+). The *striped area* denotes the mean ± S.D. of the 17-ketosteroid levels in normal pregnancies. Reprinted with permission of Excerpta Medica Foundation, Amsterdam, Intrauterine Dangers to the Fetus (1967).

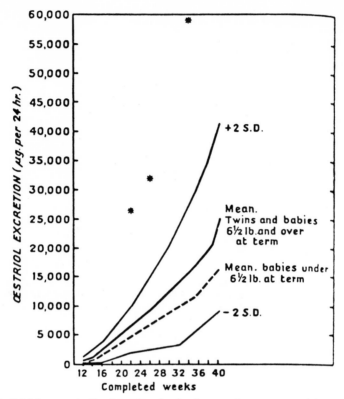

Figure 7. Estriol concentration in maternal urine in normal pregnancy and in a pregnancy which resulted in an infant with congenital adrenal hyperplasia. *Asterisks* denote values for the affected fetus. Reprinted with permission of Lancet 1:732 (1969).

Table 5. Steroid concentrations in cord blood and amniotic fluid

Steroid	Cord blood µg/1000 ml	Amniotic fluid µg/1000 ml
Dehydroisoandrosterone	1600	8.3
16α-OH-dehydroisoandrosterone	1000	797.7
Pregnenolone	1500	nondetectable
16α-OH-pregnenolone	194	119.0
Estradiol	6.0	3.1
Estriol	1000.0	1572.5

Reprinted with permission of J. Clin. Endocrinol. 28:1189–1198 (1968).

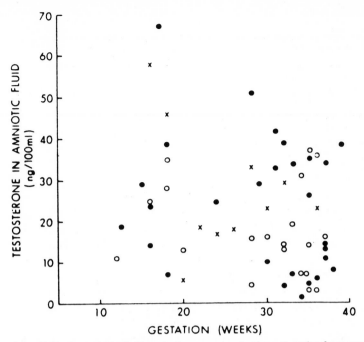

Figure 8. Individual amniotic fluid testosterone concentrations. Samples from pregnancies in which the fetus was a girl (○), a boy (●), or a male subsequently found to have CAH (✗). Reprinted with permission of J. Pediatr. 84:738–741 (1974).

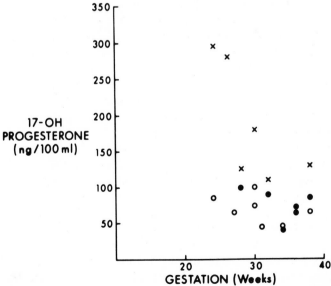

Figure 9. Individual amniotic fluid 17-OHP concentrations. Samples from pregnancies in which the fetus was a girl (○), a boy (●), or a male subsequently found to have CAH (✗). Reprinted with permission of J. Pediatr. 86:310–312 (1975).

Table 6. Feasible methods of prenatal diagnosis of CAH not yet attempted

1. Studies of steroid metabolism of cultured amniotic cells or fetal skin cells.
2. Amniography, with the use of water-soluble dye.[a]
3. Fetography, with the use of fat-soluble dye.[a]
4. Fetoscopy, direct visualization of genitalia.[a]
5. Fetal blood sampling and determination of steroid and/or ACTH level.

[a]Useful only in the diagnosis of fetuses with ambiguous genitalia.

Cultured fibroblasts obtained from skin and from amniotic cells have been used to detect several inborn errors of metabolism (Burton, Gerbie, and Nadler, 1974; Milunsky et al., 1970). Recently it has been shown that amniotic fluid cells in culture metabolized testosterone (Shanies, Hirschhorn, and New, 1971). Furthermore, a recent abstract suggested that amniotic cells in culture were capable of metabolizing several steroids (Beling and Cederqvist, 1974). Pregnenolone was converted to progesterone, 17-OHP, and 20α-dihydroprogesterone, whereas progesterone was converted to 17α-OHP, 20α-dehydroepiandrosterone, and corticosterone. This early report indicated that amniotic cells in culture demonstrated a wide variety of enzymatic activities, including 3β-ol-dehydrogenase, 17α-hydroxylase, 20α-hydroxysteroid dehydrogenase, and 21-hydroxylase. Should these studies be confirmed, then amniotic cells in culture may possibly be used to define enzyme defects of steroid synthesis as they have been used for other hereditable enzyme defects. Furthermore, fetal skin biopsy may be possible in the future (Sato and Kadotani, 1970). Fetal skin fibroblasts may prove to be more useful than amniotic cells, because they grow faster and may be more active in steroid metabolism. The maternal and fetal risk of fetal skin biopsy has yet to be evaluated.

The fetus may be visualized by amniography (Agüero and Zighelboim, 1970; Queenan and Gadow, 1970) or fetography (Agüero and Zighelboim, 1970; Erbslöh, 1942). In the former, water-soluble dye is injected into the amniotic fluid, which the fetus swallows, and in the latter, a fat-soluble dye is injected which adheres to the vernix caseosa. Thus, anatomical malformations such as ambiguous genitalia would be detectable. This technique would be applicable to the female fetus with virilized external genitalia due to congenital adrenal hyperplasia resulting from a 21-hydroxylase deficiency. It could also be applied to the male with ambiguous genitalia due to CAH with a 3β-hydroxylase deficiency or 17α-hydroxylase defect. The safety of fetography and amniography has yet to be evaluated in middle or early pregnancy.

Direct visualization of the fetus is referred to by Burton, Gerbie, and Nadler (1974). When this technique has been adequately evaluated, it also may be used to detect ambiguous genitalia for the prenatal diagnosis of CAH.

Finally, sampling of fetal blood (Valenti, 1973) may one day be sufficiently

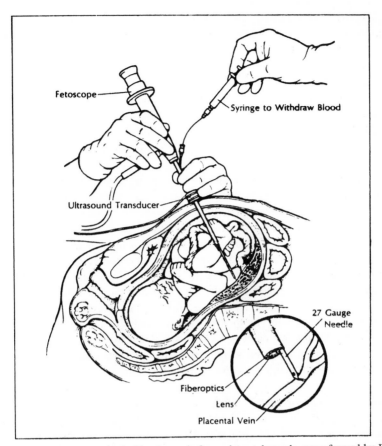

Figure 10. Fetoscopy to obtain blood sample from placental vessels, as performed by Dr. J. C. Hobbins at Yale University. *Detail,* needle about to enter vessel. Sonographic scanning is first used to locate placenta and fetus. The ultrasound transducer then provides echoes from abdominal and uterine walls and from fetus as fetoscope is inserted and pushed toward the placenta. Assistant draws blood, which is analyzed for sickle-cell disease or β-thalassemia. Reprinted with permission of Hosp. Practice June:41–51 (1975).

safe and feasible so that hormonal determination of fetal blood may provide a new tool for prenatal diagnosis of CAH (Figure 10).

ETHICS OF PRENATAL DIAGNOSIS OF CAH

Prolonged consideration of the important subject of the ethics of prenatal diagnosis of congenital adrenal hyperplasia is inappropriate here and has been extensively reviewed by experienced geneticists (Goodner, 1973; Nadler, 1975). A desirable goal for early prenatal diagnosis of CAH would presumably be prenatal treatment (Jeffcoate, 1971). Because the abnormality of sexual differentiation in the female is complete by the 14th–15th week of gestation when amniocentesis first becomes possible, prenatal treatment could only prevent progressive enlargement of the clitoris. This would be a substantial benefit not to be ignored if the pangs of clitoral surgery are considered.

Prenatal diagnosis would also allow parents of children with CAH to electively abort a pregnancy in which a positive diagnosis of CAH was made before the 20th week. However, to recommend abortion in CAH converts a nonlethal gene to a lethal gene. CAH is, after all, a disorder compatible with life if properly treated. Indeed, if a woman decides to abort a fetus with CAH should the prenatal diagnosis be possible, there might be an adverse effect on living siblings with CAH. They may learn that the reason for the abortion was the very condition for which they are being treated with an optimistic outlook by the physician. The best reason for prenatal diagnosis at present would be to decrease the anxiety of the expectant mother by exclusion of the diagnosis.

Finally, consideration must be given to the question of increasing the gene pool for CAH by abortion of those children with CAH. Patients with CAH have reduced fertility. Two-thirds of those allowed to be born will be heterozygotes as the parents replace the aborted child with a presumably normal child. These individuals, heterozygous for the recessive gene of CAH, will ultimately reproduce and give birth to a greater number of affected children.

In conclusion, the present state of the art of prenatal diagnosis of CAH does not permit unequivocal prediction of an affected or normal fetus. The most promising lead appears to be the determination of pregnanetriol or 17-OHP in the amniotic fluid near term. Out of 10 fetuses at risk, this test predicted the diagnosis correctly in 7 and did not predict the diagnosis in 3. Presently, the most that can be expected from prenatal diagnosis is that, near term, it may allow parent and physician to prepare for the advent of a newborn with CAH. Intervention seems in the distant future.

REFERENCES

Agüero, O., and I. Zighelboim. 1970. Fetography and molegraphy. Surg. Gynecol. Obstet. 130:649–654.

Beling, C., and L. L. Cederqvist. 1974. Metabolism of progesterone in cultured amniotic cells. Program and Abstracts: 56th Annual Meeting of The Endocrine Society, June, Atlanta, Georgia. Abstr. 183, pp. A–147. Endocrinol. (Suppl.) 94.

Breborowicz, H., and W. Biniszkiewicz. 1967. The relation between the urinary oestriol and 17 KS levels and the state of maternal and foetal adrenals. In J. Horsky and Z. K. Stembera (eds.), Intrauterine Dangers to the Fetus. Excerpta Medica Foundation, Amsterdam.

Burton, B. K., A. B. Gerbie, and H. L. Nadler. 1974. Present status of intrauterine diagnosis of genetic defects. Am. J. Obstet. Gynecol. 118:718–746.

Cathro, D. M., J. Bertrand, and M. G. Coyle. 1969. Antenatal diagnosis of adrenocortical hyperplasia. Lancet 1:732.

Erbslöh, J. 1942. Das intrauterine Fetogramm. Arch. Gynaekol. 173:160–162.

Frasier, S. D., I. H. Thorneycroft, B. A. Weiss, and R. Horton. 1975. Elevated amniotic fluid concentration of 17α-hydroxyprogesterone in congenital adrenal hyperplasia. J. Pediatr. 86:310–312.

Frasier, S. D., B. A. Weiss, and R. Horton. 1974. Amniotic fluid testosterone: implications for the prenatal diagnosis of congenital adrenal hyperplasia. J. Pediatr. 84:738–741.

Fuchs, F., and P. Riis. 1956. Antenatal sex determination. Nature 177:330.

Goodner, D. M. 1973. Antenatal diagnosis of genetic defects. J. Reprod. Med. 10:261–268.

Jeffcoate, N. 1971. The unborn child. Aust. N.Z. J. Obstet. Gynaecol. 11:129–138.

Jeffcoate, T. N. A., J. R. H. Fliegner, S. H. Russell, J. C. Davis, and A. P. Wade. 1965. Diagnosis of the adrenogenital syndrome before birth. Lancet 2:553–555.

Makowski, E. L., K. A. Prem, and I. H. Kaiser. 1956. Detection of sex of fetuses by the incidence of sex chromatin body in nuclei of cells in amniotic fluid. Science 123:542–543.

Merkatz, I. R., M. I. New, R. E. Peterson, and M. P. Seaman. 1969. Prenatal diagnosis of adrenogenital syndrome by amniocentesis. J. Pediatr. 75:977–982.

Milunsky, A., J. W. Littlefield, J. N. Kanfer, E. H. Kolodny, V. E. Shih, and L. Atkins. 1970. Prenatal genetic diagnosis. N. Engl. J. Med. 283:1370–1381, 1441–1447, 1498–1504.

Nadler, H. L. 1975. Prenatal diagnosis of inborn defects: a status report. Hosp. Practice 10:41–51.

New, M. I. 1972. Adrenogenital syndrome. In A. Dorfman (ed.), Antenatal Diagnosis, pp. 153–160. University of Chicago Press, Chicago.

New, M. I., and L. S. Levine. 1973. Congenital adrenal hyperplasia. In H. Harris and K. Hirschhorn (eds.), Advances in Human Genetics, pp. 251–326. Plenum Press, New York.

Nichols, J. 1969. Antenatal diagnosis of adrenocortical hyperplasia. Lancet 1:1151.

Nichols, J. 1970. Antenatal diagnosis and treatment of the adrenogenital syndrome. Lancet 1:83.

Nichols, J., and G. G. Gibson. 1969. Antenatal diagnosis of the adrenogenital syndrome. Lancet 2:1068–1069.

Oakey, R. E. 1969. Antenatal diagnosis of adrenocortical hyperplasia. Lancet 1:886–887.

Queenan, J. T., and E. C. Gadow. 1970. Amniography for detection of congenital malformations. Obstet. Gynecol. 35:648–657.

Reynolds, J. W. 1963. Isolation of 16-OH-pregnenolone from urine of newborn infants. Proc. Soc. Exp. Biol. Med. 113:980–983.

Riis, P., and F. Fuchs. 1960. Antenatal determination of foetal sex in prevention of hereditary diseases. Lancet 2:180–182.

Sato, H., and T. Kadotani. 1970. Fetal skin biopsy. J.A.M.A. 272:323.

Schindler, A. E., and P. K. Siiteri. 1968. Isolation and quantitation of steroids from normal human amniotic fluid. J. Clin. Endocrinol. 28:1189–1198.

Serr, D. M., L. Sachs, and M. Danon. 1955. Diagnosis of sex before birth using cells from the amniotic fluid. Bull. Res. Council Israel 5B:137.

Shanies, D. D., K. Hirschhorn, and M. I. New. 1971. Metabolism of testosterone-^{14}C by cultured human cells. J. Clin. Invest. 51:1459–1468.

Shettles, L. B. 1956. Nuclear morphology of cells in human amniotic fluid in relation to sex of infant. Am. J. Obstet. Gynecol. 71:834–838.

Valenti, C. 1973. Antenatal detection of hemoglobinopathies: a preliminary report. Am. J. Obstet. Gynecol. 115:851–853.

Index